Exercise, Health and Mental Health

Can a sedentary lifestyle have an adverse effect on mental health?

Does exercise help people cope better with chronic physical illness, mental health problems, sleep disorders, and smoking cessation?

What research is needed on the role of exercise for promoting mental health?

As alternative approaches to health and social care gain wider acceptance, exercise is being adopted as a strategy for mental health promotion in a variety of settings.

Exercise, Health and Mental Health provides an introduction to this emerging field and a platform for future research and practice. Written by internationally acclaimed exercise, health, and medical scientists, this is the first systematic review of the evidence for the psychological role of exercise in:

- treating and managing mental health problems including dementia, schizophrenia, and drug and alcohol dependence
- coping with chronic clinical conditions including cancer, heart disease, and HIV/AIDS
- enhancing well-being in the general population – by improving sleep, assisting in smoking cessation, and as a way of addressing broader social issues such as antisocial behavior.

Adopting a consistent and accessible format, the research findings for each topic are summarized and critically examined for their implications. For students and researchers, the book provides an authoritative guide to current issues and future research. For exercise professionals, health practitioners, and policymakers, it is a basis for the development of evidence-based practice.

Guy E. J. Faulkner is Assistant Professor in the Faculty of Physical Education and Health at the University of Toronto, Canada and coordinates the activities of the Exercise Psychology Unit. His research interests lie primarily within the field of physical activity and psychological well-being. Current funded research concerns the physical health needs of mental health service users in relation to antipsychotic medication and weight gain; mediated health messages; and the role of physical activity in harm reduction and smoking cessation.

Adrian H. Taylor is Reader in Exercise and Health Psychology in the School of Sport and Health Sciences at the University of Exeter, UK. His work has focused on three main themes: (1) Psycho-social determinants of sport and exercise behavior; (2) The effectiveness of physical activity promotion interventions; and (3) Physical activity and psychological well-being. Adrian coauthored the NHS National Quality Assurance Framework for exercise referral schemes (www.doh.gov.uk/exercisereferrals) and with coauthors published the Cochrane review on the effects of exercise on smoking cessation.

Exercise, Health and Mental Health
Emerging relationships

Edited by
Guy E. J. Faulkner and
Adrian H. Taylor

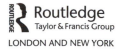
Routledge
Taylor & Francis Group

LONDON AND NEW YORK

First published 2005
by Routledge
2 Park Square, Milton Park, Abingdon, Oxon OX14 4RN

Simultaneously published in the USA and Canada
by Routledge
270 Madison Ave, New York, NY 10016

Routledge is an imprint of the Taylor & Francis Group

Typeset in Garamond by
Newgen Imaging Systems (P) Ltd, Chennai, India
Printed and bound in Great Britain by
TJ International Ltd, Padstow, Cornwall

British Library Cataloguing in Publication Data
A catalogue record for this book is available from the British Library

Library of Congress Cataloging in Publication Data
    Exercise, health and mental health: emerging relationships / edited by
Guy E. J. Faulkner and Adrian H. Taylor.
        p. cm.
    Includes bibliographical references and index.
      1. Exercise therapy. 2. Exercise – Psychological aspects.
3. Mental illness – Exercise therapy. 4. Mental health promotion.
I. Faulkner, Guy E. J., 1970– II. Taylor, Adrian H., 1955–

RC489.E9E95 2005
616.89′13–dc22   2005003834

ISBN 0–415–33430–6 (hbk)
ISBN 0–415–33431–4 (pbk)

Contents

1 Exercise and mental health promotion   1

GUY E. J. FAULKNER AND ADRIAN H. TAYLOR

2 Physical activity and dementia   11

DANIELLE LAURIN, RENÉ VERREAULT, AND JOAN LINDSAY

Figures

Tables

Notes on contributors

Fred Coalter is Professor of Sports Policy at the University of Stirling. Previously, he was Director of the Centre for Leisure Research at the University of Edinburgh. Recent work includes *The Role of Sport in Regenerating Deprived Urban Areas* (Scottish Executive), *Realising the Potential of Cultural Services* (Local Government Association), and *Sport and Community Development*, a manual (Sportscotland). He has been a member of several committees and working groups including: the Council of Europe's Working Group on Sport and Social Exclusion, the Sports Advisory Board of the Neighbourhood Renewal Unit in the Office of the Deputy Prime Minister, and Sport England's Working Group on Performance Measurement for the Development of Sport. He is also Chair of Edinburgh Leisure Ltd (the trust that manages sports provision for the City of Edinburgh Council) and is a member of the editorial board of *Managing Leisure*, an international journal.

Kerry S. Courneya is a Professor and Canada Research Chair in Physical Activity and Cancer in the Faculty of Physical Education at the University of Alberta in Edmonton, Canada. He received his BA (1987) and MA (1989) in physical education from the University of Western Ontario (London, Canada) and his PhD (1992) in kinesiology from the University of Illinois (Urbana, IL, USA). Kerry's research program focuses on the role of physical activity in cancer control including primary prevention, coping with treatments, rehabilitation after treatments, and secondary prevention and survival. His research interests include both the outcomes and determinants of physical activity for cancer control as well as behavior change interventions. His research program has been funded by the National Cancer Institute of Canada, the Canadian Breast Cancer Research Alliance, the National Institutes of Health (USA), the Alberta Heritage Foundation for Medical Research, and the Alberta Cancer Board.

Marie E. Donaghy is the Head of School of Health Sciences, Queen Margaret University College, Edinburgh. She took up her first research and teaching post 15 years ago following a 19-year career as a physiotherapist. It was during these clinical years that her interest in psychology developed, obtaining graduate membership to the British Psychological Society in 1990 and a PhD in 1997 investigating the effects of exercise on fitness and mood in recovering problem drinkers. Since then her interest in exercise has extended to include other clinical populations. In addition, she has developed and evaluated a framework for facilitating reflective practice in students. Marie has published papers and book chapters on both these topics and is a regular contributor to UK and European educational and scientific conferences. She is co-author of a recently published book on evidence-based interventions in mental health for physiotherapists and occupational therapists.

Guy E. J. Faulkner is currently an Assistant Professor in the Faculty of Physical Education and Health at the University of Toronto and coordinates the activities of the Exercise Psychology Unit. In 2001, he completed a PhD in Exercise Psychology in 2001 at Loughborough University before taking up an academic position at the University of Exeter in England. His current research concerns the physical health needs of mental health service users in relation to antipsychotic medication, weight gain, diabetes, and medication compliance; mediated health messages; and the role of physical activity in harm reduction and smoking cessation.

Julie D. Freelove-Charton is a Doctoral Student and Research Assistant in the Department of Exercise Science, Norman J. Arnold School of Public Health, at the University of South Carolina. She has an MSc in kinesiology and health promotion, and a BA in psychology. For over six years, Charton has been involved with research and community-based physical activity interventions exploring the benefits of exercise training in late life. Julie is also an accomplished cyclist, who has competed in the US Olympic Trials, the International PowerBar Women's Challenge, and the National Collegiate Cycling Championships.

Danielle Laurin received her PhD in Epidemiology from Laval University, Québec City, Canada, while studying the associations between lifestyle risk factors and the incidence of dementia using data from the Canadian Study of Health and Aging. Her postdoctoral training was performed in the Neuroepidemiology section of the Laboratory of Epidemiology, Demography, and Biometry at the National Institute on Aging, Bethesda, MD. She worked on the nutritional data from another large population-based study, the Honolulu-Asia Aging Study. Dr Laurin is now Assistant Professor at the Faculty of Pharmacy at Laval University and a new investigator at Laval University Geriatrics Research Unit at the Research Centre of the Centre Hospitalier Affilié Universitaire de Québec.

Joan Lindsay has a PhD in Epidemiology from the University of Western Ontario. She worked at Statistics Canada for several years, and has been working at Health Canada since 1987. She currently works at the newly created Public Health Agency of Canada, and at the Department of Epidemiology and Community Medicine, University of Ottawa. She also has a cross-appointment at Laval University. She has been actively involved in the overall planning, conducting, and data analysis of the three phases of the Canadian Study of Health and Aging – a large, national, multicenter study of the epidemiology of Alzheimer's disease and other dementias, and other aspects of seniors' health.

Ffion Lloyd-Williams is a Senior Research Fellow at the Institute of Health, Liverpool John Moores University. She was previously research fellow at the division of primary care at the University of Liverpool and prior to that her career was as a researcher with the National Health Service in Wales. She gained a PhD at the University of Keele and her research interests include the psychosocial aspects of heart failure. Her work has also examined patients' perceptions of heart failure, the benefits of exercise for heart failure, the role of primary care in heart failure management, and the information needs of people with heart failure.

Frances Mair is a Medical Graduate from Glasgow University. After completing her vocational training in general practice in Glasgow, she worked as a general practitioner for the US Navy within the US Embassy in London for four years. In 1993, she entered academic general practice at Liverpool University. During 1995–1996 she went to the USA on a one-year sabbatical and worked as a Research Fellow in Telemedicine/Family Medicine at the University of Kansas Medical Center. Professor Mair was appointed Professor of Primary Care Research at the University of Liverpool in May 2003 and at the same time became Director of the Mersey Primary Care Research and Development Consortium, one of the largest primary care research networks in the United Kingdom. Her major research interests are heart failure and e-health and she has published widely and holds substantial grant funding in these areas.

William W. Stringer is the chairman of the Department of Medicine at Harbor-UCLA Medical Center, and a Professor of Medicine at the David Geffen School of Medicine at UCLA. He graduated from the University of California, San Diego School of Medicine in 1984, and did his internship, residency, chief residency, and Pulmonary/Critical Care fellowship at Harbor-UCLA Medical Center. He is active in research involving HIV, chronic obstructive pulmonary disease (COPD), cardiopulmonary exercise testing, and physiological calibration of exercise systems at the Los Angeles Biomedical Institute at Harbor-UCLA Medical Center.

Adrian H. Taylor completed his PhD in Exercise Science at the University of Toronto in 1989. As a Reader in Exercise and Health Psychology in the School of Sport and Health Sciences at the University of Exeter in the United Kingdom, his main interest is in acute and chronic psychological outcomes from physical activity. He has published in prestigious journals such as Health Psychology, Ageing and Physical Activity, Epidemiology and Community Health, and Addiction with investigations on the effectiveness of interventions in primary care and from exercise counseling on physical self-perceptions and identity, CHD risk factors, and smoking abstinence. He is currently involved in a large four-year randomized trial of an exercise intervention in primary care to treat depression in the United Kingdom. He is also investigating the effects of walking on cigarette cravings, affect, and psychophysiological stress reactivity in lab-based settings. He is a Fellow of the British Association of Sport and Exercise Science and is currently Co-editor in Chief of *Psychology of Sport and Exercise*, an international journal.

Michael H. Ussher is a Lecturer in Health Psychology in the Department of Community Health Sciences at St George's Hospital Medical School, University of London. Dr Ussher conducts epidemiological, intervention and experimental research in both smoking cessation and physical activity promotion. Much of his work has focused on the role of physical activity interventions in smoking cessation and in alcohol rehabilitation and he has published numerous scientific articles on these research topics. Dr Ussher is the author of the *Cochrane Review* of "Exercise interventions for smoking cessation."

René Verreault received his PhD in Epidemiology from Laval University, Québec City, Canada, in 1988, and completed his postdoctoral training at the School of Public Health, University of Washington, Seattle, WA. He is currently Professor in the Department of Social and Preventive Medicine, Faculty of Medicine, Laval University. He holds the Laval University Chair for Geriatric Research and is Director of the Laval University Geriatrics Research Unit. He is also involved in clinical work as a practicing physician in geriatric and palliative care. His research activities focus mainly on the epidemiology of Alzheimer's disease and other types of dementia.

Shawn D. Youngstedt graduated from the University of Texas–Austin in 1982 with a BA in Psychology, and then a PhD in Exercise Psychology (1995) at the University of Georgia under the mentorship of Drs Rod K. Dishman and Patrick J. O'Connor. After a postdoctoral fellowship in the Department of Psychiatry at UCSD, Dr Youngstedt was appointed to a faculty position at UCSD. In 2003, he began his current position as Assistant Professor in the Department of Exercise Science, Norman J. Arnold School of Public Health, at the University of South Carolina, Columbia, SC. Dr Youngstedt's research has focused on the influence of exercise and bright light on sleep, circadian rhythms, and mood. Recent research examines the potential risks associated with long sleep durations.

Acknowledgments

Guy E. J. Faulkner and Adrian H. Taylor would like to thank Stuart J. H. Biddle (Loughborough University), Rod K. Dishman (University of Georgia), and all of the contributors for creating these insightful and timely overviews of their areas of research. We would also like to thank Chris Gee (University of Toronto) for his editorial work, Sara-Jane Finlay (University of Toronto at Mississauga) for her critical feedback and support, and everyone at Routledge for their hard work and assistance in the production of this book.

Adrian dedicates this work to his parents, Joyce and James, and family, Helen, Jamie, Katrina, and Duncan, who have provided insights into well-being across the lifespan, and Aidan, who has opened new doors for understanding the meaning of mental health. Thanks for all your support.

Foreword

The study of psychological processes in physical activity and health has grown considerably in recent years. "Exercise psychologists" study the psychological antecedents of physical activity and use their theoretical perspectives to inform the design and implementation of interventions to change sedentary lifestyles. In addition, involvement in physical activity can have important psychological benefits. Although we have known this for a very long time, it is only relatively recently that a systematic approach has been adopted to the accumulation of evidence. This has involved the use of experimental trials, largescale surveys, and detailed qualitative studies. Many have been brought together in well-cited meta-analytic reviews where the "effects" of exercise and physical activity have been assessed on anxiety, stress reactivity, depression, mood, and cognitive functioning. In addition, reviews exist on the links between physical activity and self-perceptions including self-esteem and health-related quality of life.

In 2000, Ken Fox, Steve Boutcher, and I pulled together this literature in an edited volume with the intention of providing a current consensus of knowledge. The feeling at the time was that we needed to summarize what we knew and needed to know about these key psychological outcomes. Less was known about the role of physical activity in important health-related conditions and behaviors such as smoking or alcohol consumption. It is here that Guy Faulkner and Adrian Taylor have done so well in bringing together an important collection of papers and provided a unique look at the role of physical activity.

These issues are far from trivial. While many accept that "exercise is good for you," mentally and physically, few understand its importance in helping people cope with debilitating and difficult conditions such as heart disease and HIV, or with common behavioral problems of alcoholism or smoking addiction. Coupled with the physical benefits, physical activity may not be the "magic bullet" we are looking for, but it comes a lot closer than most things!

Guy and Adrian, with this book, have enabled the field to take a step forward and to move from the evidence based on psychological outcomes to the newer area of the (psychological) role of physical activity in a variety of conditions including important social issues such as social inclusion. With their extensive experience and wisdom in the field, and their open-minded approach to a wide variety of research methods and questions in their own research, they are well placed to lead us onto new and exciting avenues for the role of physical activity in health-related behaviors.

Stuart J. H. Biddle, PhD
Professor of Exercise and Sport Psychology
Loughborough University
Leicestershire, UK

Foreword

Exercise psychology is the study of brain and behavior in physical activity and exercise settings. It is a new field, but it is based on old ideas. The ancient Greek physician, Hippocrates, recommended physical activity for the treatment of mental illness. In 1632 the British theologian, Robert Burton, warned about the risks of a sedentary lifestyle, "Opposite to Exercise is Idleness or want of exercise, the bane of body and minde, . . . one of the seven deadly sinnes, and a sole cause of Melancholy." William James, the father of American Psychology, stated in 1899 that . . . "muscular vigor will . . . always be needed to furnish the background of sanity, serenity, and cheerfulness to life, to give moral elasticity to our disposition, to round off the wiry edge of our fretfulness, and make us good-humored and easy of approach."

Though the study of consciousness and subjective experience is the defining feature of psychology that distinguishes it from other disciplines such as physiology and sociology, areas of modern psychology vary in their emphasis on physiological, behavioral, cognitive, or social questions and methods. Since the field of exercise psychology is concerned with mental health and health-related behaviors within both clinical settings and secular populations it also encompasses approaches from the fields of psychiatry, clinical and counseling psychology, health promotion, and epidemiology.

The aim of the current edited collection of reviews is to "consider what research evidence exists to support the emerging use of physical activity and exercise as a mental health promotion strategy in a range of conditions and populations, and how it can guide practitioners and researchers in the context of increasing concern for evidence-based practice." Rather than constraining the topics to the usual suspects of depression, anxiety, and self-esteem, editors Taylor and Faulkner rightfully expand the book's scope to other clinical concerns of contemporary importance to public health, namely, sleep disorders, smoking, alcohol and substance abuse, schizophrenia, dementia, delinquency and quality of life among cancer survivors, and patients with HIV disease or congestive heart failure. When I addressed some of these topics in a review of physical activity and mental health for the National Association of Sport and Physical Education in the USA 20 years ago, there was hardly any evidence upon which to draw conclusions or make professional recommendations. It's gratifying to now see interest in these important areas mature, and it's about time that someone accumulated the evidence in a way that can help guide practitioners and researchers alike. Well done.

Rod K. Dishman, PhD
Professor of Exercise Science and
Adjunct Professor of Psychology
The University of Georgia, Athens, USA

Exercise and mental health promotion

GUY E. J. FAULKNER AND ADRIAN H. TAYLOR

The mind–body link (e.g., healthy body ↔ healthy mind) has long been recognized but increasingly society is engaging in sedentary work, travel, domestic, and leisure activities. Many of the psychological consequences of sedentary behavior, and conversely physical activity, were identified in a previous text *Physical Activity and Psychological Well-Being* (Biddle *et al.*, 2000a). This text provided an invaluable review of the evidence for the role of exercise in improving well-being in relation to anxiety, depression, mood, self-esteem, and cognitive functioning. It also raised many issues for the researcher and practitioner concerned with both the prevention and treatment of mental health problems. The book also identified a number of emergent areas of research that were not assessed which adds further scope to the exciting and as yet untapped potential that exercise may offer within the growing field of mental health promotion and enhancement of quality of life. The current edited collection provides a unique overview of this emerging case for exercise and the promotion of mental health for all of us in general, and for individuals with mental illness and those coping with clinical conditions.

WHAT IS MENTAL HEALTH PROMOTION?

Mental health can be seen as the emotional and spiritual resilience which enables us to enjoy life and cope with adversity such as physical disability, pain, cravings, and stress, while also surviving pain, disappointment, and sadness. It is a positive sense of well-being and an underlying belief in our own and others' dignity and worth (Health Education Authority, 1997). Mental health may be central to all health and well-being, as it has been shown that how we think has a significant impact on physical health. Critically, since everyone has mental health needs, the need for mental health promotion is universal and of relevance to everyone (DoH, 2001). Mental health promotion is concerned with (1) how individuals, families, and organizations think and feel, (2) the factors which influence how we think and feel, individually and collectively, and (3) the impact that this has on overall health and well-being (Friedli, 2000). Overall, mental health promotion seeks to strengthen individuals and communities.

We now have a convincing body of literature that supports the role of physical activity and exercise as strategies for promoting mental health (see Table 1.1; Biddle *et al.*, 2000a; DoH, 2004). Physical activity may also be an innovative and effective way of enhancing the balance between physical and mental health (New Freedom Commission on Mental Health, 2003). We use physical activity as a general term that refers to any movement of the body that results in energy expenditure above that of resting level (Caspersen *et al.*, 1985). Exercise is often, but incorrectly, used interchangeably with

Table 1.1 Physical activity and psychological well-being: a research consensus

DOMAIN	WHAT WE KNOW
Anxiety and stress (Taylor, 2000)	• Exercise has a low–moderate anxiety-reducing effect • Exercise training can reduce trait anxiety and single exercise sessions can result in reductions in state anxiety • The strongest anxiety-reduction effects are shown in randomized controlled trials • Single sessions of moderate exercise can reduce short-term physiological reactivity to, and enhance recovery from, brief psychosocial stressors
Depression (Mutrie, 2000)	• There is support for a causal link between exercise and decreased depression • Epidemiological evidence has demonstrated that physical activity is associated with a decreased risk of developing clinically defined depression • Evidence from experimental studies shows that both aerobic and resistance exercise may be used to treat moderate and more severe depression, usually as an adjunct to standard treatment • The anti-depressant effect of exercise can be of the same magnitude as that found for other psychotherapeutic interventions • No negative effects of exercise have been noted in depressed populations
Emotion and mood (Biddle, 2000)	• Physical activity and exercise have consistently been associated with positive mood and affect • Meta-analytic evidence shows that aerobic exercise has a small–moderate effect on vigor (+), tension (−), depression (−), fatigue (−) and confusion (−), and a small effect on anger (−)

DOMAIN	WHAT WE KNOW
	• A positive relationship between physical activity and psychological well-being has been confirmed in several large-scale epidemiological surveys using different measures of activity and well-being • Experimental trials support a positive effect for moderate intensity exercise on psychological well-being • Meta-analytic evidence shows that adopting a goal in exercise that is focused on personal improvement, effort, and mastery has a moderate–high association with positive affect • Meta-analytic evidence shows that a group climate in exercise and sport settings that is focused on personal improvement and effort has a moderate–high association with positive affect
Self-esteem (Fox, 2000b)	• Exercise can be used as a medium to promote physical self-worth and other important physical self-perceptions such as body image. In some situations, this improvement is accompanied by improved self-esteem • Physical self-worth carries mental well-being properties in its own right and should be considered as a valuable end-point of exercise programs • Positive effects of exercise on self-perceptions can be experienced by all age groups but there is strongest evidence for change for children and middle-aged adults • Positive effects of exercise on self-perceptions can be experienced by men and women • Positive effects of exercise on self-perceptions are likely to be greater for those with initially low self-esteem • Several types of exercise are effective in changing self-perceptions but there is most evidence to support aerobic exercise and resistance training, with the latter indicating greatest effectiveness in the short-term
Cognitive functioning (Boutcher, 2000)	• The majority of cross-sectional studies show that fit older adults display better cognitive performance than less fit older adults • The association between fitness and cognitive performance is task-dependent, with most pronounced effects in tasks that are attention-demanding and rapid (e.g., reaction time tasks) • Results of intervention studies are equivocal but meta-analytic findings indicate a small but significant improvement in cognitive functioning of older adults who experience an increase in aerobic fitness
Psychological dysfunction (Szabo, 2000)	• Exercise dependence is extremely rare • Many people suffering from eating disorders undertake high levels of physical activity • The personality characteristics of anorectics are significantly different from highly committed exercisers

Source: Adapted from Biddle *et al.*, 2000b.

physical activity. However, exercise refers to a subset of physical activity in which the activity is purposefully undertaken with the aim of maintaining or improving physical fitness or health. Examples of exercise include "going to the gym," jogging, brisk walking, taking an aerobics class, or taking part in recreational sport for fitness.

This relationship between physical activity and mental health may be critical for two reasons. The literature indicates that mental health outcomes motivate people to persist in physical activity while also having a potentially positive impact on well-being (Biddle and Mutrie, 2001). Furthermore, because physical activity is an effective method for improving important aspects of physical health such as obesity, cardiovascular fitness, and hypertension (see Bouchard et al., 1994), the promotion of exercise for psychological well-being can be seen as a "win-win" situation with both mental and physical health benefits accruing (Mutrie and Faulkner, 2003). Undoubtedly, methodological concerns do exist concerning the research on the mental health benefits of exercise (e.g., Biddle et al., 2000b; Lawlor and Hopker, 2001). This is significant, as the acceptance of exercise within health care services will be based on the strength of available evidence. Indeed, the previous text, edited by Biddle et al. (2000a), emerged from a commission by health service policy makers and practitioners to identify evidence for the role of exercise in enhancing mental health.

Analysis of fairly recent mental health promotion policy documents (e.g., DoH, 2000; USDHHS, 1999) revealed rather limited inclusion of the role of physical activity, despite the fact that at least seven texts have appeared on the subject. The US Surgeon General's Report on Mental Health (USDHHS, 1999) suggests that there are multiple and complex explanations for the gap between what is known through research and what is actually practiced. Indeed, the US National Advisory Mental Health Council (1998) noted that new strategies are required to bridge the gap between research and practice. Several reasons exist for why physical activity has not been widely prescribed in the promotion of positive mental health. First, mental health practitioners may not have access to the same research. This may have been true in the past, but electronic data searches make this less likely. Second, those conducting research on the psychological benefits of exercise may have been using different criteria for judging the effects. It is, therefore, important to consider the type of evidence available.

THE EVIDENCE

It is important that any mental health promotion strategy such as the promotion of physical activity is based on sound evidence. However, it is important to recognize that what constitutes sound evidence, and how this is measured, is complex and open to debate (DoH, 2001). Evidence-based practice is defined by its adherents as the "conscientious, explicit and judicious use of current best evidence in making decisions about the care of individual patients" (Sackett et al., 1996, p. 71). Such evidence is principally gathered through randomized controlled trials (RCT):

It is when asking questions about therapy that we should try to avoid the non-experimental approaches, since these routinely lead to false-positive conclusions about efficacy. Because the randomised trial, and especially the systematic review of several randomised trials, is so much more likely to inform us and so much less likely to mislead us, it has become the 'gold standard' for judging whether a treatment does more good than harm.

(Sackett *et al.*, 1996, p. 72)

Random selection of participants and random assignment to treatments is the most effective means of controlling threats to internal and external validity, while the inclusion of a control group rules out the possibility that something other than the experimental treatment (e.g., exercise) produces the results. As a minimum, the use of a control group should "be viewed as a necessary rather than a sufficient design requirement" (Morgan, 1997, p. 12) and a comparison treatment should be included to consider the effects compared to something else, such as normal treatment, when evaluating the role of physical activity. Ideally, either the investigators, research participants, or both, should not know who is receiving what treatment option. This "blinding" helps protect the study from bias due to the Hawthorne effect or Placebo effect (see Morgan, 1997). Clearly, RCTs will play an influential role in convincing policy makers and practitioners of the relative worth of physical activity as a mental health promotion strategy.

At the same time, mental health promotion itself has lagged behind the promotion of physical health (Sainsbury, 2000) and the evidence base is accordingly less extensive. In relation to exercise, Fox (1999, 2000a) outlined a number of suggestions as to why the evidence for the mental health benefits of exercise has not been widely translated into mental health service practice. For example, the recognition of evidence-based principles has only been relatively recent, with attention on academic rather than service outcomes. More specifically, studies have rarely addressed the cost-effectiveness of treatments or used intention-to-treat analyses, which entails including dropouts from studies in final analyses. Failing to do so is likely to positively bias the results. Overall, criteria for RCTs have rarely been satisfied (Faulkner and Biddle, 2001; Lawlor and Hopker, 2001).

Unfortunately, such designs may not be well-suited for the study of exercise and mental health. For example,

- An RCT may require modification of normal treatment or exercise promotion opportunities, thereby raising the issue of what is being evaluated (NHS Executive, 2001). A wide variation in clinical settings such as outpatient, inpatient and community settings may also influence attempts at generalization (Burbach, 1997; Morgan, 1997).
- The effects of exercise are likely to be a very individual experience with each "exerciser" relying on a unique exercise formula for maximum psychological benefit (Fox, 2000a). Individuals who are allocated to their non-preferred treatment may not experience great psychological benefit and as a result may dropout. This differential attrition introduces a nonrandom element into the design, and those who complete an exercise program may be atypically receptive, reducing attempts at generalization (Roth and Parry, 1997).
- Ensuring evaluators are blind to treatment conditions may be particularly difficult during exercise interventions. Specifically, when interviewing patients to assess progress, it is difficult to avoid exposure to information when patients will often recount their experiences.

- Given the small number of mental health patients that may be available at any one time, a multicenter trial, which is often prohibitive due to cost and hard to standardize across treatment centers, makes experimental work difficult (Mutrie, 1997).
- Small-scale schemes, in which patients become familiar with the support of specific exercise professionals, may result in better adherence. Adequately powered controlled trials may not, therefore, demonstrate optimal levels of adherence (NHS Executive, 2001).
- Finally, RCT's answer "a circumscribed set of questions and issues related to outcome rather than to process, and to efficacy rather than effectiveness" (Roth and Parry, 1997, p. 370). Efficacy describes what works under ideal or optimal conditions, usually when the dose of exercise is controlled and carefully monitored, while effectiveness refers to what works in typical clinical practice settings. That is, the external validity or generalizability of RCTs has been questioned. More practically, the cost of conducting RCT's may be overly prohibitive for many researchers.

Such difficulties do not make RCTs impossible and we hope that researchers continue to examine exercise as a mental health promotion strategy using such designs. However, while urging caution, we concur with "a more flexible and forgiving approach to the interpretation of the existing literature and the planning for future research" (Biddle *et al.*, 2000b, p. 161).

QUASI-EXPERIMENTAL AND PRE-EXPERIMENTAL DESIGNS

A quasi-experimental study, like the RCT, attempts to minimize the possibility of bias in interpreting research findings. This approach is very similar to the RCT, although it lacks the random assignment of participants to treatment groups. Such designs may be particularly suited to research in applied settings, where control over the research setting is more difficult. Non-equivalent groups or time-series designs are examples of quasi-experiments.

In a pre-experimental study, only one group of participants receives the intervention. There may be a pre- and post-test but this design does not allow us to relate any changes in the variables of interest to the intervention per se. Typically, this type of design could be considered a pilot study that provides initial support for the consideration of a particular treatment that can then be tested using more rigorous research protocols.

QUALITATIVE RESEARCH

Qualitative research comprises a wide range of research approaches but it is usually characterized by rich description and designs in which narrative is used to more closely represent the experience of participants. It is ideally suited to understanding the process by which events and actions take place and how views and attitudes change over time (Maxwell, 1996). For example, longitudinal involvement in the "field" of study offers an opportunity to explore perceptions of physical activity, the motives and barriers to involvement, and its role in promoting psychological well-being alongside the narrative of participant's lives (see Faulkner and Biddle, 2004). An important objective may be to discover and "understand naturally occurring phenomena in their naturally occurring states" (Patton, 1980, p. 41). As Maykut and Morehouse (1994) remind us:

Qualitative researchers value context sensitivity, that is, understanding a phenomena in all its complexity and within a particular situation and environment. The quantitative researcher works to eliminate all of the unique aspects of the environment in order to apply the results to the largest possible number of subjects and experiments.

(p. 13)

Given the low number of research participants that a researcher may have access to in some settings, qualitative research designs may be insightful in examining the physical activity and mental health relationship. Qualitative studies concerned with how different patients perceive the role of exercise in treatment have been encouraged (Mutrie, 2000). Increasing attention has also been given to allowing patients and clients to discuss their experiences and have a voice regarding the improvement in their own quality of life (e.g., Faulkner and Layzell, 2000). Furthermore, Carless and Faulkner (2003) suggest that qualitative studies with a focus on change at the individual level do permit greater insight and understanding of person-level changes than are possible through an RCT.

Qualitative research can therefore focus on both efficacy and effectiveness questions. In terms of efficacy, participants may individually report on the effects of both acute and chronic exercise, which may reveal information about associated processes and mechanisms, and perhaps interactions with medication or other important factors such as type, frequency, intensity, and duration of exercise. In terms of effectiveness, participants may describe their experiences with the delivery of the exercise intervention, including the positive and negative role of others, and the favorability of the processes in which they enter, remain in, and exit exercise programs.

Overall, we would argue that it is the integration and awareness of this diversity of research designs and methodological approaches that will further understanding in exercise science in general, and physical activity and mental health in particular. We invite readers to critically assess the claims, made by the reviewers in this collection, in light of these methodological issues. We believe that a range of research designs, drawn from the diverse disciplines available, can all contribute to not only developing our evidence base to support the consideration of physical activity as a mental health promotion strategy but also our evidence-based *practice*.

PURPOSE OF THE BOOK

The aim of the current edited collection of reviews is to consider what research evidence exists to support the emerging use of physical activity and exercise as a mental health promotion strategy in a range of conditions and populations, and how it can guide practitioners and researchers in the context of increasing concern for evidence-based practice.

Leading researchers have been recruited to produce systematic reviews that aim to minimize bias and use clear criteria for the inclusion of interventions. Priority has been given to evidence from RCTs, large scale epidemiological studies, and meta-analytic reviews. Where such experimental studies are lacking, less rigorous research designs such as quasi- and pre-experimental designs, and qualitative studies are considered. Authors have been asked to summarize their findings in tables, identify implications for both researchers and practitioners, and provide closing sections featuring "what we know" and "what we need to know" statements. The reviews are loosely divided into three sections.

First, there is interest in the effects of exercise as a treatment or adjunct for clinically defined mental health problems. Dementia is common, costly, and highly age related. Danielle Laurin, René Verreault, and Joan Lindsay start this collection by reviewing the role of physical activity in protecting against problems of serious cognitive impairment in old age as experienced in some forms of dementia and Alzheimer's disease.

Schizophrenia is the most common serious mental illness and places a disproportionately heavy burden on resources in psychiatric care. For people with severe and enduring mental health problems, improvement in quality of life tends to enhance the individual's ability to cope with and manage their disorder. Guy Faulkner reviews the evidence suggesting that regular physical activity can improve positive aspects of mental health (such as psychological quality of life and emotional well-being) in people with mental disorders. Dependence on alcohol or drugs falls into all of the commonly used classifications of mental illness, while alcohol dependence is a common problem affecting one in six adults aged 16–24 years. Marie Donaghy and Michael Ussher consider the use of exercise as a coping strategy for these conditions and its subsequent impact on individual quality of life and overall treatment cost.

Second, there is interest in how exercise may improve mental health in individuals with common cardiovascular and immunological conditions where complete remission is difficult or unlikely. The incidence of cancer, HIV, and heart disease is rising and all are significant causes of mortality. Although once viewed as conditions progressing to death, these conditions are now often characterized by unpredictable cycles of wellness and illness. Coping with the diagnosis, impairments, and treatment of such conditions may be necessary while exercise has the potential to improve both physical and psychological functioning. Kerry Courneya, Ffion Lloyd-Williams and Frances Mair, and William Stringer review the evidence for exercise in improving the mental health of individuals coping with the clinical conditions of cancer, heart failure, and HIV/AIDS respectively.

Third, there is growing interest in the effects of exercise in enhancing mental health in the general public. Current consensus clearly supports an association between physical activity and numerous domains of mental health in the general population. This section will extend these analyses with reviews by Shawn Youngstedt and Julie Freelove-Charton examining the role of exercise in enhancing quantity and quality of sleep in good and poor sleepers, and Adrian Taylor and Michael Ussher examining the role of exercise in smoking cessation and treating nicotine addiction. Finally, contemporary claims for exercise participation serving as a forum for the alleviation of social exclusion (individuals or communities that suffer from a combination of problems such as poor education, housing, employment, and health), specifically in terms of juvenile delinquency, are critically assessed by Fred Coalter.

A closing chapter draws together key findings and identifies issues of both convergence and divergence emerging across the reviews. The most critical implications for further research and practice are discussed. Overall, we hope that this resource will be a catalyst and valuable for researchers who want to take the field of exercise and mental health further, and for practitioners in "making the case" for physical activity and mental health in a range of service delivery settings.

REFERENCES

Biddle, S. J. H. (2000). Emotion, mood and physical activity. In S. J. H. Biddle, K. R. Fox, and S. H. Boutcher (Eds). *Physical Activity and Psychological Well-being* (pp. 63–87). London: Routledge.

Biddle, S. J. H. and Mutrie, N. (2001). *Psychology of Physical Activity: Determinants, Well-being, and Interventions*. London: Routledge.

Biddle, S. J. H., Fox, K. R., and Boutcher, S. H. (Eds). (2000a). *Physical Activity and Psychological Well-being*. London: Routledge.

Biddle, S. J. H., Fox, K. R., Boutcher, S. H., and Faulkner, G. (2000b). The way forward for physical activity and the promotion of psychological well-being. In S. J. H. Biddle, K. R. Fox, and S. H. Boutcher (Eds). *Physical Activity and Psychological Well-being* (pp. 154–168). London: Routledge.

Bouchard, C. R., Shephard, R. J., and Stephens, T. (Eds). (1994). *Physical Activity, Fitness and Health: International Consensus Proceedings*. Champaign, IL: Human Kinetics.

Boutcher, S. H. (2000). Cognitive performance, fitness, and aging. In S. J. H. Biddle, K. R. Fox, and S. H. Boutcher (Eds). *Physical Activity and Psychological Well-being* (pp. 118–129). London: Routledge.

Burbach, F. R. (1997). The efficacy of physical activity interventions within mental health services: anxiety and depressive disorders. *Journal of Mental Health*, 6, 543–566.

Carless, D. and Faulkner, G. (2003). Physical activity and psychological health. In J. McKenna and C. Riddoch (Eds). *Perspectives on Health and Exercise* (pp. 61–82). London: Palgrave Macmillan.

Caspersen, C. J., Powell, K. E., and Christenson, G. M. (1985). Physical activity, exercise and physical fitness: definitions and distinctions for health-related research. *Public Health Reports*, *100*, 126–131.

DoH (Department of Health) (2000). *National Service Framework: Mental Health*. London: HMSO.

DoH (Department of Health) (2001). *Making it Happen: A Guide to Delivering Mental Health Promotion*. London: HMSO.

DoH (Department of Health) (2004). *At Least Five a Week. A Report from the Chief Medical Officer*. London: HMSO.

Faulkner, A. and Layzell, S. (2000). *Strategies for Living: A Report of User-led Research into People's Strategies for Living with Mental Distress*. London: Mental Health Foundation.

Faulkner, G. and Biddle, S. J. H. (2001). Exercise as therapy: it's just not psychology! *Journal of Sports Sciences*, *19*, 433–444.

Faulkner, G. and Biddle, S. J. H. (2004). Physical activity and depression: considering contextuality and variability. *Journal of Sport and Exercise Psychology*, *26*, 3–18.

Fox, K. R. (1999). The influence of physical activity on mental well-being. *Public Health Nutrition*, *2*, 411–418.

Fox, K. R. (2000a). Physical activity and mental health promotion: the natural partnership. *International Journal of Mental Health Promotion*, *2*, 4–12.

Fox, K. R. (2000b). The effects of exercise on self-perceptions and self-esteem. In S. J. H. Biddle, K. R. Fox, and S. H. Boutcher (Eds). *Physical Activity and Psychological Well-being* (pp. 88–117). London: Routledge.

Friedli, L. (2000). Mental health promotion: rethinking the evidence base. *The Mental Health Review*, 5, 15–18.

Health Education Authority (1997). *Mental Health Promotion: A Quality Framework*. London: Health Education Authority.

Lawlor, D. A. and Hopker, S. W. (2001). The effectiveness of exercise as an intervention in the management of depression: systematic review and meta-regression analysis of randomised controlled trials. *British Medical Journal*, 322, 763.

Maxwell, J. A. (1996). *Qualitative Research Design*. Thousand Oaks, CA: Sage.

Maykut, P. and Morehouse, R. (1994). *Beginning Qualitative Research*. London: Falmer Press.

Morgan, W. P. (1997). Methodological considerations. In W. P. Morgan (Ed.). *Physical Activity and Mental Health* (pp. 3–32). Washington, DC: Taylor and Francis.

Mutrie, N. (1997). The therapeutic effects of exercise on the self. In K. Fox (Ed.). *The Physical Self: From Motivation to Well-being* (pp. 287–314). Champaign, IL: Human Kinetics.

Mutrie, N. (2000). The relationship between physical activity and clinically defined depression. In S. J. H. Biddle, K. R. Fox, and S. H. Boutcher (Eds). *Physical Activity and Psychological Well-being* (pp. 46–62). London: Routledge.

Mutrie, N. and Faulkner, G. (2003). Physical activity and mental health. In T. Everett, M. Donaghy, and S. Fever (Eds). *Physiotherapy and Occupational Therapy in Mental Health: An Evidence Based Approach* (pp. 82–97). Oxford: Butterworth Heinemann.

National Advisory Mental Health Council (1998). *Parity in Financing Mental Health Services: Managed Care Effects on Cost, Access, and Quality: An Interim Report to Congress by the National Advisory Mental Health Council*. Bethesda, MD: Department of Health and Human Services, National Institutes of Health, and National Institute of Mental Health.

New Freedom Commission on Mental Health (2003). *Achieving the Promise: Transforming Mental Health Care in America. Final Report*. Rockville, MD: DHHS Pub. No. SMA-03-3832.

NHS Executive (National Health Service Executive) (2001). *Exercise Referral Systems: A National Quality Assurance Framework*. London: NHS Executive.

Patton, M. Q. (1980). *Qualitative Evaluation Methods*. Thousand Oaks, CA: Sage.

Roth, A. D. and Parry, G. (1997). The implications of psychotherapy research for clinical practice and service development: lessons and limitations. *Journal of Mental Health*, 6, 367–380.

Sackett, D. L., Rosenberg, W. M. C., Gray, J. A. M., Haynes, R. B., and Richardson, W. C. (1996). Evidence based medicine: what it is and what it isn't. *British Medical Journal*, 312, 71–72.

Sainsbury, P. (2000). Promoting mental health: recent progress and problems in Australia. *Journal of Epidemiology and Community Health*, 54, 82–83.

Szabo, A. (2000). Physical activity as a source of psychological dysfunction. In S. J. H. Biddle, K. R. Fox, and S. H. Boutcher (Eds). *Physical Activity and Psychological Well-being* (pp. 130–153). London: Routledge.

Taylor, A. H. (2000). Physical activity, anxiety, and stress. In S. J. H. Biddle, K. R. Fox, and S. H. Boutcher (Eds). *Physical Activity and Psychological Well-being* (pp. 10–45). London: Routledge.

USDHHS (United States Department of Health and Human Services) (1999). *Mental Health: A Report of the Surgeon General*. Rockville, MD: US Department of Health and Human Services, Substance Abuse and Mental Health Services Administration, Center for Mental Health Services, National Institutes of Health, National Institute of Mental Health.

CHAPTER 2

Physical activity and dementia

DANIELLE LAURIN, RENÉ VERREAULT, AND JOAN LINDSAY

▉ DEMENTIA

Dementia represents a very challenging public health problem affecting our aging societies, and is projected to further become one of the most preoccupying issues for social and health services over the next decades (Ernst and Hay, 1997). With few exceptions, the scientific literature on dementia and Alzheimer's disease (AD) has not yet permitted the identification of definitive etiologic hypotheses. However, little attention has been given to the identification of modifiable factors such as lifestyle habits, including physical activity.

There is an increasing body of evidence showing that fit older individuals display enhanced cognitive performance as compared with less fit older individuals, as reviewed by Boutcher (2000), and demonstrated more recently by Schuit *et al.* (2001), Tabbarah *et al.* (2002), and Yaffe *et al.* (2001). In addition, physical activity early in life could delay cognitive deficits later in life (Dik *et al.*, 2003). To date, few studies have examined the role of physical activity on the risk of developing dementia and AD in older persons. There has been some suggestion that physical activity may be protective against dementia, in particular AD, in analyses using prevalent cases, but these findings were not consistently replicated. Discordant results were also reported in longitudinal studies on dementia (Laurin *et al.*, 2001; Wilson *et al.*, 2002). Pathways through which physical activity could be involved in cognitive function and consequently dementia in late life have been proposed and tested in experimental studies.

This chapter will review published studies of the association between physical activity and the risk of dementia, AD, and vascular dementia (VaD) in older populations. Following a summary of the definitions of concepts surrounding dementia, this chapter will focus on the evidence for the relationship between physical activity and the risk of dementia from prevalence and incidence analyses in the light of their methodological limitations. A brief review of the mechanisms of action underlying these associations will be given, and further sections will identify issues for the researcher and practitioner, and identify what we know and need to know.

DEFINITIONS

According to the criteria of the *Diagnostic and Statistical Manual of Mental Disorders, fourth edition* (American Psychiatric Association, 1994), dementia is essentially characterized by the development of multiple cognitive deficits including impairment in memory, the prominent early symptom and the manifestation of at least one of four possible cognitive disturbances: deterioration of language function, impaired ability to execute motor activities, failure to recognize or identify objects, or disturbance in executive functioning. These cognitive deficits must be severe enough to cause impairment in social or occupational functioning, and represent a decline from a previous level of functioning.

AD represents the predominant subtype of dementia and accounts for 50–60% of all cases. Its onset is progressive and continues over several decades before the manifestation of clinical symptoms (American Psychiatric Association, 1994). Histopathological changes in the brain associated with AD comprise the accumulation of beta-amyloid protein to form senile plaques (Beyreuther and Masters, 1991), and of twisted protein fragments to form neurofibrillary tangles (Braak and Braak, 1991). These neuropathological hallmarks of AD have been generated in transgenic mice, a well-accepted animal model of AD (Hock and Lamb, 2001; Ishihara *et al.*, 2001). The diagnosis of probable AD is supported by the gradual deterioration of specific cognitive functions such as language, motor skills, and perceptions; impaired activities of daily living and altered patterns of behavior; family history of similar disorders; and laboratory results of normal lumbar puncture, normal pattern of nonspecific changes in electroencephalogram, and evidence of cerebral atrophy with progression documented by serial observation (McKhann *et al.*, 1984). The diagnosis of AD is made only after the elimination of other causes for dementia. Early onset of AD indicates an onset at age 65 years or before whereas late onset AD is after age 65.

VaD is the second most common subtype of dementia (approximately 20–30%), and occurs when cells in the brain are deprived of oxygen. In contrast to AD, the onset of VaD is usually unexpected and characterized by rapid modifications in functioning (American Psychiatric Association, 1994; Roman *et al.*, 1993). Computed tomography of the head and magnetic resonance imaging must reveal multiple vascular lesions of the cerebral cortex and subcortical structures. Clinical features of probable VaD include the early presence of a gait disturbance; a history of unsteadiness and frequent, unprovoked falls; an early urinary frequency, urgency, and other urinary symptoms not explained by urologic disease; speech disorder; and personality and mood changes, lack of motivation, depression, or deficits such as psychomotor retardation and abnormal executive function. VaD is most frequently the result of a single stroke or multiple strokes. A stroke occurs when a blood vessel reaching the brain is either blocked by a clot or bursts.

PREVALENCE AND INCIDENCE OF DEMENTIA

Dementia represents the most prevalent neurodegenerative disease in older persons. Estimates from the Canadian Study of Health and Aging, a large representative sample of the population aged 65 years and over, living in the community and institutions, suggested that the prevalence of dementia was 8% (Canadian Study of Health and Aging Working Group, 1994). AD and VaD were the two most prevalent subtypes, with AD leading with a prevalence of 5.1% and VaD with 1.5%. As previously demonstrated (Jorm *et al.*, 1987), the prevalence of dementia rose notably with age: the age-standardized prevalence rates ranged from 2.4%, among those aged 65–74 years, to 34.5%, among those aged 85 years and over. Using again estimates from the follow-up of the Canadian Study of Health and Aging (1991–1996), about 2% of the population developed dementia each year (21 cases per 1,000 persons aged 65 years and over) (Canadian Study of Health and Aging Working Group, 2000). The annual number of incident cases increased to 106.5 cases per 1,000 in nondemented persons aged 85 years and over. These prevalence and incidence rates tend to be positioned toward the upper end of the range reported in other studies in Europe and North America (Canadian Study of Health and Aging Working Group, 2000; McDowell, 2001; Rockwood and Stadnyk, 1994), but this may reflect the inclusion of both community and institutional samples and the addition of cases of early-stage dementia.

METHOD

Reports were drawn through electronic searches using Medline, Cinahl, and PsycLit as well as tracking the reference section of relevant papers. Search terms included study design terms: *prospective* or *trial* or *cross-sectional* or *intervention* with *exercise* or *physical activity*; and with *dementia* or *Alzheimer* or *vascular dementia* or *cognition*. Publications were considered if they were in English or French, if they included some measurement of physical activity or exercise with dementia as one of the primary outcomes, and if they were conducted in adult populations with an average or median age of 65 years and over.

CASE-CONTROL AND CROSS-SECTIONAL STUDIES

As the preliminary step toward the elucidation of a possible relationship between physical activity and the risk of dementia, researchers generally compared groups of individuals with dementia (cases) with groups of individuals without dementia (controls) in case-control studies. Case-control studies have the advantage of being relatively inexpensive to conduct but the major disadvantage of assessing a past exposure which may be biased due to recall. In cross-sectional studies, both past exposure and disease (dementia) are determined simultaneously for each subject in a sample of a defined population. The associations observed in cross-sectional studies may be related to survival after dementia rather than to the risk of developing dementia. In addition, because dementia and past exposure are assessed at the same time, the association may not reflect a causal relationship. Recall bias may also affect the exposure in cross-sectional studies. In this section, we will briefly summarize seven studies that were selected because they had a respectable sample size and included some information on the assessment of physical activity.

Broe *et al.* (1990) were one of the first to report the protective effect of physical activity against AD in an Australian study including 170 age- and sex-matched pairs of cases and controls aged 52–96 years. Informants of all newly recognized cases of AD and of their controls were administered a risk factor interview in their home by trained research assistants. The interview was developed to assess previous health, family history, lifestyle, and occupational or domestic exposures. Among the 87 variables considered, physical underactivity as a behavioral trait in the recent past (in the previous 10 years) and the more distant past (before 10 years ago) was noted to be significantly associated with the risk of AD, as shown by odds ratios (ORs) of 3.5 and 6.3, respectively. However, these two results were computed according to 85 and 84 of the initial 170 pairs of subjects, which could indicate some selection bias. Furthermore, the study population included both early- and late-onset cases of AD, which prevent us from generalizing to either subtype. On the other hand, it was noteworthy that underactivity in the more distant past was related to an increased risk of AD, thereby attenuating the argument that people with preclinical dementia would be less likely to be physically active.

Using a similar study design focusing on the impact of specific lifestyles in Japan and involving 60 cases of AD matched for age and sex with two controls aged 43–89 years, Kondo *et al.* (1994) also reported physical inactivity as a significant risk factor. Trained nurses interviewed close relatives of the cases in order to complete a structured questionnaire covering 135 questions on lifestyles. The practice (yes/no) of 10 physical activities (walking, patterned gymnastics, gardening, gate ball, jogging, hiking, dance, cycling, golf, swordsmanship) during the fifth and sixth decades of life was individually evaluated. Significant reduced risks of AD were observed for walking, gardening, dance, and cycling (ORs of 0.4, 0.5, 0.1, and 0.1, respectively). No associations between sports such as gymnastics, gate ball, jogging, hiking, or golf were found, although all results tended to show protective risk values. The inclusion of early- and late-onset cases of AD, the poor validity of the measurement of physical activity, and the fact that exposure was not assessed in the same manner in cases and controls seriously limits the interpretation of the results.

In contrast to the previous two studies, Mayeux *et al.* (1993) did not observe any differences between 138 older cases of AD and 193 controls residing in New York communities, in the frequency of reported athletic activity now and in the past. Exposure to physical activity was ascertained following a structured interview with cases and their informants together, while controls were interviewed directly without informants.

Using information collected from a mailed health survey questionnaire completed 11 and 14 years before assessment of cognitive status, Paganini-Hill and Henderson (1994, 1996) published two case-control analyses within a cohort of residents of a California retirement community initially including 8,877 women. The questionnaire comprised details of lifestyle characteristics including exercise habits. According to the authors, no association between physical activity and the prevalence of AD and related dementia was observed in either analysis. A major limitation of these analyses was that the outcomes were collected using death certificates which are known to underreport dementia (Raiford *et al.*, 1994).

More recently, Friedland *et al.* (2001) carried out a case-control study in the US including 193 cases of AD and 358 controls matched for age and sex in order to determine the association with activities during midlife. The researchers collected data on 26 nonoccupational activities from ages 20–60. Questionnaires were completed in the home by informants for cases, and by controls themselves. Activities were grouped into three categories (passive, intellectual, and physical) which were used to create three measures: diversity (total number of activities), intensity (hours per month), and percentage intensity (percentage of total activity hours for each activity category). After controlling for year of birth, sex, education, and income, a significant increased risk of AD was found in subjects having less than the mean value of activities (OR = 3.9), and in those with low physical diversity (OR = 2.7). No difference was observed on physical activity according to intensity score and percentage intensity. Despite these inconsistent results, the authors nevertheless concluded that subjects with AD were less active in midlife in terms of physical activities than controls.

Using information collected from a self-administered questionnaire completed more than 20 years ago, Yamada *et al.* (2003) also investigated the association between midlife risk factors and the prevalence of AD ($n = 51$) and VaD ($n = 38$) in 1,774 surviving members of a cohort including atomic bomb survivors and controls residing in Hiroshima and Nagasaki. No effects on the risk of AD and VaD were observed according to the physical activity index calculated from occupational and leisure activities. Although the source of information for this analysis should not be influenced by recall as in more traditional case-control studies, these results are difficult to generalize to other older populations due to the selection of the participants.

SUMMARY

These studies tend to suggest a slight beneficial influence of physical activity against AD. One major limitation is that the measurement of physical activity is based on a single question without detailed information on the frequency of the activity, its duration, or its intensity. Another frequent limitation is the fact that asymmetrical data collection was performed: exposure was collected from surrogates (e.g., spouses, children, other family members) for cases, and from controls for themselves. This procedure may have potentially introduced important misclassification biases. Data from surrogate interviews is generally considered reliable, but its validity is yet to be confirmed. It is well known that the use of a case-control design or a cross-sectional one may interfere with the interpretation of results since they could be the consequence of the onset of the disease rather than a risk factor. This is especially true since dementia is known to have a long preclinical period.

COHORT STUDIES

Cohort or prospective studies, where researchers selected samples from defined older populations, separated them according to physical activity status, and followed them up to compare the incidence of dementia, constituted the second type of study design generally used. Since exposure is collected from individuals free of dementia at baseline, this design allows a more accurate evaluation of the contribution of physical activity to the causation of dementia in the sense that it clarifies the temporal relationship between exposure and disease. However, temporality may still remain problematic because subjects in the early stages of dementia could reduce their activities due to the manifestation of symptoms during the preclinical phase, generating an overestimation of the protective effect. This limitation is particularly important when data with short follow-up periods are used. With this in mind, several studies investigated the effect of physical activity on cognitive performance, but few of them concentrated their efforts on dementia and its main subtypes. Eight studies are summarized in Table 2.1.

Using prevalence data from 1,090 community residents in an urban area of Beijing, Li *et al.* (1989) observed a small but significant correlation between physical mobility and the Mini-Mental State Examination (MMSE) score, a validated screening test for dementia (Folstein *et al.*, 1975). Information including physical mobility was obtained by interviewing subjects in their homes. Follow-up of this cohort for three years corroborated the previous finding (Li *et al.*, 1991). Subjects limited to indoor activities had a significantly higher relative risk (RR) of dementia (RR = 4.9, after adjustment for age). This follow-up analysis, however, was based on only 13 incident cases of dementia from the 739 surviving members of the cohort.

The effect of physical activity was considered in a French prospective cohort by studying the association between leisure activities and the risk of dementia (Fabrigoule *et al.*, 1995). Data on sports or gymnastics participation (yes/no) was collected during the visit of a psychologist trained for home interviews. Two follow-up examinations took place, after one year, and after three years, and included a total of 2,040 subjects. Participation in sports at baseline was related to a significantly reduced risk of dementia after adjustment for age (RR = 0.24; 95% confidence interval (CI), 0.09–0.64). However, this protective effect was no longer significant after further adjustment for baseline cognitive performance (MMSE score) (RR = 0.33; 95% CI, 0.10–1.04). Because cognitive performance is highly correlated with dementia, its inclusion in the regression model contributed to the underestimation of the association, which resulted in a nonsignificant relationship.

Table 2.1 Prospective studies examining the effects of physical activity to the risk of dementia in older persons

AUTHORS	PARTICIPANTS	FOLLOW-UP	OUTCOME	MEASUREMENTS	SIGNIFICANT RESULTS
Li et al. (1991)	726 controls 13 cases of dementia	3-year	Dementia	Limited physical activity	↑ risk of dementia
Fabrigoule et al. (1995)	1956 censored 84 events of dementia	3-year	Dementia	Leisure activities (sports and gardening)	↓ risk of dementia with gardening
Yoshitake et al. (1995)	723 censored 103 events of dementia: 42 AD, 50 VaD	7-year	AD, VaD	Daily exercise during leisure period or moderate to severe physical activity at work	↓ risk of AD
Broe et al. (1998)	252 controls 47 cases of dementia: 29 AD	3-year	Dementia, AD	Monthly practice of gardening, active sports, and walks	Nonsignificant (NS)
Laurin et al. (2001)	3679 controls 248 cases of dementia: 169 AD, 54 VaD	5-year	Dementia, AD, VaD	4-level index of regular physical activity	↓ risk of dementia, AD ↓ risk in women
Wilson et al. (2002)	622 censored 111 events of dementia	4.5-year	AD	Quartiles of physical activity score	NS
Wang et al. (2002)	437 censored 123 events of dementia	6.4-year	Dementia	Regular physical activity (swimming, walking, or gymnastics)	NS
Verghese et al. (2003)	345 censored 124 events of dementia: 61 AD, 30 VaD	5.1-year	Dementia	Weekly participation in physical activities Score of physical activity	↓ risk of dementia with dancing NS for the overall score

In a cohort study of 826 Japanese subjects followed for seven years by Yoshitake *et al.* (1995), moderate physical activity was associated with a preventive effect on AD. The active group included subjects who reported in the initial screening survey either exercising daily during the leisure period (four categories), or doing moderate to strenuous physical activity at work (four categories). No other details about physical activities are given. Physical activity (yes/no) was associated with a markedly significant 80% reduction in risk for AD after adjustment for age, sex, and initial screening score. No significant association was observed between physical activity and VaD.

In a small three-year cohort study including 299 very old subjects (i.e., 75–99) living in the community at baseline, Broe *et al.* (1998) did not find any associations between physical activity, dementia, and AD. Physical activity was ascertained by asking subjects the number of times per month they worked in the garden or yard, did active sports or exercises, and went for walks. No health habits predicted incident cases of dementia and AD after adjustment for age, sex, and education.

Significant protective effects of physical activity against dementia and AD were reported in a large-scale, multicenter, cohort study of a representative sample of the Canadian elderly population after a five-year follow-up (Laurin *et al.*, 2001). Physical activity at baseline was measured by combining two questions from a self-administered questionnaire regarding frequency and intensity of regular physical activity to create a four-level composite score which was further validated using an interview-administered version of the questionnaire (Davis *et al.*, 2001). The effect of physical activity was analyzed using a case-control approach including information from 3,679 controls and 248 incident cases of dementia of which 169 were diagnosed with AD and 54 with VaD. Moderate and high levels of physical activity were associated with significantly lower risks for AD and dementia by 30–50%. A similar nonsignificant effect was found in VaD, which may be due to a small sample size. The associations between AD and dementia were significant and stronger in women, and revealed a dose-response relationship showing decreasing risk with increasing level of physical activity. Like several studies on dementia, analyses did not include subjects who died during follow-up. However, the possibility of a selection bias due to survival was examined by the means of a variable generated using the information from death certificates, proxy interviews, and a logistic regression model estimating the probability of death due to dementia (Canadian Study of Health and Aging Working Group, 2000). Revised analyses showed that the exclusion of deceased subjects from the analysis had little effect, if anything making the estimates more conservative. In addition, the potentially confounding effect of several variables related to health status was investigated, and risk estimates remained essentially unchanged.

Wilson *et al.* (2002) tested the associations between cognitive and physical activities, and the incidence of AD based on a cohort including 733 older nuns, priests, and brothers recruited from groups across the United States and followed up for an average of 4.5 years. Assessment of cognitive activity at baseline was established by asking subjects about time spent in seven common activities involving information processing as a main component (e.g., watching television, listening to the radio). Participation in physical activities at baseline was estimated using a series of questions about the number of occasions and average minutes per occasion they had practiced five types of physical activities in the last two weeks (e.g., walking, gardening). A composite measure of physical activity was generated and divided into quartiles. Cognitive activity score was associated with a 33% reduction in risk of AD, after adjustment for age, sex, and education, whereas participation in physical activities was reported not to be associated with AD. According to the authors, these results may suggest that the association between the cognitive activity and dementia is a reflection of mental stimulation rather than a nonspecific consequence of being active. Nevertheless, the highest quartile of physical activity showed a lower risk by 39% for AD compared with the lowest quartile (RR = 0.61; 95% CI, 0.35–1.05). One limitation of this study was the fact that the cohort was self-selected, and almost certainly differed from older general populations in education, and other lifestyle habits.

Wang *et al.* (2002) also tested the hypothesis that leisure activities including intellectual, physical, social, productive, and recreational categories, could be protective against dementia using data from a population-based study in the area of Stockholm. Subjects ($n = 507$) were interviewed personally by trained nurses about recreational activities at baseline, on average 6.4 years before the diagnosis of dementia. They were also asked whether they regularly engaged in any particular activities, and if so, to specify the types of activities and the frequency of participation. Physical activity covered swimming, walking, or gymnastics. Results suggested that frequent participation in intellectual, social, or productive activity was independently associated with a lower risk of dementia. In contrast, no significant beneficial effect of physical activity on dementia was observed (RR = 0.41; 95% CI, 0.13–1.31) after controlling for several potential confounders including baseline cognitive functioning (MMSE). Only 9 incident cases of 123 had engaged in some physical activity, which restricts the statistical power of this result.

In a more recent study on the relationship of leisure (cognitive and physical) activities to dementia, Verghese *et al.* (2003) analyzed the data of a cohort of 469 volunteers residing in the Bronx community and followed up for an average of 5.1 years. Subjects were interviewed at baseline about the frequency of participation in 6 cognitive activities and 11 physical activities. Possible frequency of participation comprised: daily, several days per week, once weekly, monthly, occasionally, or never. These answers were examined individually, and recoded to create a scale with one point corresponding to participation in one activity for one day per week. An increment in the cognitive activity score was significantly associated with a reduced risk of dementia, AD, and VaD, even after adjustment for several potential confounding variables. There was no association between the physical activity score and dementia. On the other hand, dancing and walking were inversely associated with dementia (RRs = 0.24; 95% CI, 0.06–0.99, and 0.67; 95% CI, 0.45–1.05, respectively). Inclusion of volunteer subjects who were aged 75 years or over at baseline restricts the generalizability of the results.

SUMMARY

Of the previous eight studies addressed, five suggested some protective effect of physical activity on dementia or AD. Among the three studies reporting no association, two suggested a trend towards a decreased risk. The majority of studies were limited to data collected from a single question which does not allow a valid estimation of the predictive value of several physical activities. None of these studies assessed changes in physical activity or adherence during the follow-up period. Only one study investigated the role of physical activity from representative samples of older persons randomly selected, and suggested that regular physical activity might delay the onset of AD and dementia in an older population. On the other hand, the most recent prospective studies tend to highlight that physical activities with a cognitive component could be especially protective when compared to physical activity alone.

POTENTIAL MECHANISMS

Support for the role of physical activity in the prevention of cognitive impairment and dementia later in life comes from the identification of a number of mechanisms in animal and clinical studies, as reviewed by Laurin et al. (2003). One of the most frequently mentioned mechanisms pertaining to the relationship between physical activity and cognition concerns the sustenance of cerebral blood flow. Regular participation in physical activity could result in the maintenance of optimal cerebral perfusion and good cerebrovascular health. Vascular factors are part of the pathogenesis of VaD, and much evidence has suggested that they also play an important role in AD (Launer, 2002). The effects of three levels of physical activity on cerebral perfusion in three groups of 30 older volunteers each, were measured in a four-year prospective study designed by Rogers et al. (1990). Compared to working and retired-active subjects, only retired-inactive subjects exhibited significant declines in cerebral blood flow over time. Retired-inactive subjects had also significantly lower cognitive performance compared to working and retired-active subjects at the end of follow-up, but cognitive performance was not evaluated at baseline. Physical activity could help to sustain cerebral perfusion in hypertensive persons by decreasing blood pressure (Whelton et al., 2002), which has been documented as a risk factor for VaD and cognitive impairment. The presence of high blood pressure 15–20 years prior to the onset of AD, as well as an increased risk of AD, has been observed in population-based studies (Launer et al., 2000; Skoog et al., 1996). In addition, physical activity may act on cerebral blood perfusion by reducing the concentration of low-density lipoproteins (Stefanick et al., 1998). Endurance exercise training has been found to have an independent but complementary effect to hormone replacement therapy on serum lipid profiles in healthy postmenopausal women (Binder et al., 1996). Moreover, physical activity could inhibit platelet aggregability (Rauramaa et al., 1986) and enhance cerebral metabolic demands (Rogers et al., 1990).

Reduced cerebral oxygenation is another mechanism potentially associated with neuropsychological function. Although oxygen may not play the key role in brain function, it has been related to changes occurring with aging in brain chemistry. Aerobic capacity and nutrient supply to the brain could be improved in response to an exercise program. Enhanced performances on several neuropsychological tasks were observed following a four-month aerobic exercise program in three groups of 13–15 older sedentary volunteers (Dustman et al., 1984). Improvement in test scores could be linked to the increase in transport and exploitation of oxygen in the brain and tissues following the exercise program. In contrast, increased aerobic metabolism during and after physical activity has been suggested to be a source of oxidative stress (Leeuwenburgh and

Heinecke, 2001). Strenuous exercise increases oxygen consumption and causes a disturbance of intracellular prooxidant–antioxidant homeostasis (Ji, 1999). This phenomenon could promote the accumulation of reactive oxygen species (Bejma and Ji, 1999) which lead to apoptotic cell death. It has been speculated that exercise-induced apoptosis ensures optimal body function that rather serves to remove specific damaged cells without any important inflammatory responses (Phaneuf and Leeuwenburgh, 2001).

On a molecular basis, growth factors are believed to stimulate protective mechanisms in the brain following physical activity given their roles in promoting cell growth and neuronal function. Experimental studies in rodents have demonstrated that physical activity may regulate the expression of fibroblast growth factor, which indicates that growth factors could be mediators (Gómez-Pinilla *et al.*, 1997). Combined antidepressant treatment and physical activity led to the potentiation of brain-derived neurotrophic factor expression of the rat hippocampus, the most widely distributed growth factor within the brain that influences the function of several neurotransmitter systems (Russo-Neustadt *et al.*, 1999). In a review by Cotman and Berchtold (2002), it was mentioned that in addition to increasing concentrations of brain-derived neurotrophic factor, exercise induced the expression of genes that would be predicted to benefit brain plasticity processes such as vascularization, neurogenesis, functional changes in neuronal structure and neuronal resistance to injury.

SUMMARY

AD and dementia represent major health problems for our aging societies and despite much research effort, few protective factors exist. As we have shown, very few studies have been specifically designed to investigate the association between physical activity and dementia. Unfortunately, those studies that have, did not use a validated measurement of physical activity. Moreover, this measurement of physical activity would be especially valuable if it evaluated dimensions of relevance to dementia and its subtypes, in terms of type, frequency, intensity, and duration. Gradation of the mental challenge in performing the activity could be another factor to consider. For example, pedaling a stationary bike may do less for the prevention of decline in neuropsychological processes than a game of table tennis or a walk through undulating surroundings.

The fairly consistent finding of a reduced risk of dementia with physical activity tends to suggest that physical activity may have some impact on the onset of the disease in older people. Plausible biological pathways underlying the potentially protective effect of physical activity on cognition have been established. Nevertheless, a variety of methodological issues exist in the research which may limit the conclusions that can be drawn at this early stage in this work.

IMPLICATIONS FOR RESEARCHERS AND PRACTITIONERS

Further research is thus warranted to demonstrate more rigorously the relationship between physical activity and the incidence of dementia and its subtypes. Randomized trials are regarded as the best study design for evaluating the effectiveness and harmful effects of new interventions. To date, the results of a first randomized controlled trial testing physical training interventions in order to improve physical health and function and affective status of older individuals with AD have been reported (Teri *et al.*, 2003). The home-based exercise training over three months combined with caregiver training in behavioral management techniques reduced functional dependence and delayed institutionalization among subjects with AD, thus, improving their mobility and enhancing their quality of life despite progression of the disease. Although the previous study may be viewed as a convincing demonstration of secondary prevention, the role of physical activity as a primary measure of prevention would be even more important to evaluate inasmuch as older individuals are able to adapt and respond to physical training. Given the lengthy preclinical phase of dementia, it may be argued that primary prevention in clinical trials is difficult to ascertain. Despite major constraints of design conceptualization, results from these experimental studies could have important public health implications.

The finding of some positive effects on cognitive function (e.g., delayed risk of onset of dementia or delayed institutionalization rate with physical activity) suggests that physical activity may have significant protective effects in older persons. Benefits of physical training interventions on cognitive performance have already been reported in older individuals – even in the very old, healthy or frail, living in the community or in institutions (Boutcher, 2000). Before randomized trials provide invalid or confirmatory evidence between physical activity and dementia, a fair recommendation for the majority of older people would be to remain physically active as much as possible. Physical activity has been shown to be beneficial in several chronic disease associated with aging (Mazzeo *et al.*, 1998), and dementia could soon be another one more to add to the list.

WHAT WE KNOW SUMMARY

- Physical activity has been shown to be inversely associated with cognitive decline, as measured by the drop in cognitive performance over time, in older persons.
- Case-control studies tend to show a slight beneficial influence of physical activity against AD.
- Prospective analyses tend to show a more convincing protective effect of physical activity against AD and all forms of dementia combined.
- No association is evident between physical activity and VaD.
- Physical activity has been shown to improve the functional status in frail nursing home residents with dementia including AD.
- There is no evidence that physical activity or exercise (including vigorous) is harmful.

WHAT WE NEED TO KNOW SUMMARY

- Is lower intensity physical activity as effective as higher intensity physical activity? Are there risks from very high intensity exercise?
- Could physical activity in midlife prevent the onset of dementia in late life?

- What are the benefits of short-term programs of exercise? How long does it take for an exercise program to show any protective effects?
- Is the intensity of less physical activities categorized as recreational or leisure activities, substantial enough to contribute to the overall aerobic capacity?
- Do physical activities that require concentration, or concurrent mental activity, have a stronger protective effect than physical activity alone?
- What are the bio-physical and psycho-social mechanisms underlying the protective effect of physical activity against dementia?
- Are there any interactions between medication and physical activity?

REFERENCES

American Psychiatric Association (1994). *Diagnostic and Statistical Manual of Mental Disorders* (4th edn). Washington, DC: APA.

Bejma, J. and Ji, L. L. (1999). Aging and acute exercise enhance free radical generation in rat skeletal muscle. *Journal of Applied Physiology, 87*, 465–470.

Beyreuther, K. and Masters, C. L. (1991). Amyloid precursor protein (APP) and beta A4 amyloid in the etiology of Alzheimer's disease: precursor product relationships in the derangement of neuronal function. *Brain Pathology, 1*, 241–251.

Binder, E. F., Birge, S. J., and Kohrt, W. M. (1996). Effects of endurance exercise and hormone replacement therapy on serum lipids in older women. *Journal of the American Geriatrics Society, 44*, 231–236.

Boutcher, S. H. (2000). Cognitive performance, fitness, and ageing. In S. J. H. Biddle, K. R. Fox, and S. H. Boutcher (Eds). *Physical Activity and Psychological Well-being* (pp. 118–129). London: Routledge.

Braak, H. and Braak, E. (1991). Neuropathological stageing in Alzheimer-related changes. *Acta Neuropathologica, 82*, 239–259.

Broe, G. A., Henderson, A. S., Creasey, H., McCusker, E., Korten, A. E., Jorm, A. F., *et al.* (1990). A case-control study of Alzheimer's disease in Australia. *Neurology, 40*, 1698–1707.

Broe, G. A., Creasey, H., Jorm, A. F., Bennett, H. P., Casey, B., Waite, L. M., *et al.* (1998). Health habits and risk of cognitive impairment and dementia in old age: a prospective study on the effects of exercise, smoking and alcohol consumption. *Australian and New Zealand Journal of Public Health, 22*, 621–623.

Canadian Study of Health and Aging Working Group (1994). Canadian study of health and Aging: study methods and prevalence of dementia. *Canadian Medical Association Journal, 150*, 899–913.

Canadian Study of Health and Aging Working Group. (2000). The incidence of dementia in Canada. *Neurology, 55*, 66–73.

Cotman, C. W. and Berchtold, N. C. (2002). Exercise: a behavioral intervention to enhance brain health and plasticity. *Trends in Neurosciences, 25*, 295–301.

Davis, H. S., MacPherson, K., Merry, H. R., Wentzel, C., and Rockwood, K. (2001). Reliability and validity of questions about exercise in the Canadian study of health and aging. *International Psychogeriatrics, 13*(Suppl. 1), 177–182.

Dik, M. G., Deeg, D. J. H., Visser, M., and Jonker, C. (2003). Early life physical activity and cognition at old age. *Journal of Clinical and Experimental Neuropsychology, 25*, 643–653.

Dustman, R. E., Ruhling, R. O., Russell, E. M., Shearer, D. E., Bonekat, H. W., Shigeoka, J. W., *et al.* (1984). Aerobic exercise training and improved neuropsychological function of older individuals. *Neurobiology of Aging, 5*, 35–42.

Ernst, R. L. and Hay, J. W. (1997). Economic research on Alzheimer disease: a review of the literature. *Alzheimer Disease and Associated Disorders*, *11*(Suppl. 6), 135–145.

Fabrigoule, C., Letenneur, L., Dartigues, J. F., Zarrouk, M., Commenges, D., and Barberger Gateau, P. (1995). Social and leisure activities and risk of dementia: a prospective longitudinal study. *Journal of the American Geriatrics Society*, *43*, 485–490.

Folstein, M. F., Folstein, S. E., and McHugh, P. R. (1975). "Mini-mental state." A practical method for grading the cognitive state of patients for the clinician. *Journal of Psychiatric Research*, *12*, 189–198.

Friedland, R. P., Fritsch, T., Smyth, K. A., Koss, E., Lerner, A. J., Chen, C. H., *et al.* (2001). Patients with Alzheimer's disease have reduced activities in midlife compared with health control-group members. *Proceedings of National Academy of Sciences of the United States of America*, *98*, 3440–3445.

Gómez-Pinilla, F., Dao, L., and So, V. (1997). Physical exercise induces FGF-2 and its mRNA in the hippocampus. *Brain Research*, *764*, 1–8.

Hock, B. J., Jr. and Lamb, B. T. (2001). Transgenic mouse models of Alzheimer's disease. *Trends in Genetics*, 17, S7–S12.

Ishihara, T., Zhang, B., Higuchi, M., Yoshiyama, Y., Trojanowski, J. Q., and Lee, V. M. (2001). Age-dependent induction of congophilic neurofibrillary tau inclusions in tau transgenic mice. *American Journal of Pathology*, *158*, 555–562.

Ji, L. L. (1999). Antioxidants and oxidative stress in exercise. *Proceedings of the Society for Experimental Biology and Medicine*, *222*, 283–292.

Jorm, A. F., Korten, A. E., and Henderson, A. S. (1987). The prevalence of dementia: a quantitative integration of the literature. *Acta Psychiatrica Scandinavica*, *76*, 465–479.

Kondo, K., Niino, M., and Shido, K. (1994). A case-control study of Alzheimer's disease in Japan – significance of life-styles. *Dementia*, *5*, 314–326.

Launer, L. J. (2002). Demonstrating the case that AD is a vascular disease: epidemiologic evidence. *Ageing Research Reviews*, *1*, 61–77.

Launer, L. J., Ross, G. W., Petrovitch, H., Masaki, K., Foley, D., White, L. R., *et al.* (2000). Midlife blood pressure and dementia: the Honolulu–Asia aging study. *Neurobiology of Aging*, *21*, 49–55.

Laurin, D., Verreault, R., Lindsay, J., MacPherson, K., and Rockwood, K. (2001). Physical activity and risk of cognitive impairment and dementia in elderly persons. *Archives of Neurology*, *58*, 498–504.

Laurin, D., Verreault, R., and Lindsay, J. (2003). Impact of physical activity on prevention of Alzheimer's disease. In R. W. Richter and B. Z. Richter (Eds). *Alzheimer's disease: A Physician's Guide to Practical Management* (pp. 281–286). Totowa, NJ: Humana Press Inc.

Leeuwenburgh, C. and Heinecke J. W. (2001). Oxidative stress and antioxidants in exercise. *Current Medicinal Chemistry*, *8*, 829–838.

Li, G., Shen, Y. C., Chen, C. H., Zhao, Y. W., Li, S. R., and Lu, M. (1989). An epidemiological survey of age-related dementia in an urban area of Beijing. *Acta Psychiatrica Scandinavica*, *79*, 557–563.

Li, G., Shen, Y. C., Chen, C. H., Zhau, Y. W., Li, S. R., and Lu, M. (1991). A three-year follow up study of age-related dementia in an urban area of Beijing. *Acta Psychiatrica Scandinavica*, *83*, 99–104.

McDowell, I. (2001). Alzheimer's disease: insights from epidemiology. *Aging (Milano)*, *13*, 143–162.

McKhann G., Drachman, D., Folstein, M., Katzman, R., Price, D., and Stadlan, E. M. (1984) Clinical diagnosis of Alzheimer's disease: report of the NINCDS-ADRDA Work Group under the auspices of Department of Health and Human Services Task Force on Alzheimer's Disease. *Neurology*, *34*, 939–944.

Mayeux, R., Ottman, R., Tang, M. X., Noboa Bauza, L., Marder, K., Gurland, B., *et al.* (1993). Genetic susceptibility and head injury as risk factors for Alzheimer's disease among community-dwelling elderly persons and their first-degree relatives. *Annals of Neurology, 33,* 494–501.

Mazzeo, R. S., Cavanagh, P., Evans, W. J., Fiatarone, M., Hagberg, J., McAuley, E., *et al.* (1998). ACSM Position Stand: exercise and physical activity for older adults. *Medicine and Science in Sports and exercise, 30,* 992–1008.

Paganini-Hill, A. and Henderson, V. W. (1994). Estrogen deficiency and risk of Alzheimer's disease in women. *American Journal of Epidemiology, 140,* 256–261.

Paganini-Hill, A. and Henderson, V. W. (1996). Estrogen replacement therapy and risk of Alzheimer disease. *Archives of Internal Medicine, 156,* 2213–2217.

Phaneuf, S. and Leeuwenburgh, C. (2001). Apoptosis and exercise. *Medicine and Science in Sports and Exercise, 33,* 393–396.

Raiford, K., Anton-Johnson, S., Haycox, Z., Nolan, K., Schaffer, A., Caimano, C., *et al.* (1994). CERAD part VII: accuracy of reporting dementia on death certificates of patients with Alzheimer's disease. *Neurology, 44,* 2208–2209.

Rauramaa, R., Salonen, J. T., Seppanen, K., Salonen, R., Venalainen, J. M., Ihanainen, M., *et al.* (1986). Inhibition of platelet aggregability by moderate-intensity physical exercise: a randomized clinical trial in overweight men. *Circulation, 74,* 939–944.

Rockwood, K. and Stadnyk, K. (1994). The prevalence of dementia in the elderly: a review. *Canadian Journal of Psychiatry, 39,* 253–257.

Rogers, R. L., Meyer, J. S., and Mortel, K. F. (1990). After reaching retirement age physical activity sustains cerebral perfusion and cognition. *Journal of the American Geriatrics Society, 38,* 123–128.

Roman, G. C., Tatemichi, T. K., Erkinjuntti, T., Cummings, J. L., Masdeu, J. C., Garcia, J. H., *et al.* (1993). Vascular dementia: diagnostic criteria for research studies. Report of the NINDS-AIREN International Workshop. *Neurology, 43,* 250–260.

Russo-Neustadt, A., Beard, R. C., and Cotman, C. W. (1999). Exercise, antidepressant medications, and enhanced brain derived neurotrophic factor expression. *Neuropsychopharmacology, 21,* 679–682.

Schuit, A. J., Feskens, E. J. M., Launer, L. J., and Kromhout, D. (2001). Physical activity and cognitive decline, the role of the apolipoprotein e4 allele. *Medicine and Science in Sports and Exercise, 33,* 772–777.

Skoog, I., Lernfelt, B., Landahl, S., Palmertz, B., Andreasson, L. A., Nilsson, L., *et al.* (1996). 15-year longitudinal study of blood pressure and dementia. *Lancet, 347,* 1141–1145.

Stefanick, M. L., Mackey, S., Sheehan, M., Ellsworth, N., Haskell, W. L., and Wood, P. D. (1998). Effects of diet and exercise in men and postmenopausal women with low levels of HDL cholesterol and high levels of LDL cholesterol. *New England Journal of Medicine, 339,* 12–20.

Tabbarah, M., Crimmins, E. M., and Seeman, T. E. (2002). The relationship between cognitive and physical performance: MacArthur studies of successful aging. *Journal of Gerontology: Medical Sciences, 57A,* M228–M235.

Teri, L., Gibbons, L. E., McCurry, S. M., Logsdon, R. G., Buchner, D. M., Barlow, W. E., *et al.* (2003). Exercise plus behavioral management in patients with Alzheimer disease. *Journal of the American Medical Association, 290,* 2015–2022.

Verghese, J., Lipton, R. B., Katz, M. J., Hall, C.B., Derby, C. A., Kuslansky, G., *et al.* (2003). Leisure activities and the risk of dementia in the elderly. *New England Journal of Medicine, 348,* 2508–2516.

Wang, H. X., Karp, A., Winblad, B., and Fratiglioni, L. (2002). Late-life engagement in social and leisure activities is associated with a decreased risk of dementia: a longitudinal study from the Kungsholmen project. *American Journal of Epidemiology, 155,* 1081–1087.

Whelton, S. P., Chin, A., Xin, X., and He, J. (2002). Effect of aerobic exercise on blood pressure: a meta-analysis of randomized controlled trials. *Annals of Internal Medicine, 136,* 493–503.

Wilson, R. S., Mendes de Leon, C. F., Barnes, L. L., Schneider, J. A., Bienias, J. L., Evans, D.A., and Bennett, D. A. (2002). Participation in cognitively stimulating activities and risk of incident Alzheimer disease. *Journal of the American Medical Association, 287,* 742–748.

Yaffe, K., Barnes, D., Nevitt, M., Lui, L. Y., and Covinsky, K. (2001). A prospective study of physical activity and cognitive decline in elderly women: women who walk. *Archives of Internal Medicine, 161,* 1703–1708.

Yamada, M., Kasagi, F., Sasaki, H., Masunari, N., Mimori, Y., and Suzuki, G. (2003). Association between dementia and midlife risk factors: the radiation effects research foundation adult health study. *Journal of the American Geriatrics Society, 51,* 410–414.

Yoshitake, T., Kiyohara, Y., Kato, I., Ohmura, T., Iwamoto, H., Nakayama, K., *et al.* (1995). Incidence and risk factors of vascular dementia and Alzheimer's disease in a defined elderly Japanese population: the Hisayama study. *Neurology, 45,* 1161–1168.

CHAPTER 3

Exercise as an adjunct treatment for schizophrenia

GUY E. J. FAULKNER

SCHIZOPHRENIA

Schizophrenia is a serious mental illness characterized by severe personality disorganization, distortion of reality, and an inability to function in daily life. The clinical features of schizophrenia typically include changes in thinking, changes in perception, blunted or inappropriate affect, and a reduced level of social functioning. Schizophrenia is often regarded as one of the most debilitating psychiatric disorders as it imposes a heavy burden on patients, caregivers, the health service, and wider society, far in excess of its prevalence (Knapp, 1997). For example, nearly 3% of the total burden of human disease globally is attributed to schizophrenia despite a commonly reported prevalence of only 1% (Murray and Lopez, 1996). Estimates suggest CAN$4.35 billion is spent annually on the direct and indirect costs of schizophrenia in Canada (Goeree *et al.*, 1999), and AUS$740 million on direct costs in Australia between 1997 and 1998 (Andrews *et al.*, 2003).

The symptoms of schizophrenia can be divided into positive and negative symptoms because of their impact on diagnosis and treatment, although it is important to highlight that the range and nature of symptoms vary widely between individuals (USDHHS, 1999). Positive symptoms are those that appear to reflect an excess or distortion of normal functions and are manifested in symptoms such as delusions, hallucinations, and thought disorder. Negative symptoms are those that appear to reflect a reduction or loss of normal functions and reflect symptoms such as affective flattening, apathy, social withdrawal, and cognitive impairments.

The cause of schizophrenia has not yet been determined although typically medical science considers schizophrenia as a disease of the brain (Health Canada, 2002). However, psychiatric consensus points to the onset and course of schizophrenia being most likely the result of an interaction between genetic and environmental influences (e.g., Puri *et al.*, 2002). In terms of onset, the disorder often appears earlier in men, usually in the late teens or early twenties, than in women, who are generally affected in the twenties to early thirties (USDHHS, 1999). However, with respect to prevalence rates, schizophrenia affects men and women with equal frequency. The course and outcome of schizophrenia is again highly unpredictable. Long-term follow-up studies indicate that one-half to two-thirds of individuals with schizophrenia significantly improve or recover, some completely, and that less than a quarter remain permanently affected (Ciompi, 1984; Harding *et al.*, 1992; Tsuang *et al.*, 1979).

Optimal treatment of schizophrenia includes some form of pharmacotherapy with antipsychotic medication. However, pharmacological treatment is typically not considered sufficient by itself due to problems with medication compliance and concerns about the effectiveness of such medication. For example, up to 40% of patients have a poor response to antipsychotic medication and continue to show moderate to severe psychotic symptoms (Kane, 1996). Moreover, there is even doubt as to whether more recent pharmacological developments such as atypical antipsychotics are more effective or better tolerated than conventional antipsychotics (Geddes *et al.*, 2000). Additionally, antipsychotic drugs have little impact on the negative symptoms of schizophrenia which may make occupational and social rehabilitation difficult. Drug treatment is consequently often combined with a variety of psychosocial interventions. Cognitive behavior therapy (CBT) and family interventions are two treatments that may be potentially effective (Pilling *et al.*, 2002a) while social skills training and cognitive remediation have no reliable support (Pilling *et al.*, 2002b). In general, the treatment of schizophrenia is far from perfected and other strategies that may reduce relapse, and the residual symptoms or negative symptoms associated with schizophrenia, require examination.

THE CASE FOR PHYSICAL ACTIVITY/EXERCISE

For people with mental health disorders such as schizophrenia, improvement in quality of life tends to enhance the individual's ability to cope with and manage their disorder. As such, physical activity has the potential to improve quality of life for people with mental health disorders through two inter-related routes: physical and psychological (Carless and Faulkner, 2003). In terms of physical quality of life, individuals with mental health disorders have the same physical health needs as the general population.

Physical benefits

Individuals with serious mental illness are more likely to be sedentary than the general population (Brown *et al.*, 1999; Chamove, 1986; Davidson *et al.*, 2001; Farnam *et al.*, 1999) and are consequently at high risk for chronic medical conditions associated with sedentariness. Epidemiological surveys demonstrate an excess of physical morbidity and premature mortality in individuals with mental disorders (e.g., Harris and Barraclough, 1998). For example, rates of physical comorbidities such as hypertension, diabetes, respiratory disease, and cardiovascular disease are as high as 60% in people with serious mental illness while premature mortality rates are 2.4 times higher than in the general population (Bartsch *et al.*, 1990; Berren *et al.*, 1994; Koran *et al.*, 1989). There is a marked increase in standardized mortality ratios in schizophrenia in both natural and unnatural causes of death with the largest single cause of death being cardiovascular diseases (Osby *et al.*, 2000). Much of the increase in chronic medical illness among individuals with serious mental illness may be attributed to the increased prevalence of obesity in this population (Green *et al.*, 2000; McCreadie, 2003; McIntyre *et al.*, 2001) and the excessive weight gain associated with antipsychotic medication (Allison *et al.*, 1999).

While it is difficult to identify the relative contributions of disease-specific factors such as genetics, the side-effects of medications, or lifestyle factors such as diet, to the prevalence of obesity and increased mortality, it is clear that helping individuals with serious mental illness become more physically active can decrease their health risks. For example, patients with schizophrenia are generally likely to develop type 2 diabetes mellitus up to two times greater than age-corrected general population rates (Lean and Pajonk, 2003) yet we know from large randomized intervention trials that lifestyle interventions including physical activity can reduce its incidence (e.g., Knowler *et al.*, 2002; Tuomilehto *et al.*, 2001). Given inconsistent results regarding pharmacological interventions for weight loss, programs that include physical activity provision may play a critical role in limiting weight gain in this population (Faulkner *et al.*, 2003).

Good physical health is a realistic goal for people with mental illness and lifestyle programs that consider both physical activity and diet are essential (Le Fevre, 2001; Osborn, 2001). Recovery from serious mental illness and reintegration into the community is fundamentally threatened by ignoring the physical health needs of these patients. For example, the weight gain induced by many antipsychotic agents is likely to have important deleterious effects on mortality, health, quality of life, and physical functioning, and may reduce compliance to treatment regimens (Fontaine *et al.*, 2001; Kawachi, 1999; Kurzthaler and Fleischhacker, 2001; Weiden *et al.*, 2004). If we ignore these physical health needs then we will continue to see people with severe mental illness dying 10–15 years earlier than the general population (Goldman, 1999). The physical benefits alone from regular physical activity in reducing morbidity and mortality in this population are sufficient justification for the inclusion of exercise in programs of rehabilitation (Faulkner and Biddle, 1999).

Psychological benefits

Given the clear health benefits to be derived for this population if exercise was a regular "habit," any psychological benefit can almost be seen as a bonus, although not a prerequisite before promoting the use of exercise as an adjunct treatment for schizophrenia.

However, positive psychological effects from physical activity in clinical populations have been reported even among those individuals who experience no objective diagnostic improvement (Faulkner and Biddle, 1999; Plante, 1993), and improved quality of life is particularly important for individuals with severe and enduring mental health problems when complete remission may be unrealistic (Faulkner and Sparkes, 1999). Simply, individuals with a severe mental illness such as schizophrenia can attain positive mental health benefits (Carless and Faulkner, 2003). Exercise may be an appropriate and inexpensive form of secondary preventive/rehabilitative medicine in schizophrenia (Pelham *et al.*, 1993). The aim of the following review is to identify and critically evaluate the existing research that has utilized exercise as an adjunct therapy for schizophrenia.

METHOD

Published studies investigating exercise/physical activity as a therapeutic intervention for adults with schizophrenia were identified using Social Science Citation Index and Embase via BIDS, PsychLit, MEDLINE, and Sport Discus. Keywords included exercise, physical activity, fitness, and schizophrenia. Three decades of literature were searched from 1974 to 2004 with only English language studies selected. The search was supplemented by examining the references from the retrieved papers and handsearching. There was no exclusion criteria related to study design, and studies using qualitative or quantitative methodologies were included. Studies were excluded if exercise/physical activity was not the specific intervention examined and/or the sample used did not specifically consist of individuals with schizophrenia (Auchus *et al.*, 1995; Chastain and Shapiro, 1987; Clark *et al.*, 1975; Conroy *et al.*, 1982; Hannaford *et al.*, 1988; Hutchinson and Skrinar, 1994; Hutchinson *et al.*, 1999; Kaplan *et al.*, 1983; Netz *et al.*, 1994; Powell, 1974; Skrinar and Hutchinson, 1994; Skrinar *et al.*, 1992; Sule, 1987). These studies fail to distinguish relative effects of exercise on different diagnostic groups and apply a nomothetic approach to widely diverse and heterogeneous diagnoses. Overall, fifteen studies were included in the review.

The results are presented in three sections and classified by means of Campbell and Stanley's (1963) pre-experimental, quasi-experimental, and experimental categories. Additionally, a number of other categories are included. "Participants" describes the general nature of participants involved; "Design" expands on the research design that was used; "Treatment" describes the content of the exercise program offered; "Psychological instruments" refers to the dependent measures assessed at pre- and post-treatment including self-report and qualitative methods; and "Outcome" describes the effects of exercise participation for the participants. Statistical significance criteria are presented where available.

RESULTS

Pre-experimental research

Nine studies (60% of all studies in the review) were located in this section and were predominantly of a one group pretest–posttest design. A summary of the pre-experimental research can be found in Table 3.1.

The participants were generally adult males and females representing both inpatient and outpatient populations. All had diagnoses of chronic schizophrenia, which is characterized by the existence of more negative than positive features of schizophrenia. Standardized psychological instruments used included the Beck Depression Inventory (BDI; Beck *et al.*, 1961), the Mental Health Inventory (MHI; Veit and Ware, 1983), Brief Psychotic Rating Scale (BPRS; Overall and Gorham, 1962), and the Nurses' Observation Scale for In-Patient Evaluation (NOSIE; Honigfeld *et al.*, 1965).

Qualitative measures ranged from more in-depth ethnography (including participant observation) (Faulkner and Sparkes, 1999) to standard interviewing techniques (Carter-Morris and Faulkner, 2003; Pelham *et al.*, 1993). Submaximal predicted oxygen uptake tests were included in three studies. Exercise programs were generally of a moderate intensity, each session of at least 30 min duration, during a program of eight, ten, or twelve weeks. Frequency was less consistent, ranging from once a week to two or four sessions a week. Cycle ergometer, walking, swimming, football, weight training, and movement (stretching) sessions were reported.

Outcome results indicated all studies reported some improvement on psychometric outcome variables (i.e., body image, mental health, depression, components of NOSIE and BPRS). Where measured, increased aerobic fitness was reported. Additionally, there was a significant negative correlation between predicted aerobic fitness and level of depression in one study (Pelham *et al.*, 1993).

The qualitative studies reported antidepressant, anxiety-reduction, mood elevating effects, increased social interaction, self-esteem, and improved concentration. Three small case studies reported individuals who self-reported exercise as a useful strategy for reducing auditory hallucinations (Belcher, 1988; Carter-Morris and Faulkner, 2003; Faulkner and Sparkes, 1999). Improved behavior and sleep patterns were also reported in one study (Faulkner and Sparkes, 1999).

Conversely, Faulkner and Sparkes (1999) described one participant who did not experience any psychological improvement, self-reported or observed, during participation in the exercise program. Adams (1995), in his single subject case study, also reported that while there were changes on certain items of the BPRS, overall the total psychopathology score suggested the participant became "less well mentally."

Quasi-experimental research

Four studies in this category were located, with two using control group comparisons and two with a repeated measures and/or cross-over design. A summary can be found in Table 3.2.

The participants were predominantly adult males and females representing both inpatient and outpatient populations. All had diagnoses of chronic schizophrenia. One study examined adolescent boys and girls (Bergman *et al.*, 1993) and is perhaps the first to consider the role of exercise after the initial onset of schizophrenia. Standardized psychological instruments used included the Brief Symptom Inventory (BSI; Derogatis and Melisaratos, 1983), BPRS, the NOSIE, the Profile of Mood States (POMS; McNair *et al.*, 1971), the State-Trait Anxiety Inventory (STAI; Spielberger *et al.*, 1983), the Physical Estimation and Attraction Scales (PEAS; Sonstroem, 1978), Physical

Table 3.1 Pre-experimental research examining psychological effects of exercise for individuals with schizophrenia

STUDY	PARTICIPANTS	DESIGN	TREATMENT	PSYCHOLOGICAL INSTRUMENTS	OUTCOME
Rosenthal and Beutell (1981)	9 outpatients (age mean = 45.4 yrs) (4 f; 5 m)	Pre-experimental	Ten 30-min "movement" sessions over 10 wks. Adherence not described	Draw-a-person	Movement improved body image ($p < 0.05$)
Belcher (1988)	1 male inpatient (60 yrs old)	Pre-experimental	Guided "rapid" walking at onset of hallucinatory episode	Staff observation	Mild contingent exercise decreased overt hallucinatory behavior
Pelham and Campagna (1991)	3 outpatients (1 f; 2 m; age range 18–45 yrs)	Pre-experimental Single subject case studies	30-min cycle ergometer, 65–75% HR reserve, 4/wk for 12 wks. Adherence not described	BDI, MHI, submaximal predicted oxygen test	General trend of reduced BDI scores, increased mental health (MHI) scores and increased aerobic fitness
Pelham, Campagna, Ritvo and Birnie (1993a) Note: 3 studies described (a, b, c)	11 outpatients (age range 18–45 yrs)	Pre-experimental Structured interview ($n = 5$ aerobic; $n = 6$ non-aerobic)	Aerobic: 30-min bike ergometer, 65–75% HR reserve, 4/wk for 8 wks. Non-aerobic: muscle tone/strengthening exercises, 30 min, 4/wk for 8 wks. Adherence not clearly described	Interviews videotaped Keyword ratios measured	9 clients identified either moderate or significant benefits. Anxiolytic, antidepressant, and energizing effects reported. Aerobic group had higher ratio of +ve to −ve keywords in endorsing treatment
Pelham et al. (1993c)	15 outpatients (age range 18–45 yrs)	Pre-experimental Correlational	Clients not involved in a formal exercise program but had exercised for the last 12 months or more	Predicted VO$_2$max test, BDI	Significant −ve correlation ($r = -0.731, p < 0.005$) between predicted aerobic fitness and level of depression

Study	Participants	Design	Intervention	Measures	Results
Adams (1995)	1 male outpatient	Pre-experimental Single subject case study	Progressive 12-wk exercise program, from 2–4/wk, 20–50 min, weight training	NOSIE-30, BPRS observation and interview	Physical fitness improved On NOSIE, marked improvement on social interest, competence, and personal neatness No signs of psychosis and fewer signs of irritability On BPRS, total pathology score suggested patient less mentally well
Mrazek and Hatlova (1995) (Czech study in English)	17 male inpatients	Pre-experimental Ambiguous design	3-month program, 2/wk for 30 min Activity unclear – sport? Adherence not described	BPRS	Participants improved by 8.7% on BPRS
Faulkner and Sparkes (1999)	3 (2 m; 1 f) individuals with chronic schizophrenia in sheltered accommodation	Pre-experimental Ethnography	10-wk program, 2/wk 30 min of walking/ jogging Adherence not clearly described	Participant observation and interviews	No change for 1 participant Antidepressant, anxiolytic, mood elevating effects Reduced auditory hallucinations reported by 2 participants Improved sleep and behavior observed
Carter-Morris and Faulkner (2003)	3 male individuals with chronic schizophrenia (age mean = 41 yrs)	Pre-experimental Qualitative	Ongoing sport participation	Interview	Social benefits prominent and coping strategy for auditory hallucinations self-reported

Notes: f = female; m = male; yrs = years; wk = week; min = minutes.

Table 3.2 Quasi-experimental and experimental research examining psychological effects of exercise for individuals with schizophrenia

STUDY	PARTICIPANTS	DESIGN	TREATMENT	PSYCHOLOGICAL INSTRUMENTS	OUTCOME
Gimino and Levin (1984)	80 inpatients	Quasi-experimental 40 in treatment 40 in control matched for sex, age, and diagnosis Expected to participate but did not	10 wks of 40 min jogging, and 3/wk Adherence not described	POMS, SCL-90, STAI, PEAS	Significant decrease on depression ($p < 0.05$) and tension ($p < 0.02$) of POMS for exercise group only; depression, anxiety, phobic anxiety, obsessive-compulsive ($p < 0.05$) symptoms of SCL-90; A-scale of STAI ($p < 0.05$) No difference in self-image scores
Chamove (1986)	40 outpatients (21 m; 19 f; M = 51 yrs)	Quasi-experimental Rated blindly by nurses on days of inactivity for at least 2 days of each	Normal variations in participation in one of the following: swimming, gardening, keep fit, occupational therapy	NOSIE	All patients rated better on all NOSIE measures on active days; less psychotic features, less irritable, less tense, less depressed, more social interest/competence Greatest benefits for less severely disturbed, sedentary, over-weight and female subjects
Lukoff et al. (1986)	28 male inpatients	Experimental Randomly assigned to a social skills or holistic treatment intervention (including exercise	Holistic intervention included 30 min of walking/running each weekday for 9 wks Adherence not clearly described	Cooper 12-min fitness test Symptom Checklist-90; Psychiatric Assessment Scale	Significant increase in fitness in holistic group Significant improvement in both groups on psycho-pathology measures but no differences between groups

Study	Sample	Design	Intervention	Measures	Results
			and education in stress management)	(PAS), Nurses Global Impressions Scale (NGI), and Tennessee Self-Concept Test (TSC)	No change for either group in self-concept. No significant difference in either group in incidence of relapse at 2 years
Bergman et al. (1993)	15 adolescent inpatients (9 m; 6 f; M = 19.13 years)	Quasi-experimental Cross-over design	3 wks, 5/wk, 45 min low-intensity activity. Adherence not described. Alternative educational group activity	Brief Symptom Inventory (BSI), Visual Analogue Scale (VAS), Physical Self-Efficacy Scale (PSE), Perceived Competence Scale	No improvement in clinical measures. Significant improvements in physical self-efficacy
Pelham et al. (1993b)	10 outpatients (18–45 years)	Experimental. Fitness assessed, randomly assigned to aerobic/non-aerobic condition	Aerobic: 30 min bike ergometer, 65–75% HR reserve, 4/wk for 8 wks. Non-aerobic: muscle tone/strengthening exercises, 30 min, 4/wk for 8 wks. Adherence not described	Predicted VO_2max tests, BDI	Significant increase in VO_2max of aerobic group, 20.9% by wk 12. Significant reductions in BDI ($p < 0.05$) from baseline. No change in predicted aerobic fitness and insignificant reductions in BDI of non-aerobic group
Hatlova and Basny sen (1995)	70 inpatients (45 m; 25 f)	Quasi-experimental Ambiguous design	3 groups: (1) warmup/stretching exercises (2) more active; games for men, aerobics for women (3) no exercise. Groups 1 and 2, 6 months, 2/wk, 30–50 min. Adherence not described	BPRS	Group 1 improved by 12.3% on BPRS, Group 2 by 8.8%, and Group 3 by 1.3%. Greater acceptance of program by participants in group 2

Notes: f = female; m = male; yrs = years; wks = weeks; min = minutes.

Self-Efficacy (PSE; Ryckman *et al.*, 1982) and Perceived Competence Scales (PCS; Harter, 1982), Visual Analogue Scale (VAS; Carlsson, 1983), and the Symptoms Check List-90 (SCL-90; Derogatis *et al.*, 1974). No study examined physiological change.

Exercise programs lasted from three weeks to six months and consisted of 40 min jogging three times a week, 45 min of moderate skills-based physical activity five times a week, or 30–50 min of light or moderate activity twice a week. The study reported by Hatlova and Basny sen (1995), was one of a series of Czech studies (Mrazek and Hatlova, 1995; Petra and Hatlova, 1995) that poorly described the delivery of exercise programs for patients at a Psychiatric Hospital in Prague. Problems in translation may be a cause, but only vague descriptions of the exercise program and research design are given, with little discussion of the findings and limitations of their work. Three groups were established including a light callisthenics group, a more active sport/aerobics group, and a control group. In the study conducted by Gimino and Levin (1984) a control group was matched for sex, age, and diagnosis. No mention was made about whether participants were randomly allocated to each condition. Finally, Chamove (1986) used participants as their own control by comparing behavior on days of activity and inactivity. Additionally, nurses and patients were blind to the true purpose of this study.

Outcome results indicated that all studies reported some improvement on the inventory measures used (components of NOSIE, POMS, SCL-90, STAI, PSE, and the BPRS) except for the PEAS scale where no change was reported on perceived self-image scores. Changes on BPRS measures in the Czech studies imply reductions in a "total pathology" score; however, it does not specify which items of the BPRS changed. This information would provide greater insight as to what the "exercise" possibly influenced, such as the positive symptoms of hallucinations and delusions or the negative symptoms of social withdrawal and depressed mood. In contrast, Bergman and colleagues (1993) found no improvement in psychopathological characteristics among their adolescent sample.

Experimental research

Two studies incorporated an element of randomization into their research design although randomization procedures are not described (Lukoff *et al.*, 1986; Pelham *et al.*, 1993). In Pelham and colleagues' (1993) study, a time-series analysis showed that five chronic outpatients randomly assigned to a twelve week aerobic exercise group had significant reductions in depression scores (BDI), along with increases in aerobic fitness (see Table 3.2). Conversely, five clients assigned to a non-aerobic 12-week training group did not improve in aerobic fitness or BDI scores. No explanation was offered for the difference in BDI scores across the two conditions.

Lukoff and colleagues (1986) found that both a social skills group and an exercise group (which included education) showed similar but substantial and significant reductions in overall psychopathology over the course of their nine-week program (as measured by the SCL-90, Psychiatric Assessment Scale (PAS; Krawiecka *et al.*, 1977), Nurses Global Impressions Scale (NGI; Guy, 1976), and the Tennessee Self-Concept Test (TSC; Fitts, 1965)). There were no dropouts in the exercise group and an increase in fitness, as measured by the Cooper 12-min aerobic fitness test, was reported. However, there was a high rate of relapse (79%) in the exercise group during the two-year follow-up. The authors suggest that participants had difficulty transferring the skills obtained during the highly structured inpatient program to the community. Given the multiple components within this intervention it would be impossible to attribute any outcomes specifically to exercise.

DISCUSSION

Research on the effects of physical activity on the physical and mental health of individuals with schizophrenia is relatively scarce and existing research is weak. Small samples of self-selected participants, lack of control groups, or inadequately selected control groups are common methodological weaknesses. Also, adherence rates were rarely reported. Neither randomized controlled physical activity intervention trials nor cost-effectiveness studies have been conducted to evaluate physical activity interventions in people with serious mental illness. Accordingly, any conclusions drawn from these studies must be treated with caution. At the very least, the existing research clearly demonstrates that physical activity interventions are possible with this population group. Furthermore, tentative evidence also suggests that physical activity participation is associated with the alleviation of some of the positive and negative symptoms of schizophrenia.

Positive symptoms

Very few research studies have attempted to directly investigate the effects of exercise on psychotic symptoms. This has subsequently led researchers such as Folkins and Sime (1981) and Plante (1993, 1996) to conclude that it was not possible to draw any conclusions regarding the effect of exercise training on psychotic symptomatology. When psychometrically validated measures of such symptomatology were used, four of six studies reported improvement (Chamove, 1986; Hatlova and Basny sen, 1995; Lukoff et al., 1986; Mrazek and Hatlova, 1995). For example, findings from Chamove (1986) that less psychotic features were displayed on days of activity, Belcher's (1988) single subject case study, and descriptions by Faulkner and Sparkes (1999) and Carter-Morris and Faulkner (2003) of participants self-reporting the use of exercise to control auditory hallucinations are tentative indications that exercise can alleviate some of the more chronic psychotic symptoms.

However, more conclusive evidence does exist that individuals with schizophrenia can develop effective means of dealing with their illness (Carr, 1988; Lee et al., 1993; Tarrier, 1994). Further inferences can be drawn from research that has explored the general coping strategies of individuals with schizophrenia. For example, as many as 78% of individuals with schizophrenia report that they have used exercise in some way to reduce hallucinations (Falloon and Talbot, 1981). Similarly, Yagi et al. (1991) analyzed coping strategies of a sample of patients with schizophrenia and depression and concluded that "in comparison with depressive patients [that] most schizophrenic patients might successfully cope with their acute psychosis by an increase in activity" (p. 88). It is unclear, as with general coping research, whether the symptoms themselves, or merely the patient's reports of them, have been reduced (Tarrier *et al.*, 1993).

One element of CBT is the investigation of "coping strategies." Exercise is suggested as a *behavioral* strategy (Tarrier, 1994), but as yet has received no systematic investigation in the psychological literature as a strategy in its own right. Links between the process of exercise and CBT have been suggested (Faulkner and Biddle, 2001), and using exercise and physical activity as an experiential context for challenging disturbing hallucinations or delusions might be appropriate for some individuals with schizophrenia (Carter-Morris and Faulkner, 2003).

Negative symptoms

The research has been more illuminating in terms of the effects of exercise on the negative symptoms associated with schizophrenia. Caution again is required in coming to any firm conclusions given the limited research. On a more optimistic note, all of the research reports a positive trend in relation to the negative symptoms of schizophrenia. Reductions in depression, greater social interest, improved behavior on days of activity, and improvements in self-esteem are also reported, albeit inconsistently.

Depression and anxiety are not uncommon among schizophrenia sufferers. All studies incorporating measures of depression have reported reductions from baseline. Additionally, drawing from the "encouraging" research evidence into the positive benefits of exercise on clinical depression and anxiety (see Burbach, 1997; Mutrie, 2000) such benefits may be extended to individuals with schizophrenia who are also experiencing such symptoms. Future research should clearly target such negative symptoms and assess the impact of exercise on depression, self-esteem, anxiety, and even levels of social interaction.

By alleviating these symptoms, overall quality of life may be improved and the possibility of relapse reduced. Conversely, ignoring these symptoms may cause further social withdrawal and increase direct costs of treatment (Knapp, 1997). Moreover, "satisfactory outcome may be more dependent on the modification of such disturbances than the psychotic phenomena themselves" (Hemsley, 1995, p. 309). Overall, it is evident that the existing research does not allow any firm conclusions to be made as to the psychological benefits of exercise for individuals with schizophrenia. It does, however, support the potential efficacy of exercise in alleviating the negative symptoms of schizophrenia and as a coping strategy for the positive symptoms.

Dosage and mechanisms

No research has directly investigated the potential mechanisms underpinning the positive benefits reported. Qualitative case studies tend to infer that any benefit is largely related to hypothesized psychosocial mechanisms such as increased social interaction, physical self-esteem, and competence (Carter-Morris and Faulkner, 2003; Faulkner and Sparkes, 1999) while exercise may also provide short-term distraction and relief from positive symptoms (Faulkner and Sparkes, 1999). However, there is no reason to assume that commonly hypothesized physical, biochemical, and psychosocial mechanisms (see Mutrie and Faulkner, 2003) are also not applicable to individuals with schizophrenia. In acknowledging the huge diversity of potential triggers (i.e., exercise type, environment, social context) and individual circumstances (i.e., state of mental health, needs, preferences, and personal background), Fox (1999) suggests that several mechanisms most likely operate in concert with the precise combination being highly individual-specific. That is, different processes operate for different people at different times. The isolation of a specific mechanism cannot realistically address the large number of potential psychological influences that may be experienced through physical activity (Carless and Faulkner, 2003).

One particularly pertinent process may be the development of social inclusion (see Chapter 10). Individuals who use mental health services, such as individuals with schizophrenia, are likely to be poor, unemployed, living in substandard housing, and socially isolated by their experiences of stigma and discrimination (Sainsbury Centre for Mental Health, 2002). Opportunities for services, such as exercise programing, that are meaningful and relevant to people's lives, separate from "mainstream" mental health services, and staffed by non-specialist mental health staff, may be particularly beneficial (Raine et al., 2002). It may be that physical activity is no more than a highly valued activity of daily living (ADL), that offers a route to social inclusion by making accessible opportunities for social interaction within the context of a "normalizing" activity (Carter-Morris and Faulkner, 2003).

Identifying an optimum dosage or mode of physical activity for mental health in general, and for individuals with schizophrenia, is not yet possible. Further research will be needed comparing different types of activity in order to identify which program works best for this population and in what way. In the absence of a single generic mechanism, a range of exercise modes and intensities should be recommended based on the participant's previous exercise experiences, preferences, and goals. Current guidelines for lifestyle activity and exercise appear just as acceptable to individuals with schizophrenia in terms of potential mental health benefit. That is, accumulating 30 min of moderate physical activity on most or all days should apply equally to this population. In terms of short-term goals, sedentary individuals could be encouraged to participate in two 30-min sessions of moderate activity a week. This target informed the chosen "exercise dosage" in the Faulkner and Sparkes (1999) study.

IMPLICATIONS FOR RESEARCHERS

Faulkner and Biddle (1999) described a range of methodological concerns that are particularly relevant to the study of exercise as an adjunct treatment for schizophrenia. These may make more rigorous research designs exceedingly difficult – although not impossible – to conduct. For example, given the heterogeneity of schizophrenia, common comorbidity, the wide variation in clinical settings, and the often vastly differing individual pharmacological interventions, ascertaining base levels or generalizing results is always tenuous. Particularly problematic is the small number of patients available at any one time. This makes experimental work difficult and may explain the dearth of material related to exercise and schizophrenia in comparison to other less troublesome groups of participants (e.g., depression or nonclinical populations) (Faulkner and Sparkes, 1999).

A notable barrier may also include gaining access to such individuals to deliver an exercise intervention. Given the lack of "scientific" evidence linking exercise and psychological benefits for individuals with schizophrenia, there must be greater methodological diversity in examining the relationship between exercise and mental health in conjunction with an inclusive rather than exclusive acceptance of existing and future research (Faulkner and Biddle, 1999). Clearly, attempts should be made to conduct rigorous experimental designs, particularly utilizing a randomized control treatment when possible. Specifically, the comparison of varying types of exercise (e.g., aerobic/non-aerobic), both against and in combination with other therapies, such as CBT, is needed. At all times, the exact nature of the exercise program must be clearly defined with the duration, frequency, and intensity of exercise reported. Adherence must also be clearly reported. Changes in fitness levels should also be documented as well as the incorporation of follow-up measures in research designs. The participants should be clearly described in terms of their age, sex, diagnosis, duration of illness, and medication regimen. Outcome measures should include measures relevant to schizophrenia-related symptomatology, particularly the negative symptoms, and consider broader clinical outcomes such as use of health services, medication compliance, and rate of relapse. However, given the difficulties inherent in conducting RCTs, qualitative case studies may provide further insight into the process of exercise participation for individuals with schizophrenia. Experimentally, time-series before and after designs may be more appropriate and feasible.

Examining barriers and strategies to increase physical activity are needed. A lack of motivation has been commonly reported (Archie et al., 2003). Research must first examine the barriers faced by individuals with schizophrenia in becoming more active and identify the most effective strategies for increasing their participation in physical activity. Comparison of lifestyle and structured interventions to increase physical activity should also be conducted as we do not know whether less structured interventions can work with this population. Their flexibility, lower cost, and easy integration into daily schedules might be particularly appealing to individuals with schizophrenia.

IMPLICATIONS FOR THE HEALTH PROFESSIONAL AND HEALTH SERVICE DELIVERY

Given the inherent physical health benefits of regular physical activity participation, the opportunity for consistent and structured exercise experiences should be integrated within mental health service delivery. Ensuring such provision through the interdisciplinary and collaborative coordination of appropriate personnel, resources, and facilities will remain a challenge. Physical activity behavior change strategies that have been successful in healthier populations can be adopted for those with serious mental illness (Richardson et al., 2005). Richardson and colleagues (2005) have described examples of structured, supervised, facility-based exercise programs as well as lifestyle physical activity interventions that encourage participants to incorporate walking into their everyday life, and discuss a range of practical issues related to physical activity promotion with this population.

Most notably, the majority of participants with schizophrenia who have undertaken an exercise or sport program (e.g., Carter-Morris and Faulkner, 2003; Faulkner and Sparkes, 1999; Pelham *et al.*, 1993) have valued the role of exercise. Reviewing the literature on exercise and mental health, Martinsen (1995) highlighted the consistency of patients evaluating the usefulness of exercise in a positive way. If programs are made available as part of psychiatric services, individuals will choose to enrol. Furthermore, adherence to exercise programs among individuals with schizophrenia appears comparable to that of the general population, although such observations are primarily based on clinical experience as opposed to empirical evidence (Martinsen, 1993, 1995; Richardson *et al.*, 2005).

Meyer and Broocks (2000) suggest there are almost no contraindications for psychiatric patients to participate in exercise programs provided they are free from cardiovascular disease. Screening for risk factors must be undertaken and medical clearance should be sought prior to participation in an exercise program. Attention should be given to making physical activity opportunities easily accessible and consistently available. There is some indication that any positive benefits associated with exercise may be rapidly lost when exercise provision is withdrawn (Faulkner and Sparkes, 1999; Lukoff *et al.*, 1986).

Another concern may be related to antipsychotic medication, but little research exists on the extent to which the use of medication interacts with the effects of exercise (Martinsen and Stanghelle, 1997). Carlsson and colleagues (1967, 1968a,b) performed several studies on the physiological effects of medication on patients receiving chlorpromazine (1.5–3.6 g/day). They found that large doses of chlorpromazine tended to reduce stroke volume, leading to a reduction of cardiac output and arterial blood pressure during exercise. For this reason, Martinsen and Stanghelle believed that exercise was even more important for such patients, both to increase physical work capacity and to reduce the level of noradrenaline in blood plasma through regular aerobic training. However, chronic exercise may affect the pharmacokinetics of pharmacological interventions that may require further individualization of dosing regimens (Persky *et al.*, 2003). Overall, the potential of psychological benefits accruing through exercise far outweighs the potential risk that no effect or even harm will occur (Mutrie and Faulkner, 2003).

WHAT WE KNOW SUMMARY

- There is a high incidence of obesity and other morbid conditions strongly related to physical inactivity in this population.
- Exercise interventions are possible.
- The existing research examining the psychological benefits of exercise participation does have many methodological flaws and tends to be of pre-experimental design.
- There is some tentative support that participating in exercise is associated with an alleviation of negative symptoms associated with schizophrenia, such as depression, low self-esteem, and social withdrawal.
- There is less evidence that exercise may be a useful coping strategy for dealing with positive symptoms, such as auditory hallucinations.

WHAT WE NEED TO KNOW SUMMARY

- Are the determinants of exercise different in this population?
- How should interventions be best designed to help individuals with schizophrenia adopt and maintain adherence to exercise programs?
- Are the psychological benefits of exercise participation supported by stronger research designs such as RCTs?
- How does exercise interact with medication and other common therapeutic strategies such as CBT?
- What is the effect of regular exercise participation on other important outcomes such as use of health services, medication compliance, and rate of relapse?

REFERENCES

Adams, L. (1995). How exercise can help people with mental health problems. *Nursing Times, 91*, 37–39.

Allison, D. B., Mentore, J. L., Heo, M., Chandler, L. P., Cappelleri, J. C., Infante, M. C. *et al.* (1999). Antipsychotic-induced weight gain: a comprehensive research synthesis. *American Journal of Psychiatry, 156*, 1686–1689.

Andrews, G., Sanderson, K., Corry, J., Issakidis, C., and Lapsley, H. (2003). Cost-effectiveness of current and optimal treatment for schizophrenia. *British Journal of Psychiatry, 183*, 427–435.

Archie, S., Wilson, J. H., Osborne, S., Hobbs, H., and McNiven, J. (2003). Pilot study: access to fitness facility and exercise levels in Olanzapine-treated patients. *Canadian Journal of Psychiatry, 48*, 628–632.

Auchus, M. P., Wood, K., and Kaslow, N. (1995). Exercise patterns of psychiatric patients admitted to a short-term inpatient unit. *Psychosocial Rehabilitation Journal, 18*, 137–140.

Bartsch, D. A., Shern, D. L., Feinberg, L. E., Fuller, B. B., and Willett, A. B. (1990). Screening CMHC outpatients for physical illness. *Hospital and Community Psychiatry, 41*, 786–790.

Beck, A. T., Ward, C. H., Mendelson, M., Mock, J., and Erbangh, J. (1961). An inventory for measuring depression. *Archives of General Psychiatry, 4*, 561–571.

Belcher, T. L. (1988). Behavioral reduction of overt hallucinatory behavior in a chronic schizophrenic. *Journal of Behavior Therapy and Experimental Psychiatry, 19*, 69–71.

Bergman, U., Hutzler, Y., Stein, D., Avidan, G., and Wozner, Y. (1993). Therapeutic physical activity for adolescents in a closed psychiatric ward. *Issues in Special Education and Rehabilitation, 8*, 41–54.

Berren, M. R., Hill, K. R., Merikle, E., Gonzalez, N., and Santiago, J. (1994). Serious mental illness and mortality rates. *Hospital and Community Psychiatry, 45*, 604–605.

Brown, S., Birtwhistle, J., Roe, L., and Thompson, C. (1999). The unhealthy lifestyle of people with schizophrenia. *Psychological Medicine, 29*, 697–701.

Burbach, F. R. (1997). The efficacy of physical activity interventions within mental health services: anxiety and depressive disorders. *Journal of Mental Health, 6*, 543–566.

Campbell, D. and Stanley, J. (1963). *Experimental and Quasi-experimental Designs for Research.* Chicago, IL: Rand McNally.

Carless, D. and Faulkner, G. (2003). Physical activity and psychological health. In C. Riddoch and J. McKenna (Eds). *Critical Perspectives in Physical Activity and Health* (pp. 61–82). London: Macmillan.

Carlsson, A. M. (1983). Assessment of chronic pain: aspects of reliability and validity of the visual analogue scale. *Pain*, *16*, 87–101.

Carlsson, C., Dencker, S., Grimby, G., and Heggendal, J. (1967). Noradrenaline in human blood plasma and urine during exercise in patients receiving large doses of chlorpromazine. *Acta Pharmacology et Toxicology*, *25*, 97–106.

Carlsson, C., Dencker, S., Grimby, G., and Heggendal, J. (1968a). Circulatory studies during physical exercise in mentally disordered patients. I. Effects of large doses of chlorpromazine. *Acta Medica Scandinavica*, *184*, 499–509.

Carlsson, C., Dencker, S., Grimby, G., and Heggendal, J. (1968b). Circulatory studies during physical exercise in mentally disordered patients. II. Effects of physical training in patients with and without administration of chlorpromazine. *Acta Medica Scandinavica*, *184*, 511–516.

Carr, V. (1988). Patients' techniques for coping with schizophrenia: an exploratory study. *British Journal of Medical Psychology*, *61*, 339–352.

Carter-Morris, P., and Faulkner, G. (2003). A football project for service users: the role of football in reducing social exclusion. *Journal of Mental Health Promotion*, *2*, 24–31.

Chamove, A. S. (1986). Positive short-term effects of activity on behavior in chronic schizophrenic patients. *British Journal of Clinical Psychology*, *25*, 125–133.

Chastain, P. B. and Shapiro, G. E. (1987). Physical fitness program for patients with psychiatric disorders: a clinical report. *Physical Therapy*, *67*, 545–548.

Ciompi, L. (1984). Is there really a schizophrenia? The long-term course of psychotic phenomena. *British Journal of Psychiatry*, *145*, 636–640.

Clark, B. A., Wade, M. G., Massey, B. H., and Van Dyke, R. (1975). Response of institutionalized geriatric mental patients to a twelve-week program of regular physical activity. *Journal of Gerontology*, *30*, 565–573.

Conroy, R. W., Smith, K., and Felthous, A. R. (1982). The value of exercise on a psychiatric hospital unit. *Hospital and Community Psychiatry*, *33*, 641–645.

Davidson, S., Judd, F., Jolley, D., Hocking, B., Thompson, S., and Hyland B. (2001). Cardiovascular risk factors for people with mental illness. *The Australian and New Zealand Journal of Psychiatry*, *35*, 196–202.

Derogatis, L. R. and Melisaratos, N. (1983). The brief symptom inventory: an introduction report. *Psychological Medicine*, *13*, 595–605.

Derogatis, L. R., Lipman, R. S., Rickels, K., Uhlenhuth, E. H., and Covi, L. (1974). The Hopkins Symptom Checklist (HSLC): a self report symptom inventory. *Behavioural Science*, *19*, 1–15.

Falloon, I. R. H. and Talbot, R. E. (1981). Persistent auditory hallucinations: coping mechanisms and implications for management. *Psychological Medicine*, *11*, 329–339.

Farnam, C. R., Zipple, A. M., Tyrrell, W., and Chittinanda, P. (1999). Health status and risk factors of people with severe and persistent mental illness. *Journal of Psychosocial Nursing*, *37*, 16–21.

Faulkner, G. and Biddle, S. (1999). Exercise and schizophrenia: a review. *Journal of Mental Health*, *8*, 441–457.

Faulkner, G. and Biddle, S. J. H. (2001). Exercise and mental health: it's just not psychology! *Journal of Sports Sciences*, *19*, 433–444.

Faulkner, G. and Sparkes, A. (1999). Exercise as therapy for schizophrenia: an ethnographic study. *Journal of Sport and Exercise Psychology*, *21*, 52–69.

Faulkner, G., Soundy, A., and Lloyd, K. (2003). Weight control and schizophrenia: a systematic review. *Acta Psychiatrica Scandinavica*, *108*, 324–332.

Fitts, W. H. (1965). *Tennessee Self-Concept Scale: Manual*. Los Angeles, CA: Western Psychological Services.

Folkins, C. and Sime, W. (1981). Physical fitness and mental health. *American Psychologist*, *36*, 373–389.

Fontaine, K. R., Heo, M., Harrigan, E. P., Shear, C. L., Lakshminarayanan, M., Casey, D. E. *et al.* (2001). Estimating the consequences of anti-psychotic induced weight gain on health and mortality rate. *Psychiatry Research, 101*, 277–288.

Fox, K. R. (1999). The influence of physical activity on mental well-being. *Public Health Nutrition, 2*, 411–418.

Geddes, J., Freemantle, N., Harrison, P., and Bebbington, P., National Schizophrenia Guideline Development Group (2000). Atypical antipsychotics in the treatment of schizophrenia: systematic overview and meta-regression analysis. *British Medical Journal, 321*, 1371–1376.

Gimino, F. A. and Levin, S. J. (1984). The effects of aerobic exercise on perceived self-image in post-hospitalized schizophrenic patients. *Medicine and Science in Sports and Exercise, 16*, 139.

Goeree, R., O'Brien, B. J., Goering, P., Blackhouse, G., Agro, K., Rhodes, A., and Watson, J. (1999). The economic burden of schizophrenia in Canada. *Canadian Journal of Psychiatry, 44*, 464–472.

Goldman, L. S. (1999). Medical illness in patients with schizophrenia. *Journal of Clinical Psychiatry, 60*(Suppl. 21), 10–15.

Green, A., Patel, J., and Goisman, R. (2000). Weight gain from novel antipsychotic drugs: need for action. *General Hospital Psychiatry, 22*, 224–235.

Guy, W. (1976). *ECDEU Assessment Manual for Psychopharmacology: Nurses' Global Impressions Scale*. Washington, DC: US Government Printing Office.

Hannaford, C. P., Harrell, E. H., and Cox, K. (1988). Psychophysiological effects of a running program on depression and anxiety in a psychiatric population. *The Psychological Record, 38*, 37–48.

Harding, C., Strauss, J. S., and Zubin, J. (1992). Chronicity in schizophrenia: revisited. *British Journal of Psychiatry, 161*, 27–37.

Harris, E. C. and Barraclough, B. (1998). Excess mortality of mental disorder. *British Journal of Psychiatry, 173*, 11–53.

Harter, S. (1982). The perceived competence scale for children. *Child Development, 53*, 87–97.

Hatlova, B. and Basny sen, Z. (1995). Kinesiotherapy-therapy using two different types of exercises in curing schizophrenic patients. In the Proceedings of the 9th Biennial Conference of the International Society of Comparative Physical Education and Sport. *Physical Activity for Life: East and West, South and North* (pp. 426–429). Aachen Germany: Meyer and Meyer Verlag.

Health Canada (2002). *A Report on Mental Illnesses in Canada*. Ottawa, ON: Health Canada.

Hemsley, D. (1995). Schizophrenia: treatment. In S. Lindsay and G. Powell (Eds). *The Handbook of Clinical Adult Psychology* (pp. 309–328). London: Routledge.

Honigfeld, G., Gillis, R. D., and Klett, C. J. (1965). Nurses' observation scale for inpatient evaluation: a new scale for measuring improvement in chronic schizophrenia. *Journal of Clinical Psychology, 21*, 65–71.

Hutchinson, D. and Skrinar, G. S. (1994). Exercise and self-esteem: the implications for persons with severe mental illness. *Medicine and Science in Sports and Exercise, 26*(Suppl. 5), S76.

Hutchinson, D. S., Skrinar, G. S., and Cross, C. (1999). The role of improved physical fitness in rehabilitation and recovery. *Psychiatric Rehabilitation Journal, 22*, 355–359.

Kane, J. M. (1996). Treatment resistant schizophrenic patients. *Journal of Clinical Psychiatry, 57*(Suppl. 9), 35–40.

Kaplan, K., Mendelson, L. B., and Dubroff, M. P. (1983). The effect of a jogging program on psychiatric inpatients with symptoms of depression. *Occupational Therapy Journal of Research, 3*, 173–175.

Kawachi, I. (1999). Physical and psychological consequences of weight gain. *Journal of Clinical Psychiatry, 60*(Suppl. 21), 5–9.

Knapp, M. (1997). Costs of Schizophrenia. *British Journal of Psychiatry, 171*, 509–518.

Knowler, W. C., Barrett-Connor, E., Fowler, S. E., Hamman, R. F., Lachin, J. M., Walker, E. A., Nathan, D. M., Diabetes Prevention Program Research Group (2002). Reduction in the incidence of type 2 diabetes with lifestyle intervention or metformin. *New England Journal of Medicine, 346*, 393–403.

Koran, L. M., Sox, H. C., Morton, K. I., Moltzen, S., Sox, C. H., Kraemer, H. C. *et al.* (1989). Medical evaluation of psychiatric patients. *Archives of General Psychiatry, 36*, 414–447.

Krawiecka, M., Goldberg, D., and Vaughn, M. (1977). A standardized psychiatric assessment scale for rating chronic psychotic patients. *Acta Psychiatrica Scandinavica, 55*, 299–308.

Kurzthaler, I. and Fleischhacker, W. W. (2001). The clinical implications of weight gain in schizophrenia. *Journal of Clinical Psychiatry, 62*(Suppl. 7), 32–37.

Lean, M. E. and Pajonk, F. G. (2003). Patients on atypical antipsychotic drugs: another high-risk group for type 2 diabetes. *Diabetes Care, 26*, 1597–1605.

Lee, P. W. H., Lieh-Mak, F., Yu, K. K., and Spinks, J. A. (1993). Coping strategies of schizophrenic patients and their relationship to outcome. *British Journal of Psychiatry, 163*, 177–182.

Le Fevre, P. D. (2001). Improving the physical health of patients with schizophrenia: therapeutic nihilism or realism? *Scottish Medical Journal, 46*, 11–31.

Lukoff, D., Wallace, C. J., Liberman, R. P., and Burke, K. (1986). A holistic program for chronic schizophrenic patients. *Schizophrenia Bulletin, 12*, 274–282.

McCreadie, R. G. (2003). Diet, smoking and cardiovascular risk in people with schizophrenia. *British Journal of Psychiatry, 183*, 534–539.

McIntyre, R. S., Mancini, D. A., and Basile, V. S. (2001). Mechanisms of antipsychotic-induced weight gain. *Journal of Clinical Psychiatry, 62*(Suppl. 23), 23–29.

McNair, D. M., Lorr, M., and Droppleman, L. F. (1971). *Manual for the Profile of Mood States.* San Diego, CA: Educational and Industrial Testing Service.

Martinsen, E. G. (1993). Therapeutic implications of exercise for clinically anxious and depressed patients. *International Journal of Sport Psychology, 24*, 185–199.

Martinsen, E. W. (1995). The effects of exercise on mental health in clinical populations. In S. J. H. Biddle (Ed.). *European Perspectives on Exercise and Sport Psychology* (pp. 71–84). Champaign, IL: Human Kinetics.

Martinsen, E. W. and Stanghelle, J. K. (1997). Drug therapy and physical activity. In W. P. Morgan (Ed.). *Physical Activity and Mental Health* (pp. 81–90). New York: Taylor and Francis.

Meyer, T. and Broocks, A. (2000). Therapeutic impact of exercise on psychiatric diseases: guidelines for exercise testing and prescription. *Sports Medicine, 30*, 269–279.

Mrazek, K. and Hatlova, B. (1995). Socialising effects of kinesiotherapy in a group of long-term hospitalized psychiatric patients. In the Proceedings of the 9th Biennial Conference of the International Society of Comparative Physical Education and Sport. *Physical Activity for Life: East and West, South and North* (pp. 475–476). Aachen, Germany: Meyer and Meyer.

Murray C. J. L. and Lopez, A. D. (Eds) (1996). *The Global Burden of Disease.* Cambridge, MA: Harvard School of Public Health.

Mutrie, N. (2000). The relationship between physical activity and clinically defined depression. In S. J. H. Biddle, K. R. Fox, and S. H. Boutcher (Eds). *Physical Activity and Psychological Well-being* (pp. 46–62). London: Routledge.

Mutrie, N. and Faulkner, G. (2003). Physical activity and mental health. In T. Everett, M. Donaghy, and S. Fever (Eds). *Physiotherapy and Occupational Therapy in Mental Health: An Evidence Based Approach* (pp. 82–97). Oxford: Butterworth Heinemann.

Netz, Y., Yaretzki, A., Salganik, I., Jacob, T., Finkeltov, B., and Argov, E. (1994). The effect of supervised physical activity on cognitive and affective state of geriatric and psychogeriatric in-patients. *Clinical Gerontologist, 15*, 47–56.

Osborn, D. P. J. (2001). The poor physical health of people with mental illness. *Western Journal of Medicine*, *175*, 329–332.

Osby, U., Correia, N., Brandt, L., Ekbom, A., and Sparen, P. (2000). Mortality and causes of death in schizophrenia in Stockholm County, Sweden. *Schizophrenia Research*, *45*, 21–28.

Overall, J. E. and Gorham, D. R. (1962). The Brief Psychotic Rating Scale. *Psychological Reports*, *10*, 799–812.

Pelham, T. W. and Campagna, P. D. (1991). Benefits of exercise in psychiatric rehabilitation of persons with schizophrenia. *Canadian Journal of Rehabilitation*, *4*, 159–168.

Pelham, T. W., Campagna, P. D., Ritvo, P. G., and Birnie, W. A. (1993). The effects of exercise therapy on clients in a psychiatric rehabilitation program. *Psychosocial Rehabilitation Journal*, *16*, 75–84.

Persky, A. M., Eddington, N. D., and Derendorf, H. (2003). A review of the effects of chronic exercise and physical fitness on resting pharmacokinetics. *International Journal of Clinical Pharmacology and Therapeutics*, *41*, 504–516.

Petra, Z. and Hatlova, B. (1995). Kinesiotherapeutic intervention in cure of schizophrenic patients-women. In the Proceedings of the 9th Biennial Conference of the International Society of Comparative Physical Education and Sport. *Physical Activity for Life: East and West, South and North* (pp. 530–532). Aachen, Germany: Meyer and Meyer Verlag.

Pilling, S., Bebbington, P., Kuipers, E., Garety, P., Geddes, J., Orbach, G. *et al.* (2002a). Psychological treatments in schizophrenia: meta-analysis of family intervention and cognitive behaviour therapy. *Psychological Medicine*, *32*, 763–782.

Pilling, S., Bebbington, P., Kuipers, E., Garety, P., Geddes, J., Martindale, B. *et al.* (2002b). Psychological treatments in schizophrenia: meta-analyses of randomized controlled trials of social skills training and cognitive remediation. *Psychological Medicine*, *32*, 783–791.

Plante, T. G. (1993). Aerobic exercise in prevention and treatment of psychopathology. In P. Seraganian (Ed.). *Exercise Psychology* (pp. 358–379). London: Wiley-Interscience.

Plante, T. G. (1996). Getting physical. Does exercise help in the treatment of psychiatric disorders? *Journal of Psychosocial Nursing and Mental Health*, *34*, 38–43.

Powell, R. R. (1974). Psychological effects of exercise therapy upon institutionalized geriatric mental patients. *Journal of Gerontology*, *29*, 157–161.

Puri, B. K., Laking, P. J., and Treasaden, I. H. (2002). *Textbook of Psychiatry* (2nd edn). London: Elsevier Science.

Raine, P., Truman, C., and Southerst, A. (2002). The development of a community gym for people with mental health problems: influences on psychological accessibility. *Journal of Mental Health*, *11*, 43–53.

Richardson, C., Faulkner, G., McDevitt, J., Skrinar, G. S., Hutchison, D. S., and Piette, J. D. (2005). Integrating physical activity into mental health services for individuals with serious mental illness. *Psychiatric Services*, *56*, 324–331.

Rosenthal, M. M. and Beutell, N. J. (1981). Movement and body-image: a preliminary study. *Perceptual and Motor Skills*, *53*, 758.

Ryckman, R. M., Robbins, M. A., Thornton, B., and Cantrell, P. (1982). Development and validation of a physical self-efficacy scale. *Journal of Personality and Social Psychology*, *42*, 891–900.

Sainsbury Centre for Mental Health (2002). *Working for Inclusion*. London: SCMH.

Skrinar, G. S. and Hutchinson, D. (1994). Exercise training and perceptual responses in adults with chronic mental illness. *Medicine and Science in Sports and Exercise*, *26*(Suppl. 5), S76.

Skrinar, G. S., Unger, K. V., Hutchinson, D. S., and Faigenbaum, A. D. (1992). Effects of exercise training in young adults with psychiatric disabilities. *Canadian Journal of Rehabilitation*, *5*, 151–157.

Sonstroem, R. J. (1978). Physical estimation and attraction scales: rationale and research. *Medicine and Science in Sports, 10*, 97–102.

Spielberger, C. D., Gorsuch, R. L., Lushene, R., Vagg, P. R., and Jacobs, G. A. (1983). *Manual for the State-Trait Anxiety Inventory (Form Y1)*. Palo Alto, CA: Consulting Psychologists Press.

Sule, F. (1987). Therapeutic use of sports in psychiatry and clinical psychology. *Journal of Sports Medicine, 27*, 79–84.

Tarrier, N. (1994). Management and modification of residual positive psychotic symptoms. In M. Birchwood and N. Tarrier (Eds). *Psychological Management of Schizophrenia* (pp. 109–128). Chichester, West Sussex, UK: Wiley.

Tarrier, N., Beckett, R., Harwood, S., Baker, A., Yusupoff, L., and Ugarteburu, I. (1993). A trial of two cognitive-behavioural methods of treating drug resistant residual psychotic symptoms in schizophrenic patients: outcome. *British Journal of Psychiatry, 162*, 524–532.

Tsuang, M., Woolson, R. F., and Fleming, J. A. (1979). Long-term outcome of major psychoses: I. Schizophrenia and affective disorders compared with psychiatrically symptom-free surgical conditions. *Archives of General Psychiatry, 36*, 1295–1301.

Tuomilehto, J., Lindstrom, J., Eriksson, J. G., Valle, T. T., Hamalainen, H., Ilanne-Parikka, P. et al. (2001). Prevention of type 2 diabetes mellitus by changes in lifestyle among subjects with impaired glucose tolerance. *New England Journal of Medicine, 344*, 1343–1350.

United States Department of Health and Human Services (1999). *Mental Health: A Report of the Surgeon General*. Atlanta, GA: US Department of Health and Human Services, Centers for Disease Control and Prevention, National Center for Chronic Disease Prevention and Health Promotion.

Veit, C. T. and Ware, J. E. (1983). The structure of psychological distress and well-being in general populations. *Journal of Consulting and Clinical Psychology, 51*, 730–742.

Weiden, P. J., Mackell, J. A., and McDonnell, D. D. (2004). Obesity as a risk factor for antipsychotic noncompliance. *Schizophrenia Research, 66*, 51–57.

Yagi, G., Kinoshita, F., and Kanba, S. (1991). Coping style of schizophrenic patients in the recovery from acute psychotic state. *Schizophrenia Research, 6*, 87–88.

Exercise interventions in drug and alcohol rehabilitation

MARIE E. DONAGHY AND
MICHAEL H. USSHER

This chapter provides a review of studies which have included exercise as part of the treatment intervention for those who are dependent on alcohol or illicit drugs. The review focuses on the potential of exercise for influencing the use of alcohol and drugs, psychological variables (e.g., depression, cravings), and physical fitness.

PREVALENCE, MORTALITY, AND MORBIDITY

Use of illegal drugs and alcohol is a global public health problem (World Health Organization, 2004). In 2000, alcohol abuse was responsible for the death of 5,796 males and 3,371 females in the United Kingdom alone (Office of National Statistics, 2000; Registrar General for Scotland, 2000). This is a 100% increase over 20 years (Office of National Statistics, 2004), with the highest increase occurring in the

25–44 age group; suggesting a link between early onset drinking and mortality. Among problem drinkers, chronic liver disease is the major cause of death (Office of National Statistics, 2004). Mexico and the United States have the highest mortality rates from alcoholic liver disease per capita with 13,581 and 12,109 deaths, Japan the sixth highest with 3,151 deaths, Canada lies in tenth place with 1,104 deaths, and the United Kingdom fourteenth with 866 deaths (Nationmaster, 2004). Those who are dependent on alcohol also have an increased risk of cancer of the larynx and esophagus, cerebrovascular disease, and injuries through accidents (Ritson, 1994). In addition, alcohol abuse is linked to poor physical fitness, skeletal muscle damage, loss of bone mass, increased depression and anxiety, and low self-esteem (see Donaghy and Mutrie, 1999). The cost in providing medical and social services for problem drinkers runs into billions of pounds, accounting for as much as 12% of the total NHS expenditure on hospitals in the United Kingdom (Royal College of Physicians, 2001).

Mortality figures for drug misuse are difficult to assess because many deaths are recorded as suicide, accidents, or are HIV related. In 1999, 1,711 male and 260 female drug related deaths were reported in the United Kingdom, with drug dependency and poisoning accounting for the highest mortality rates (Office of National Statistics, 2000). In addition, morbidity from drug abuse is associated with the spread of infectious diseases, such as hepatitis and HIV (Health Advisory Service, 1996).

In the United Kingdom, guidelines on drinking are exceeded by 44% of men over the age of 16 and 30% of women (Office of National Statistics, 2004). The general household survey (Office of National Statistics, 2004) indicates that the heaviest drinkers are in the age group 16–24, with 49% of men and 39% of women exceeding the guidelines on one or more days of the week. Of these, 13% of the men and 6% of the women are defined as heavy drinkers. These levels of prevalence are not unique to the United Kingdom. In the United States alcohol dependence is one of the most common psychiatric disorders affecting approximately 20% of the population (Kessler et al., 1994).

In the United Kingdom, alcohol use in pre-adolescents and adolescents is increasing. In 1996, 29% of 12–13-year-old boys and 26% of age-similar girls admitted drinking alcohol in the past week. In 1999 these rates increased to 38% and 30%, respectively (Royal College of Physicians, 2001). Studies undertaken in the last 10 years suggest that adolescents are frequently binge drinking (Goddard, 1996; Miller and Plant, 1996; Newbury-Birch et al., 2000). In the United Kingdom, higher levels of intoxication among adolescents has been reported when compared with teenagers in most other European countries (Hibell et al., 1997). This is of particular concern, as early age onset of regular drinking is associated with heavy consumption and alcohol-related problems in later life (Newbury-Birch et al., 2000).

The British Crime Survey (Home Office, 2003) reports that 12% of 16–59 year olds have taken an illicit drug and 3% have used a Class A drug in the last year. Use of illegal drugs is similarly widespread throughout Europe and North America, and among other nations, and there is evidence that use of these substances is on the increase (European Monitoring Centre for Drugs and Drug Addiction, 2003; Johnson and Gerstein, 1998). The use of illicit drugs tends to be lower in early adolescent years but increases by the age of 16. Sutherland and Shepherd (2001), in a survey of 9,742 adolescents in England, found that the prevalence of illicit drug use increased from 0.9% in 11-year olds to 14.5% at age 16.

These surveys suggest a pattern of drinking and illicit drug use in the United Kingdom that starts in school with a third of 12–13-year olds regularly consuming alcohol (Royal College of Physicians, 2001). This increases at age 15 to 50%, with binge drinking prevalent among teenagers (Newbury-Birch *et al.*, 2000) and one in five of 15-year olds in the United Kingdom taking illicit drugs (Office of National Statistics, 2004; Scottish Executive, 2003). Evidently, in many nations, the number of young problem drinkers and illicit drug users is likely to increase in the foreseeable future, leading to health and social problems that require cost-effective programs of intervention.

TREATMENT

Treatment for alcohol and drug addiction includes cognitive-behavioral approaches (Read *et al.*, 2001), pharmacological agents, including the use of naltrexone to prevent relapse and methadone to aid withdrawal from heroin (Department of Health, 1999). While these treatments may provide short-term relief, the relapse rates are high, ranging from 60–80% (Chick, 1993). Despite increasing expenditure in the last decade, treatment of drug and alcohol abuse has poor long-term outcomes with no treatment approach or context, inpatient versus outpatient, having been found to be more effective than another (Donaghy, 1997). It has long been recognized that addictions are multifaceted disorders (Cook and Gurling, 1990; Sutton, 1987) and multifaceted treatments are required, including global lifestyle changes (Read and Brown, 2003).

There is a need to provide treatment for both acute care needs and chronic needs. Three major stages of treatment are recognized (Institute of Medicine, 1990). Stage one: detoxification; emergency treatment and screening. Stage two: rehabilitation, evaluation, and assessment; primary care and extended care. Stage three: maintenance aftercare; relapse prevention; and domiciliary care. Some studies have indicated that exercise as an adjunct to treatment has been beneficial in recovery, mostly during stage two, with only two studies showing benefits for relapse prevention (Donaghy, 1997; Sinyor *et al.*, 1982).

POTENTIAL MECHANISMS OF EXERCISE

Despite the association between exercise and health and psychological well-being (Department of Health, 2004), only a few studies have investigated exercise for people with an addiction to alcohol or illegal drugs. Potential mechanisms of exercise presented in previous reviews include achievement of a pleasurable state without the use of drugs, changes in lifestyle behavior, increased social support, and improved psychological well-being including improved physical self-perceptions and achieving skills to decrease stress-reactivity, and to improve coping (Donaghy and Mutrie, 1999; Read and Brown, 2003; Tkachuk and Martin, 1999). More recently it has been argued that exercise may produce similar pleasurable experiences to drugs and alcohol through activation of the opiod systems (Biddle and Mutrie, 2001; Froelich, 1997), and therefore may provide an alternative reinforcer to drug or alcohol use (Cosgrove *et al.*, 2002).

While not mentioned specifically in the alcohol or drug literature, exercise may also act as a distraction. Moreover, distraction has been linked to exercise and reductions in depression (Biddle and Mutrie, 2001) and is plausible in this context where there is a need to break away from previous routine behavior.

THE EVIDENCE FOR EXERCISE

All studies from 1970 onwards which were located by standard search methods (Firstsearch, MEDLINE, PsychInfo, Embase, SPORTDiscus, Cinahl, Social Citation Index) and which included an exercise intervention for a clinically defined population of alcohol use disorders or illegal drug misuse were reviewed. The search words "alcohol," "problem drinking," "drinking patterns," "drugs," "illicit drugs," "substance misuse," and "substance abuse" combined with "exercise" or "physical activity" were used to conduct the review. A summary of the findings of studies included in the review is presented in Tables 4.1 and 4.2.

In total, 16 intervention studies were included, 10 relating to the treatment of alcohol addiction and six relating to drug addiction. Two studies were not included in the review, as the populations sampled had no evidence of alcohol or drug abuse (Murphy *et al.*, 1986; Scott and Myers, 1988). While the focus was on intervention studies, a survey of exercise attitudes in people undergoing rehabilitation for alcohol addiction (Read *et al.*, 2001) was also included as the findings informed the debate on the acceptance of exercise as a suitable intervention.

SUMMARY OF STUDIES

Ten intervention studies were identified which examined exercise as an adjunct to an alcohol rehabilitation program for adults (Table 4.1). The details of the study under-taken by Anstiss (1991) are limited as it is only available as a published abstract. Two of the studies investigated people attending outpatient clinics (Donaghy *et al.*, 1991; Ussher *et al.*, 2000), seven focused on inpatients, and one multi-site study included both inpatients and outpatients (Donaghy, 1997). In addition, a survey examined self-report of exercise behavior and attitudes towards exercise among those attending an alcohol rehabilitation program (Read *et al.*, 2001). Only four of the studies were ran-domized controlled trials (RCTs); however, only Anstiss (1991) and Donaghy (1997) had a sufficient sample size to provide conclusive findings. Both of these studies had a high number of dropouts and only Donaghy used intention-to-treat analysis. One study included control groups at a different center (Sinyor *et al.*, 1982), and another had a control group at a different time point (Palmer *et al.*, 1988).

The majority of the studies included group-based exercise; Ussher *et al.* (2000) tailored an individual program, and Donaghy (1997) included both group-based exer-cise and a home-based program. The length of the exercise intervention varied from three weeks to 10 months with no clear rationale for the extended timescale. The frequency of exercise varied from daily to once a week and the type of exercise was mostly aerobic. Only three studies indicated that they followed American College of

Table 4.1 Characteristics of the studies on exercise interventions with problem drinkers

STUDY	DESIGN	n	SEX	CLINICAL SETTING	TYPE OF EXERCISE	DURATION (MIN)	FREQUENCY	LENGTH OF TRAINING	OUTCOME MEASURES AND OUTCOME
Gary and Guthrie (1972)	Random control	20	M	USA inpatient	Aerobic	Not reported	5× week	4 weeks	Schneider fitness, Jourard body Cathexis ↑ fitness and self-esteem in exercise group only
Frankel and Murphy (1974)	Single group pre-post	214	M	North America inpatient	Aerobic	60	5× week	12 weeks	Illinois fitness submax step MMPI. ↑ fitness and ↓ anxiety and depression
Tsukue and Shohoji (1981)	Single group pre-post	25	M	Japan inpatient	Aerobic	Not reported	3× week	10 months	BP, skinfold, balance, grip strength ↑ coordination and fitness
Sinyor et al. (1982)	Quasi-experimental control at different center	58	M, F	Canada inpatient	Aerobic	60	5× week	6 weeks	Estimated max VO$_2$, skinfold, drinking report. In experimental group at posttest ↑ fitness and abstinence at 3-month follow-up ↑ abstinence maintained
Palmer et al. (1988)	Quasi-experimental control at different time point	27	M, F	North America inpatient	Aerobic ACSM guidelines	20–30	3× week	4 weeks	Estimated max VO$_2$, Zung depression inventory, STAI, in experimental group ↓ anxiety and depression no change in fitness

Study	Design	N	Sex	Setting	Exercise type	Duration (min)	Frequency	Length	Outcomes
Donaghy et al. (1991)	Random control 3 groups	37	M	Scotland outpatient	Aerobic and non-aerobic ACSM guidelines	30	3× week	8 weeks	Estimated max VO₂, BDI Depression Inventory, Leeds Scale, strength and flexibility ↓ anxiety and depression ↑ strength in both exercise groups change in fitness in aerobic group only
Anstiss (1991)	Random control 2 groups	166	M, F	England inpatient	Exercise bicycle aerobic high intensity and aerobic below training zone	Not stated	Daily	4 weeks	Unspecified fitness test, BDI Depression Inventory, STAI, ↓ depression in both groups ↑ fitness in both groups. No between group difference on VO₂ max, BDI, STAI, relapse rate, drinking behavior or psychosocial functioning. Increased drop out in high intensity exercise group
Ermalinski et al. (1997)	Quasi-experimental 2 treatment groups	90	M	USA Texas inpatient	Aerobic stretching and body-mind component	10 stretching 5 ↑ to 20 jogging	5× week	6 weeks	Improved training effect in exercise group only. Higher internal LOC in exercise group. No between group difference in depression or self-esteem

(Table 4.1 continued)

Table 4.1 Continued

STUDY	DESIGN	n	SEX	CLINICAL SETTING	TYPE OF EXERCISE	DURATION (MIN)	FREQUENCY	LENGTH OF TRAINING	OUTCOME MEASURES AND OUTCOME
Donaghy (1997)	Multi-site random control 2 groups	117	M, F	Scotland outpatient and inpatient	Aerobic and strength ACSM guidelines	30	3× week	3 weeks + 12 week home-based program	Estimated max VO_2, strength and flexibility, PSPP, BDI, Zung anxiety, 7-day recall physical activity, Serum CDT. At 1 month ↑ strength, ↑ fitness, ↑ physical self-perceptions in condition, strength and self-worth in exercise group only ↓ anxiety and depression both groups. At 2 month, ↑ fitness, ↑ strength, ↑ physical activity levels, ↑ physical self-perceptions in condition and strength in exercise group only ↓ anxiety and depression both groups, no between

Study	Design	N	Gender	Location	Intervention	Duration	Frequency	Weeks	Outcomes
Ussher et al. (2000)	Multiple case studies	5	M, F	England outpatient	Exercise counseling and supervised aerobic strength	75 mins	2× week 1× week	3 weeks 3 weeks	group difference in abstinence levels. At 5 months ↑ fitness maintained Field diary and self-report measures were used to create case studies. Benefits included ↑ self image ↑ body image balance hand grip and fitness ↓ weight loss, depression, and quit reduce smoking, make exercise part of everyday life
Read et al. (2001)	Survey	105	M	North America outpatient	N/A	N/A	N/A	N/A	47% engaged in regular physical activity. Level of alcohol dependency was not related to physical activity levels. Stress reduction was linked to physical activity levels

Notes: MMPI = minnesota multiphasic personality inventory; BP = blood pressure; Estimated max VO$_2$ = estimated maximum oxygen consumption; LOC = locus of control; BDI = Beck depression inventory; STAI = Spielberger state and trait anxiety inventory; CDT = carbohydrate deficiency transferrin blood analysis; PSPP = physical self-perception profile.

Table 4.2 Characteristics of the studies on exercise interventions and substance misuse

STUDY	DESIGN	n	SEX	CLINICAL SETTING	TYPE OF EXERCISE	DURATION (MIN)	FREQUENCY	LENGTH OF TRAINING	OUTCOME MEASURES AND OUTCOME
Burling et al. (1992)	Quasi-experimental control at different time point	116	M, F	North America inpatient	Softball	Not stated	3× week	Not stated	Abstinence, living situation, employment status. ↑ abstinence at 3 months post-discharge in exercise group versus control
Collingwood et al. (1991)	Single group pre-post	74	M, F	North America outpatient inpatient community	Aerobic strength flexibility	60–90	3–5× week	9 weeks	Aerobic power, strength, skinfolds, flexibility, PCSCS, GWS, substance use, abstinence ↑ fitness, self-esteem ↓ anxiety, depression, body fat, multiple drug users
Collingwood et al. (1994)	Single group pre-post	297	M, F	North America outpatient inpatient community	Not stated	Not stated	Not stated	8–16 weeks	Aerobic power, strength, skinfolds, flexibility, BIAV, GWS, substance use ↑ fitness, self-esteem ↓ substance use, anxiety, depression
Collingwood et al. (2000)	Single group pre-post	329	M, F	North America outpatient inpatient community	Aerobic strength flexibility	30–60	3× week	9–12 weeks	Aerobic power, strength, skinfolds, flexibility, BIAV, PCSCS, GWS, substance use ↑ fitness, self-esteem ↓ anxiety, depression
Li et al. (2002)	Random control 3 groups	86	M	China inpatient	Qigong	25–30	4–5× day	10 days	Urine morphine, SESWS, HAS for qigong group versus both controls: ↓ withdrawal, anxiety, morphine
Palmer et al. (1995)	Random control 3 groups	45	M, F	North America inpatient	Aerobic strength circuit-training	30–40	3× week	4 weeks	Aerobic power, CES–D, skinfolds, resting pulse rate, blood pressure, strength: ↓ depression in strength group only

Notes: GWS = General Well-Being Scale; PCSCS = Piers-Harris Children's Self-Concept Scale; BIAV = Bills Index of Adjustment and Values; SESWS = Standard Evaluation Scale of Withdrawal Symptoms; HAS = Hamilton Anxiety Scale; CES–D = Centre of Epidemiological Studies–Depression; BCFSEI = Battles Culture Free Self-Esteem Inventory; PSES = Physical Self-Efficacy Scale; BCS = Body Cathexis Scale.

Sports Medicine guidelines (1990) on the frequency, duration, and intensity of exercise required for developing and maintaining aerobic and strength fitness (1990). The most frequently used fitness outcome was estimated maximum VO_2. Other physical measures included strength, flexibility, balance, and coordination. Various measures were used for psychological outcomes relating to depression, anxiety, and perceived body image. Overall, due to the small number of RCTs and lack of consistency in the use of outcome measures, it is difficult to make firm conclusions about the role of exercise in alcohol rehabilitation.

Six studies were identified which examined the effect of an exercise intervention on use of illicit drugs (see Table 4.2). Three of the studies targeted adults who were receiving inpatient treatment for substance misuse (Burling *et al.*, 1992; Li *et al.*, 2002; Palmer *et al.*, 1995) and three studies recruited a combination of adolescents in treatment for substance misuse and adolescents from the general community (Collingwood *et al.*, 1991, 1994, 2000). The study by Li (2002) targeted heroin addicts and the other studies targeted misuse for a range of substances. All of the studies employed group-based exercise as an adjunct to a traditional drug rehabilitation and education program.

Only two of the studies were RCTs (Li *et al.*, 2002; Palmer *et al.*, 1995). One of these studies (Palmer *et al.*, 1995) had an insufficient sample size ($n = 15$ per group) to have a realistic chance of observing any significant effects of exercise. In addition, the findings of Palmer were not analyzed on an intention-to-treat basis. Of the 80 patients initially recruited to this study, 35 patients were excluded from the analysis as they did not complete the intervention program. The RCT carried out by Li *et al.* (2002) used a qigong intervention, a traditional Chinese form of exercise which combines meditation, relaxation, guided imagery, physical exercises, and breathing exercises; therefore, it was not possible to distinguish the effect of physical exercise versus the effect of the other components of qigong. Moreover, Li's intervention was highly intensive, involving 2–3 hours a day of qigong for 10 days and it is not clear whether this intervention would be attractive beyond this specific population of Chinese, inpatient heroin users.

Only two of the drug studies reported the level of compliance with the exercise regimen (Collingwood *et al.*, 1994, 2000). Also, in both cases the adherence data had limited validity as exercise levels were reported retrospectively by two questions, rather than by a detailed questionnaire or by interview (see Pereira *et al.*, 1997). Only one of the studies reported the intensity of the exercise; 60% of estimated maximum heart rate (Palmer *et al.*, 1995). In the absence of data relating to exercise adherence and exercise intensity it is difficult to make any conclusions concerning the optimum dose of exercise during drug rehabilitation. Furthermore, without measures of exercise adherence it is not possible to confirm whether any observed effects of the interventions are related to increased levels of physical activity.

EFFECTS ON ALCOHOL AND SUBSTANCE MISUSE

Maintaining abstinence or controlled drinking is the goal of alcohol rehabilitation. The goal of drug rehabilitation is to increase abstinence from drugs. The majority of the alcohol studies reviewed in this chapter examined the effects of exercise on abstinence and this was most frequently measured by self-report. Self-report has been found to be a poor outcome measure for alcohol abstinence (Stibler, 1991) and only one study included a biochemical marker of alcohol consumption (Donaghy, 1997). Thus, it is not possible to confirm any of the observed effects of increased physical activity or fitness on maintaining abstinence or controlled drinking. Only Donaghy (1997) and Sinyor *et al.* (1981) included a follow-up to examine the potential of exercise to maintain abstinence. At three-month post intervention, Sinyor *et al.* (1981) reported that abstinence had been maintained; however, Donaghy (1997) found no between group differences at either two or five-month follow-ups.

All but one of the drug studies (Palmer *et al.*, 1995) assessed the impact of an exercise intervention on the use of drugs. Only one study included biochemical validation of abstinence (Li *et al.*, 2002). The three studies conducted by Collingwood and associates (1991, 1994, 2000) used a questionnaire to assess types and amounts of use for a range of illicit substances. In their 1991 study, Collingwood reported no effect of the exercise intervention on the use of any specific substance or on levels of abstinence, although they did report a significant reduction in the number of multiple drug users. In their 1994 study, Collingwood observed a significant reduction in the number of users for marijuana, uppers, cocaine, hallucinogens, steroids, and designer drugs. However, both Collingwood studies must be treated with caution as no control group was utilized. Collingwood's 2000 study did not report any significant changes in the use of drugs following the exercise intervention. However, the chances of detecting any changes were minimal since only a very small percentage of the sample reported using these substances at the outset.

The study by Burling and associates (1992) showed increased rates of abstinence from drugs in a softball group compared to a control group, but this outcome was confounded by the observation that the softball group remained in treatment longer than the control group. Finally, one study showed that during 10 days of detoxification from heroin, those in a qigong group showed a significantly more rapid reduction in urine morphine levels compared to the controls (Li *et al.*, 2002). This study did not take measures beyond the 10 days of the intervention; therefore, it is not possible to assess the impact of qigong on relapse to heroin.

ROLE OF FITNESS

Improving fitness in a population where physical health has been damaged by continual excessive use of alcohol may be important in enabling participation in a range of new or previously enjoyed activities. Increased fitness is also an indicator of exercise adherence. All but one of the studies assessing fitness showed that exercise improves cardiovascular fitness during alcohol rehabilitation. The frequency and duration of supervised exercise programs varied between studies; most notably, the length of the training period ranged from three weeks to 10 months (Table 4.1). These differences in exercise interventions make it difficult to make comparisons across studies and to determine the optimum frequency, duration, and intensity of exercise necessary to achieve fitness gains. At this time, the evidence suggests that short three-and four-week exercise programs are as effective as longer programs in improving physical fitness and strength (Donaghy, 1997). Donaghy was the only researcher to follow-up a three-week supervised exercise program with a 12-week home-based program and found improved levels of fitness were maintained at five-month follow-up. In addition, increased levels of physical activity found at two-month follow-up were maintained at three-month follow-up, suggesting a shift towards a more active lifestyle.

The inclusion of a well-designed randomized controlled study (Donaghy, 1997) provides much needed evidence, for this population, of a causal link between exercise and improved aerobic fitness in both the short- and medium-term. More importantly, it highlights that aerobic fitness can be quickly improved in problem drinkers with poor fitness levels and that this can be sustained by undertaking a home-based program on discharge from an alcohol rehabilitation clinic. In Donaghy's (1997) study, self-report at five-month follow-up included running half marathons, returning to the sport of boxing, hill walking, and cycling to work, with the majority reporting increased daily walking. Several people reported a renewed confidence to return to activities previously enjoyed. In the qualitative study presented by Ussher *et al.* (2000), an increase in levels of independent physical activity was reported by four of the five people studied, with comments from participants indicating that greater independence was achieved through improvements in confidence and through structuring the day with physical activities. Read *et al.* (2001) indicated that of those people in alcohol treatment who were surveyed, 47% engaged in regular physical exercise (three times per week or more); however, the level of alcohol dependence was not significantly associated with reported levels of physical activity.

Four studies in drug rehabilitation included measures of cardiovascular fitness and strength and three of these reported significant gains in both fitness and strength following the exercise intervention (Collingwood *et al.*, 1991, 1994, 2000). All of the studies by Collingwood lacked a control group; therefore, it is not clear whether the observed increases in fitness are related to the exercise intervention or whether elevated fitness is a normal consequence of returning to a more active lifestyle during drug rehabilitation. The study in which exercise had no effect upon fitness or strength (Palmer *et al.*, 1995) had an exercise program lasting only four weeks. This may have been of insufficient length to obtain detectable results across either of these indices.

There are specific biological explanations that may account for the observed fitness benefits of exercise for problem drinkers. Donaghy (1997) suggests that improved aerobic fitness in problem drinkers may initially be related to peripheral vascular changes. Damage to Type IIb muscle fibers has been shown to occur with long-term alcohol abuse. More specifically, structural alterations have been found in the muscle fibers leading to atrophy (Peters *et al.*, 1985).

Participation in an exercise program may be beneficial for problem drinkers by increasing chemical activity of the muscles (Terjung and Hood, 1986) countering some of the alcohol-related damage to the muscle fibers (Donaghy and Mutrie, 1999). In addition, it is likely that other cardiovascular and respiratory changes associated with aerobic exercise will provide benefits to this clinical population, similar to those experienced within the general population.

EFFECTS ON PSYCHOLOGICAL MEASURES

Examining the effects of exercise interventions on psychological variables such as depression, anxiety, and self-esteem is important since these variables are risk factors for alcohol and substance misuse and are associated with relapse (Marlatt and Gordon, 1980).

Anxiety and depression

High levels of anxiety and depression have been found among problem drinkers on entry to alcohol rehabilitation, with clinical levels of depression frequently reported (Donaghy *et al.*, 1991). The findings from the studies in Table 4.1 offer some support for the role of exercise in reducing anxiety and depression to levels commonly found among the general population. The study by Palmer *et al.* (1995) supports the earlier findings of Frankel and Murphy (1974), suggesting that trait and state anxiety and depression are significantly reduced during exercise. However, Frankel and Murphy had no control group and the control group in Palmer *et al.*'s (1995) study was assessed at a different time point from the experimental group; therefore, the findings in these studies, with regard to anxiety and depression, could be the result of experimental bias, peripheral effects of time spent with the therapist, effects over time, or the effects from other therapeutic interventions.

In the most recent studies of exercise for problem drinkers no between group differences on anxiety or depression were found (Donaghy, 1997; Ermalinski *et al.*, 1997), although there was a significant reduction in levels of anxiety and depression for both control and intervention groups. Whether the exercise had any effect on anxiety and depression over and above the effect of other treatment components, for example psychotherapy, may be concealed by the floor effect in the reduction of these symptoms. Read *et al.* (2001) reported that tension and stress reduction were among the most strongly endorsed of the perceived benefits of physical activity during alcohol rehabilitation. Similarly, Ussher *et al.* (2000) found changes in scores from the General Health Questionnaire (GHQ; Goldberg *et al.*, 1997) that confirmed the study participants' verbal reports of improved psychological well-being.

Five studies in drug rehabilitation included measures of anxiety or depression. All the studies by Collingwood and associates observed a significant decrease in reports of depression and anxiety following exercise programs ranging from 8 to 16 weeks. However, as none of these studies included a comparison group, it is not clear whether the observed reductions in depression and anxiety were due to participation in the exercise program or were related to other elements of the process of rehabilitation. Among those receiving treatment for heroin addiction, Li (2002) observed significantly lower reports of anxiety on day five and day ten of a 10-day qigong intervention relative to anxiety levels for a medication group and a no-treatment group. This finding must be treated with caution since the qigong group had more social contact with their peers than did the other two groups; therefore, it is not clear whether the reduction in anxiety is due to qigong practice or due to social support.

Interestingly, Palmer and colleagues (1995) found a significant decrease in reports of depression following a strength-training program relative to changes in reports of depression following an aerobic step program or a circuit-training program. However, as with the study by Li, this finding is limited in that the strength-training group had more social contact with their peers than did the other two groups. Further research is required to compare the effect of different modes of exercise on psychological outcomes in those undergoing alcohol or drug rehabilitation. On balance, there is currently limited evidence to suggest that participation in regular exercise will have a positive influence in reducing depression or anxiety among those undergoing rehabilitation for alcohol or drug addiction.

Physical self-perception, self-esteem, and self-efficacy

Low self-esteem has been linked to problem drinking (McMahon and Davidson, 1986). Gary and Guthrie (1972) found that self-esteem improved following a four-week jogging program. Neither Ermalinski *et al.* (1997) nor Palmer (1988) reported improvements in self-esteem following an exercise program. Read *et al.* (2001) found that the perceived benefits of exercise, among those surveyed, included a more positive outlook and increased self-esteem.

Donaghy (1997) showed that the inclusion of a three-week exercise program in an abstinence treatment program improved perceptions of physical self-worth, physical condition and strength, as measured by the Physical Self Perception Profile (Fox and Corbin, 1989), with the latter two benefits being maintained at the two-month follow-up. In another study, Ussher *et al.* (2000), using the same measure as above, observed enhanced body image for three of the five people studied. Donaghy (1997) found that improved fitness related to improved perceptions of physical condition and physical self-worth, and improvement in actual physical strength was matched by improved perceptions of strength. While these associations are of interest, we do not know how changes in physical self-perceptions will impact on global self-esteem and subsequently on decisions made in relation to changing toward a healthier lifestyle. Self-report (Donaghy, 1997) suggests that these perceptions may have an impact on self-efficacy toward continuing to exercise and returning to previous activities. However, there is a need for further research, with this population, in order to clarify the relationship between exercise, physical self-perceptions, and global self-esteem.

Four studies in drug rehabilitation assessed the influence of an exercise program on self-esteem. All three studies by Collingwood and colleagues (1991, 1994, 2000) showed an increase in reports of self-esteem following an exercise intervention ranging from 8 to 16 weeks. As there was no comparison group in these studies, it is possible that the increases in self-esteem were a response to the normal process of rehabilitation rather than due to the effects of exercise.

Effects on drug and alcohol withdrawal symptoms and cravings

Cravings for alcohol or drugs are considered a defining characteristic of substance dependence (Pickens and Johanson, 1992) and have been related to severity of dependence

(Bohn *et al.*, 1995; Glautier and Drummond, 1994; Greeley *et al.*, 1992) and negative affect (Cooney *et al.*, 1997; Greeley *et al.*, 1992). Moreover, severe cravings and withdrawal symptoms are likely to be a discomfort for those who are substance-dependent and for some individuals these symptoms may contribute to relapse following treatment (Litt *et al.*, 2000; Marlatt and Gordon, 1980). Little is known about the moderators of urges for alcohol or drugs and few interventions are available which target these urges (Drummond *et al.*, 2000).

Exercise has been shown to have an acute and chronic effect on reducing tobacco withdrawal symptoms and urges to smoke in abstinent smokers (Ussher *et al.*, 2001, 2003). Additionally, brief cardiovascular exercise has been shown to suppress appetite (Blundell and King, 2000) and to reduce cravings for sugary foods (Thayer *et al.*, 1993). On this basis one might hypothesize that exercise would also be useful for managing withdrawal and cravings among those who misuse drugs and alcohol. Moreover, there is evidence from animal studies that exercise, as an alternative reinforcer to drug use, is related to reductions in drug consumption. For example, among rats, access to a running wheel attenuates intravenous cocaine self-administration (Cosgrove *et al.*, 2002), oral intake of amphetamines (Kanarek *et al.*, 1995), and ethanol drinking (McMillan, 1995).

Only one of the six studies examining the role of an exercise intervention on drug use included specific measures of withdrawal symptoms and cravings (Li *et al.*, 2002). In Li's study of abstinent heroin users it was shown that during a 10 day intervention, withdrawal symptoms and cravings were reduced more rapidly in the qigong group relative to the group receiving detoxification medication (Lofexidine) or to the group receiving no treatment (except for treatment of acute physical symptoms such as pain or diarrhea). Further studies are required to assess the impact of more conventional exercise on the process of detoxification. Exercise has potential advantages over medication aimed at detoxification. For example, exercise does not have the side effects associated with these medications. In addition, exercise has many general health benefits, which may assist with the process of recovery.

None of the studies in Table 4.1 examined the effect of exercise on alcohol withdrawal or cravings. However, there is some experimental evidence to suggest that exercise might help alleviate urges for alcohol. Ussher *et al.* (2004) recruited males and females following 10 days of alcohol detoxification. Using a within-subjects design, on the first day of experimentation 20 participants were randomized to undergo either a single bout of 10-minutes of moderate intensity cycling or a bout of 10-minutes of very light intensity cycling (control). On the following day they underwent the other condition. Relative to baseline, there was a significant decline in alcohol urges (Alcohol Urge Questionnaire; Bohn *et al.*, 1995) for moderate intensity exercise versus control, during exercise (after five minutes of exercise). A brief bout of moderate intensity exercise may provide short-term relief from alcohol urges during exercise. Further studies are required to confirm whether the moderating effect of exercise on alcohol urges is sustained following exercise. It would also be useful to investigate whether exercise has any beneficial effects during alcohol detoxification and to assess how exercise interacts with antiwithdrawal medications and with other medications used during alcohol and drug rehabilitation.

WHAT WE KNOW SUMMARY

- There is unequivocal support that physical exercise regimens have a positive effect on aerobic fitness and strength if administered as an adjunct in alcohol rehabilitation.
- There is unsubstantial evidence for the benefits of exercise on fitness during drug rehabilitation.
- The link between improvements in self-esteem and exercise with alcohol and drug rehabilitation at this time is equivocal.
- There is limited support that exercise regimens have a positive effect on reducing anxiety and depression if administered as an adjunct in alcohol and drug rehabilitation.
- There is experimental evidence from one study to suggest that alcohol cravings may be alleviated during exercise.
- The evidence for exercise improving abstinence levels or controlled drinking levels is at this time equivocal.

WHAT WE NEED TO KNOW SUMMARY

The final section of this chapter highlights implications for both researchers and practitioners, the points raised are intended to promote discussion around current interventions as well as to promote and influence further research.

Barriers to exercise There is some evidence to suggest that the large majority of intravenous drug users are likely to identify positive benefits of sport and exercise (Powers *et al.*, 1999). Other evidence suggests that those with substance misuse problems may be particularly concerned about the hazards of exercise, such as injury, and that they are fearful of becoming addicted to exercise (Collingwood *et al.*, 1994). It has also been suggested that, for adolescents, appropriate fitness program leadership and the proximity of the fitness program to the at-risk youth are important considerations (Collingwood *et al.*, 1994).

- Further studies are needed to systematically examine the barriers to exercise, and other psychosocial determinants of exercise among drug users and problem drinkers.

Changing several health behaviors simultaneously Most of the interventions reviewed required the patient to alter their substance misuse behavior and exercise behavior simultaneously; yet, it is not clear that this is the optimum strategy. For some individuals the demands of changing several health behaviors simultaneously may be too demanding and may result in failure for changing one or both behaviors. In order to understand the relationship between intentions to change alcohol or substance misuse behavior and intentions to change exercise behavior psychological theories such as the Theory of Planned Behavior or the Transtheoretical model need to be tested with this population (Ussher, in press). For example, it is not clear whether involvement in physical activity increases motivation toward managing substance intake or vice versa.

In addition, we do not know whether involvement of a spouse or family in exercise programs will increase motivation and participation. Ultimately, such research may lead to guidelines stating, for specific substance misuse populations, whether it is optimum to introduce exercise before, during, or following the reduction or abstinence from drugs or alcohol use and whether it is best to focus exercise participation on the individual or the family.

- What is the optimum strategy for changing multiple health behaviors?

Medical screening   Exercise screening tools may be required which address the specific needs of those with substance misuse problems. For example, those undergoing treatment for amphetamine and cocaine misuse are often undernourished and their metabolism may be distorted and these factors may impact on their ability to take up an exercise program. Problem drinkers have been found to have weakened muscle tissue and loss of bone mass with increased risk of fractures (Peris *et al.*, 1992; Preedy and Peters, 1990). This appears to be a result of the direct effects of alcohol on the Type IIb muscle fibers themselves (Peters *et al.*, 1985). Similarly, excessive amounts of alcohol may have a negative effect on the laying down of new bone (Rico, 1990). Screening can identify those most at risk of injury and allow a graded program of activity designed to stop the progression of these changes and to minimize their impact on health. Nutritional advice may need to be integrated as part of the exercise intervention and for those who are undernourished we need to determine the optimum duration, frequency, and intensity of exercise.

- Exercise screening may be necessary. How should practitioners and researchers tailor the exercise 'dosage' in relation to the physical health complications common in this population?

Exercise counseling   Only two of the intervention studies for drug users incorporated exercise counseling (Collingwood, 1991, 2000), and only one of the alcohol studies (Ussher *et al.*, 2000) including cognitive behavioral techniques such as goal setting, self-monitoring, contracting, social support, and reinforcement. Studies are needed to examine the impact of exercise alone versus exercise plus exercise counseling during alcohol and drug treatment. There is also a need to consider how the beneficial effects of exercise on self-perceptions and improved physical well-being among problem drinkers (Donaghy, 1997) can be translated into relapse prevention strategies. This requires a more explicit link to be made between exercise participation and cognitive strategies such as self-awareness, self-evaluation, stimulus control, and expectations. This approach needs to be evaluated in relation to maintaining abstinence or controlled intake.

- What is the potential role of exercise counseling in improving adherence and abstinence?

Exercise as a preventative intervention   Recent work has shown that, among adolescents, higher levels of physical activity significantly reduced the odds of progressing to smoking or to higher level of smoking (Audrain-McGovern *et al.*, 2003; see Chapter 8).

Evidently, exercise programs targeted at young people have the potential to reduce smoking uptake. Research is needed to establish whether participation in physical activity, among young children or adolescents, has a similar effect on reducing progression to heavy drinking or the use of illicit substances. Evidence for the association between participation in physical activity and drug/alcohol misuse among adolescents is equivocal and further studies, especially prospective studies, are needed in this area. For example, some large cross-sectional studies of adolescents have found a negative association between substance use and physical activity (Duncan *et al.*, 2002; Ferron *et al.*, 1999; Pate *et al.*, 1996), whereas other studies have observed no significant relationship between physical activity involvement and substance use (Dinger and Vesely, 2002; Harrison and Narayan, 2003), or have shown a negative association between these behaviors only for females (Kulig *et al.*, 2003) or only for males (Winnail *et al.*, 1995). These studies suggest a complex relationship between substance use and exercise which is mediated by gender, personality, mode of physical activity, and type of drug used.

- What is the preventative role of physical activity in alcohol and drug use?

Drug and alcohol addiction is a growing global problem among adolescents and adults of all ages. It is a multifaceted problem that is fuelled by sub-culture, and which crosses cultural and class boundaries and impacts on the education, health, and economy of many nations. The limited evidence to support the application of exercise interventions in drug and alcohol rehabilitation can partly be explained by the small number of studies that have been carried out and by the flawed research methodology of many of these studies. Exercise has been shown to be a beneficial intervention for the treatment of many physical and psychological illnesses (Department of Health, 2004) and in the context of alcohol and drug rehabilitation exercise has the potential to be an alternative reinforcer to these substances, to encourage a healthy lifestyle which is incompatible with substance misuse, to provide valuable social support, and to enhance psychological well-being and coping skills. It is hoped that the potential benefits of exercise for the treatment of the addictions promotes much needed research among physiotherapists, occupational therapists, sports scientists, and other healthcare professionals involved with this population.

REFERENCES

American College of Sports Medicine (1990). Position stand: the recommended quality and quantity of exercise for developing and maintaining cardiorespiratory and muscular fitness in healthy adults. *Medicine and Science in Sports and Exercise, 22*, 265–274.

Anstiss, T. J. (1991). A randomised controlled trial of aerobic exercise in the treatment of the alcohol dependent. *Medicine and Science in Sports and Exercise, 23*, S118.

Audrain-McGovern, J., Rodriguez, D., and Moss, H. B. (2003). Smoking progression and physical activity. *Cancer Epidemiology Biomarkers and Prevention, 12*, 1121–1129.

Biddle, S. J. H. and Mutrie, N. (2001). *Psychology of Physical Activity: Determinants, Well-being and Interventions*. London: Routledge.

Blundell, J. E. and King, N. A. (2000). Exercise, appetite control, and energy balance. *Nutrition, 16*, 519–522.

Bohn, M. J., Krahn, D. D., and Staehler, B. A. (1995). Development and initial validation of a measure of drinking urges in abstinent alcoholics. *Alcohol Clinical and Experimental Research*, *19*, 600–606.

Burling, T. A., Seidner, A. L., Robbins-Sisco, D., Krinsky, A., and Hanser, S. B. (1992). Batter up! Relapse prevention for homeless veteran substance abusers via softball team participation. *Journal of Substance Abuse*, *4*, 407.

Chick, J. (1993). Alcohol dependence: an illness with a treatment? *Addiction*, *88*, 1481–1492.

Collingwood, T. R., Reynolds, R., Kohl, H. W. III., Smith, W., and Sloan, S. (1991). Physical fitness effects on substance abuse risk factors and use patterns. *Journal of Drug Education*, *21*, 73–84.

Collingwood, T. R., Sunderlin, J., and Kohl, H. W. III. (1994). The use of a staff training model for implementing fitness programming to prevent substance abuse with at-risk youth. *American Journal of Health Promotion*, *9*, 20–33.

Collingwood, T. R., Sunderlin, J., Reynolds, R., and Kohl, H. W. III. (2000). Physical training as a substance abuse prevention intervention for youth. *Journal of Drug Education*, *30*, 435–451.

Cook, C. and Gurling, H. (1990). The genetic aspects of alcoholism and substance abuse: a review. In G. Edward and M. Lader (Eds). *The Nature of Drug Dependence* (pp. 75–111). Oxford: Oxford University Press.

Cooney, N. L., Litt, M. D., Morse, P. A., Bauer, L. O., and Gaupp, L. (1997). Alcohol cue reactivity, negative-mood reactivity, and relapse in treated alcoholic men. *Journal of Abnormal Psychology*, *106*, 243–250.

Cosgrove, K. P., Hunter, R. G., and Carroll, M. E. (2002). Wheel-running attenuates intravenous cocaine self-administration in rats: sex differences. *Pharmacology and Biochemical Behavior*, *73*, 663–671.

Department of Health (1999). *Drug Misuse and Dependence: Guidelines on Clinical Management*. London: DOH publications.

Department of Health (2004). *At Least Five a Week: Evidence on the Impact of Physical Activity and its Relationship to Health, a Report from the Chief Medical Officer*. London: DOH publication.

Dinger, M. K. and Vesely, S. K. (2001). Relationships between physical activity and other health-related behaviors in a representative sample of US college students. *American Journal of Health Education*, *3*, 83–88.

Donaghy, M. E. (1997). *An Investigation into the Effects of Exercise as an Adjunct to the Treatment and Rehabilitation of the Problem Drinker*. Unpublished doctoral dissertation, University of Glasgow, Glasgow.

Donaghy, M. E. and Mutrie, N. (1999). Is exercise beneficial in the treatment and rehabilitation of the problem drinker? A critical review. *Physical Therapy Review*, *4*, 153–166.

Donaghy, M., Ralston, G., and Mutrie, N. (1991). Exercise as a therapeutic adjunct for problem drinkers. *Journal of Sports Sciences*, *9*, 440.

Drummond, D. C., Litten, R. Z., Lowman, C., and Hunt, W. A. (2000). Craving research: future directions. *Addiction*, *95*(Suppl. 2), S247–S255.

Duncan, S. C., Duncan, T. E., Strycker, L. A., and Chaumeton, N. R. (2002). Relations between youth antisocial and prosocial activities. *Journal of Behavioral Medicine*, *5*, 425–438.

Ermalinski, R., Hanson, P. G., Lubin, B., Thornby, J. I., and Nahormek, P. A. (1997). Impact of a body-mind treatment component on alcoholic inpatients. *Journal of Psychosocial Nursing*, *35*, 39–45.

European Monitoring Centre for Drugs and Drug Addiction (2003). *Annual Report on the State of the Drugs Problem in the European Union and Norway*. Luxembourg: Office for Official Publications of the European Communities.

Ferron, C., Narring, F., Cauderay, M., and Michaud, P. A. (1999). Sport activity in adolescence: associations with health perceptions and experimental behaviours. *Health Education Research*, *14*, 225–233.

Fox, K. R. and Corbin, C. B. (1989). The physical self-perception profile: development and preliminary validation. *Journal of Sport and Exercise Psychology*, *11*, 408–430.

Frankel, A. and Murphy, J. (1974). Physical fitness and personality in alcoholism: canonical analysis of measures before and after treatment. *Quarterly Journal of the Study of Alcohol*, *35*, 1271–1278.

Froelich, J. C. (1997). Opiod peptides. *Alcohol Health and Research World*, *21*, 132–135.

Gary, V. and Guthrie, D. (1982). The effect of jogging on physical fitness and self concept on hospitalized alcoholics. *Quarterly Journal of Studies in Alcohol*, *33*, 1073–1078.

Glautier, S. and Drummond, D. C. (1994). Alcohol dependence and cue reactivity. *Journal of Studies on Alcohol*, *55*, 224–229.

Goddard, E. (1996). *Drinking in 1994*. London: HMSO publications.

Goldberg, D. P., Gater, R., Sartorius, N., Ustun, T. B., Piccinelli, M., Gureje, O. *et al.* (1997). The validity of two versions of the GHQ in the WHO study of mental illness in general health care. *Psychological Medicine*, *27*, 191–197.

Greeley, J., Swift, W., and Heather, N. (1992). Depressed affect as a predictor of increased desire for alcohol in current drinkers of alcohol. *British Journal of Addiction*, *87*, 1005–1012.

Harrison, P. A. and Narayan, G. (2003). Differences in behavior, psychological factors, and environmental factors associated with participation in school sports and other activities in adolescence. *Journal of School Health*, *73*, 113–120.

Health Advisory Service (1996). *Children and Young People*. London: Substance Misuse Services.

Hibell, B., Andersson, B., and Bjarnason, T. (Eds). (1997). *The 1995 ESPAD Report. Alcohol and Other Drug Use Among Students in 26 European Countries*. Stolkholm: Modin Tryck.

Home Office (2003). *Prevalence of Drug Use: Key Findings from the 2003/03 British Crime Survey: Research and Development Statistics Directorate*. London: Home Office.

Institute of Medicine (1990). *Broadening the Base of Treatment for Alcoholism*. New York: Wiley.

Johnson, R. A. and Gerstein, D. R. (1998). Initiation of use of alcohol, cigarettes, marijuana, cocaine, and other substances in US birth cohorts since 1919. *American Journal of Public Health*, *88*, 27–33.

Kanarek, R. B., Marks-Kaufman, R., D'Anci, K. E., and Przypek, J. (1995). Exercise attenuates oral intake of amphetamine in rats. *Pharmacology and Biochemical Behavior*, *51*, 725–729.

Kessler, R. C., McGonagle, K. S., and Shanyang, Z. (1994). Lifetime and 12-month prevalence of *DSM-III* psychiatric disorders in the United States: results from the National Co-morbidity Survey. *Archives of General Psychiatry*, *51*, 8–19.

Kulig, K., Brener, N. D., and McManus, T. (2003). Sexual activity and substance use among adolescents by category of physical activity plus team sports participation. *Archives of Pediatric and Adolescent Medicine*, *157*, 905–912.

Li, M., Chen, K., and Mo, Z. (2002). Use of qigong therapy in the detoxification of heroin addicts. *Alternative Therapies in Health and Medicine*, *8*, 50–59.

Litt, M. D., Cooney, N. L., and Morse, P. (2000). Reactivity to alcohol-related stimuli in the laboratory and in the field: predictors of craving in treated alcoholics. *Addiction*, *95*, 889–900.

McMahon, R. C. and Davidson, R. S. (1986). An examination of depressed versus nondepressed alcoholics in inpatient treatment. *Journal of Clinical Psychology*, *42*, 177–184.

McMillan, D. E., McClure, G. Y., and Hardwick, W. C. (1995). Effects of access to a running wheel on food, water and ethanol intake in rats bred to accept ethanol. *Drug and Alcohol Dependence*, *40*, 1–7.

Marlatt, G. A. and Gordon, J. R. (1985). *Relapse Prevention: Maintenance Strategies in the Treatment of Addictive Behaviors*. New York: Guildford.

Miller, P. and Plant, M. (1996). Drinking, smoking and illicit drug use among 15 and 16 year olds in the United Kingdom. *British Medical Journal, 7054*, 394–398.

Miller, P. and Plant, M. (2001). Drinking and smoking among 15–16 year olds in the United Kingdom: a re-examination *Journal of Substance Use, 5*, 285–289.

Murphy, T. J., Pagano, R. R., and Marlatt, G. A. (1986). Lifestyle modification with heavy alcohol drinkers: effects of aerobic exercise and meditation. *Addictive Behaviors, 11*, 175–186.

Nationmaster Countries by Mortality (2004). *National Mortality Rates*. Retrieved July 29, 2004, from the nationmaster database: http://www.nationmaster.com/graph-T/mor_alc_liv_dis

Newbury-Birch, D., White, M., and Kamali, F. (2000). Factors influencing alcohol and illicit drug use amongst medical students. *Drug and Alcohol Dependence, 59*, 125–130.

Office of National Statistics (2000). *Mortality Statistics Cause*. London: The Stationery Office.

Office of National Statistics (2004). *Social Trends 32*. London: The Stationery Office.

Palmer, J., Palmer, L. K., Michiels, K., and Thigpen, B. (1995). Effects of type of exercise on depression in recovering substance abusers. *Perceptual and Motor Skills, 80*, 523–530.

Palmer, J., Vacc, N., and Epstein, J. (1988). Physical exercise as a treatment intervention. *Journal of Studies in Alcohol, 49*, 418–429.

Pate, R. R., Heath, G. W., Dowda, M., and Trost, S. G. (1996). Associations between physical activity and other health behaviors in a representative sample of US adolescents. *American Journal of Public Health, 86*, 1577–1581.

Pereira, M. A., Fitzgerald, S. J., Gregg, E. W., Joswaik, M. L., Ryan, W. J., Suminsk, R. R. *et al.* (1997). A collection of physical activity questionnaires for health related research: seven day physical activity recall. *Medicine and Science in Sport and Exercise, 29*(Suppl. 6), S89–S103.

Peris, P., Pares, A., Guanabens, N., Pons, F., Martinez-De Osaba, M. J., Caballeria, J. *et al.* (1992). Reduced spinal and femoral bone mass and deranged bone mineral metabolism in chronic alcoholics. *Alcohol and Alcoholism, 27*, 619–625.

Peters, T. J., Martin, F., and Ward, K. (1985). Chronic alcoholic skeletal myopathy common and reversible. *Alcohol, 2*, 485–489.

Pickens, R. W. and Johanson, C. E. (1992). Craving: consensus of status and agenda for future research. *Drug and Alcohol Dependence, 30*, 127–131.

Powers, J. M., Woody, G. E., and Sachs, M. L. (1999). Perceived effects of exercise and sport in a population defined by their injection drug use. *American Journal of Addiction, 8*, 72–76.

Preedy, V. R. and Peters, T. J. (1990). Alcohol and skeletal muscle disease. *Alcohol and Alcoholism, 25*, 177–187.

Read, J. P. and Brown, R. A. (2003). The role of physical exercise in alcoholism treatment and recovery. *Professional Psychology: Research and Practice, 34*, 49–56.

Read, J. P., Kahler, C. W., and Stevenson, J. F. (2001). Bridging the gap between alcoholism treatment research and practice: identifying what works and why. *Professional Psychology: Research and Practice, 32*, 227–238.

Registrar General for Scotland (2000). *1999 Annual Report*. Edinburgh: Common Services Agency.

Rico, H. (1990). Alcohol and bone disease. *Alcohol and Alcoholism, 25*, 345–352.

Ritson, B. (1994). Epidemiology and primary prevention of alcohol misuse. In J. Chick and R. Cantwell (Eds). *Alcohol and Drug Misuse College Seminars Series* (pp. 75–93). London: Royal College of Psychiatrists.

Royal College of Physicians (2001). *Alcohol can the NHS Afford it? Recommendations for a Coherent Alcohol Strategy for Hospitals*. Salisbury: Sarum Colour View Group.

Scott, K. A. and Myers, A. M. (1988). Impact of fitness training on native adolescents' self-evaluations and substance use. *Canadian Journal of Public Health, 79*, 424–429.

Scottish Executive (2003). *Scotland's Health 2002*. Edinburgh: HMSO.

Sinyor, D., Brown, T., Rostant, L., and Seraganian, P. (1982). The role of a physical fitness programme in the treatment of alcoholism. *Journal of Studies on Alcohol, 43*, 380–386.

Stibler, H. (1991). Carbohydrate-deficient transferrin in serum: a new marker of potentially harmful alcohol consumption reviewed. *Clinical Chemistry*, *37*, 2029–2037.

Sutherland, I. and Shepherd, J. P. (2001). The prevalence of alcohol, cigarette, and illicit drug use in a stratified sample of English adolescents. *Addiction*, *96*, 637–640.

Sutton, S. (1987). Social-psychological approaches to understanding addictive behaviours: attitude behaviour and decision-making models. *British Journal of Addiction*, *82*, 355–370.

Terjung, R. L. and Hood, D. A. (1986). Biochemical adaptations in skeletal muscle induced by exercise training. In D. K. Layman (Ed.). *Nutrition and Aerobic Exercise* (pp. 8–26). Washington, DC: American Chemical Society.

Thayer, R. E., Peters, D. P., Takahashi, P. J., and Birkhead-Flight, A. M. (1993). Mood and behavior (smoking and sugar snacking) following moderate intensity exercise: a partial test of self-regulation theory. *Personality and Individual Differences*, *14*, 97–104.

Tkachuk, G. A. and Martin, G. L. (1999). Exercise therapy for patients with psychiatric disorders: research and clinical implications. *Professional Psychology: Research and Practice*, *30*, 275–282.

Ussher, M. (in press). Physical activity interventions. In S. Ayers, A. Baum, C. McManus, S. Newman, K. Wallston, J. Weinmann, and R. West (Eds). *Handbook of Psychology, Health and Medicine* (2nd edn). Cambridge: Cambridge University Press.

Ussher, M., McCusker, M., Morrow, V., and Donaghy, M. (2000). A physical activity intervention in a community alcohol service. *British Journal of Occupational Therapy*, *63*, 598–604.

Ussher, M., Nunziata, P., Cropley, M., and West, R. (2001). Effect of a short bout of exercise on tobacco withdrawal symptoms and desire to smoke. *Psychopharmacology*, *158*, 66–72.

Ussher, M., West, R., McEwen, A., Taylor, A., and Steptoe, A. (2003). Efficacy of exercise counseling as an aid for smoking cessation: a randomized controlled trial. *Addiction*, *98*, 523–532.

Ussher, M., Sampuran, A. K., Doshi, R., West, R., and Drummond, D. C. (2004). Acute effect of a brief bout of exercise on alcohol urges. *Addiction*, *99*, 1542–1547.

Winnail, S. D., Valois, R. F., McKeown, R. E., Saunders, R. P., and Pate, R. R. (1995). Relationship between physical activity level and cigarette, smokeless tobacco, and marijuana use among public high school adolescents. *Journal of School Health*, *65*, 438–442.

World Health Organization (2004). *The Global Burden*. Retrieved July 24, 2004, from the World Health Organization's website: http://www.who.int/substance_abuse/facts/global_burden/en/accesse

The role of exercise in recovery from heart failure

FFION LLOYD-WILLIAMS AND FRANCES MAIR

Over the past 30 years, the effectiveness of rehabilitation for patients with coronary heart disease (CHD) has been established (Wenger *et al.*, 1995). Positive outcomes from exercise programs include improvements in exercise tolerance, skeletal muscle strength, psychological status, and quality of life (QOL) (Buselli and Stuart, 1999; Dugmore *et al.*, 1999; Lavie and Milani, 1995, 1997; Stewart *et al.*, 1999). Cardiac rehabilitation for CHD patients has been shown to reduce mortality by as much as 20–25% when compared with CHD patients not enrolled in such programs (Linden *et al.*, 1996; O'Connor *et al.*, 1989; Oldridge *et al.*, 1988). In recent years however, the effect size of outcomes from cardiac rehabilitation studies have been declining because of improving standards of conventional treatments, for example, medication and surgery, offered to control group patients (Oldridge *et al.*, 2002). This raises important issues relating to the assessment of exercise effects within a multicomponent rehabilitation program.

Although many papers have been published concerning the physiological effects of exercise training on patients with Congestive Heart Failure (CHF), the role of exercise as a form of rehabilitation for patients with CHF is yet to be established. This chapter describes a review of the literature pertaining to the effects of exercise training with heart failure patients, in order to ascertain the current strength of evidence underlying the growing belief in the benefits of exercise for this patient population. However, the main focus is on evidence relating to the impact of these programs upon patients' QOL and psychological status, and what further research is required to ascertain the benefits of exercise upon these important health characteristics.

WHAT IS HEART FAILURE?

Heart failure is a chronic disorder resulting from cardiac disease that comprises ventricular systolic or diastolic function or both. The condition results when the heart is unable to generate a cardiac output sufficient to meet the demands of the body without unduly increasing diastolic pressure. It may be manifested by symptoms of poor tissue perfusion alone (e.g., fatigue, poor exercise tolerance, confusion) or by both symptoms of poor tissue perfusion and congestion of vascular beds (e.g., dyspnoea, orthopnoea, paroxysmal nocturnal dyspnoea or peripheral oedema). CHF, the focus of this chapter, can develop as a result of myocardial infarction and other chronic conditions including hypertension, ischaemia without infarction, toxic metabolic, and endocrine disorders. It is characterized by breathlessness and abnormal sodium and water retention, resulting in oedema and increased fatigue. Controversy exists in the literature with regard to whether psychosocial factors (i.e., Type A behavior, anger, hostility) predict the development of CHD (Eaker *et al.*, 2004). To date, CHF literature has examined the role of psychosocial factors as predictors of functional status, rehospitalization and mortality of patients with CHF, and evidence indicates an association (Clarke *et al.*, 2000; Moser, 2002; Moser and Worster, 2000; Schwarz and Elman, 2003). However, there has been no examination of the association between psychosocial factors and the development of CHF.

PREVALENCE, MORTALITY, AND MORBIDITY

CHF is a significant health problem worldwide, affecting 0.4–3.9% of the general population and 8–10% of the elderly (Davies *et al.*, 2001; Mair *et al.*, 1996). It is a disease with a poor prognosis and well recognized adverse effects upon patients' QOL (Hobbs *et al.*, 2002). It has been estimated that the prevalence of heart failure in western European countries may increase by as much as 70% by the year 2010 (Bonneux *et al.*, 1994). The increasing incidence and prevalence is likely to be due to multiple factors including:

- Improved survival of patients with angina, hypertension, and acute myocardial infarction. For example, modern treatments for myocardial infarction prolong life resulting in a greater number of post myocardial infarction patients developing heart failure (McMurray and Davie, 1996), while newer therapies for heart failure such as angiotensin converting enzyme inhibitors lengthen life expectancy (Rodriguez-Artalejo *et al.*, 1997).

- Increases in the general standard of living resulting in a greater proportion of the population reaching older age. Despite therapeutic advances in its treatment, the prognosis of CHF is worse than many of the common cancers, fewer than 50% of patients survive five years from the time of initial diagnosis (Kannel, 1989). Also, subsequent to a first hospital admission, CHF patients have a median survival time of 16 months with only 25% of men and women surviving to five years (Stewart *et al.*, 2001).

CHF results in high levels of health care utilization, being responsible for approximately 120,000 hospital admissions annually in the United Kingdom (McMurray and Dargie, 1992). It is therefore, a disease of major economic significance with the direct annual cost of heart failure estimated to be approximately £905 million, equivalent to 1.91% of total National Health Service (NHS) expenditure, with the predominant cost being hospitalization (Stewart *et al.*, 2002).

THE CASE FOR EXERCISE

In light of the increasing incidence of heart failure, its negative impacts on quality of life (Hobbs *et al.*, 2002) and associated high levels of morbidity and mortality, there has been increasing interest in optimizing its management. Cardiac rehabilitation programs have been traditionally limited to patients recovering from myocardial infarction, coronary revascularization, or cardiac transplantation. However, over the past 15 years evidence has accumulated suggesting that such programs can also benefit individuals with CHF. Treatment of heart failure has altered substantially over the last 10 years and in recent times a plethora of guidelines relating to diagnosis and management have been published (Canadian Cardiovascular, 1994; Konstam *et al.*, 1994; Report of the American College of Cardiology/American Heart Association Task Force on Practice Guidelines, 1995; The National Heart Foundation of New Zealand, 1997; The Task Force on Heart Failure of the European Society of Cardiology, 1995; The Task Force of the Working Group on Heart Failure of the European Society of Cardiology, 1997). However, while these guidelines provide clear advice regarding pharmacotherapy of the illness, they provide little practical help to the health care professional seeking guidance regarding the best advice to give heart failure patients concerning the subject of exercise. Traditionally, patients with CHF were recommended rest, and it was widely believed that they should refrain from physical activity due to the potential damaging results it could cause (Braunwald, 1988). This is certainly not the case today. Nowadays there is an increasing consensus among practitioners that exercise benefits the physical health of heart failure patients. Nevertheless, current clinical guidelines provide little in the way of explicit guidance with regard to the issue of exercise and CHF, while some have suggested that there is insufficient evidence to promote supervised rehabilitation programs (Konstam *et al.*, 1994).

Based upon the poor prognosis for CHF it is not surprising that patients report diminished QOL, reduced social functioning, and psychological distress.

MEASURING QOL IN CHF PATIENTS

Assessment of QOL is increasingly becoming a component of evaluating the impact of interventions for patients with CHF (Albanese *et al.*, 1999; Dracup *et al.*, 1992; Gorkin *et al.*, 1993; Grady *et al.*, 1995; Hobbs *et al.*, 2002; Jaarsma *et al.*, 1999; Rogers *et al.*, 1994; Steptoe *et al.*, 2000; Stewart *et al.*, 1989; van Jaarsveld *et al.*, 2001; Walden *et al.*, 1994). However, the inclusion of QOL measurements in evaluating the benefits of exercise for patients with CHF is still variable. In order to understand the importance of measuring QOL and to assess the relevance and application of the measures that have been used in studies of exercise for CHF patients, it is necessary in the first instance to describe the various QOL assessment approaches.

QOL is a multidimensional concept describing a patient's physical, social, and psychological health. To evaluate QOL effectively, multiple domains are assessed, including symptoms of the disease, physical function, social function, and emotional well-being. Five general approaches have been used to assess QOL, these are global, generic, condition-specific, battery, and preference-based (Leidy *et al.*, 1999). Global evaluation considers a patient's overall well-being and evaluates the impact of a treatment on general aspects of QOL. Examples include the Psychological General Well-Being (PGWB; Andrews and Withey, 1974) and the Life Satisfaction Questionnaire (LSQ; Dupuy, 1984). Generic instruments such as the Medical Outcomes Study 36-Item Short Form (SF-36; Stewart and Ware, 1992), the Nottingham Health Profile (NHP; Hunt, 1986), and Sickness Impact Profile (SIP; Deyo *et al.*, 1982) allow the comparison of baseline and end-point QOL data in CHF studies.

Condition-specific instruments enable an understanding of the effect of a treatment or intervention in relation to the specific disease state. Examples of instruments used for patients with CHF include: the Minnesota Living with Heart Failure Questionnaire (MLWHFQ); the Chronic Heart Failure Questionnaire (CHFQ); and the Kansas City Cardiomyopathy Questionnaire (Patrick Green *et al.*, 2000). The battery approach utilizes multiple QOL instruments in order to assess either generic or condition-specific QOL. For example, the SF-36, a generic measure of subjective health status, is combined with the CHFQ, which measures physical and emotional health status specific to patients with CHF. This approach can produce a comprehensive QOL profile, but the use of multiple measures disallows the use of a single summary score and increases the probability of conflicting results (Leidy *et al.*, 1999). Preference-based instruments tend to be used to assess quality adjusted life years (QALYS) in cost-utility studies. Utility values can be obtained through standard gamble or time-trade off methods or through a psychometrically based instrument such as the European Quality of Life Index (EuroQoL Group, 1990).

Given the plethora of approaches to the measurement of QOL, the question arises as to which is the most appropriate for assessing the QOL of patients with CHF. Berry and McMurray (1999) reviewed the design and validation of a number of generic and disease-specific QOL questionnaires used in clinical trials in CHF, and also evaluated their performance in recent clinical trials in CHF in relation to other outcome measures. They identified several important differences among these QOL questionnaires. The authors concluded that the choice of an appropriate QOL questionnaire was related to both patient compliance and the outcomes being measured in a CHF clinical trial.

The 36-Item Short Form (SF-36) Health Survey and SIP were regarded as the best generic instruments, and the MLWHFQ, and CHFQ were acknowledged as being the best disease-specific measurements at that time. They recommended that the optimal method for assessing QOL in CHF trials should be a combination of one of the aforementioned generic and disease-specific questionnaires, together with a patient's self-reported global health response.

Although evaluation of QOL is becoming an integral component of interventions for patients with heart failure, examination and evaluation of psychological factors in the management of heart failure is still being neglected. QOL measurements are not necessarily adequate to examine depression, and the diagnosis of depression in CHF patients is not standardized. Although the use of conventional questionnaires may indicate depressive symptoms, it has been advocated that a formal interview may more accurately determine the presence of clinical depression (Miller, 2002).

CHF AND PSYCHOLOGICAL HEALTH

Evidence suggests there are several factors that seem to link depression with the development of CHD and with a worse outcome in patients with established CHD (Zellweger et al., 2004), but it has only recently been recognized that patients with CHF often experience clinical depression (Havranek et al., 1999; Jiang et al., 2001; Rumsfeld et al., 2003; Skotzko et al., 2000), albeit these aspects of the condition are often undiagnosed and untreated. More recently, several studies have found that depressive symptoms are a strong predictor of worsening CHF symptoms, functional status, and QOL over time (Carels, 2004; Martensson et al., 2003; van Jaarsveld et al., 2001). In addition, Jiang et al. (2001) showed an increase in mortality and hospital readmissions in CHF patients with major depression. Patients with moderate to severe CHF are at a high risk for major depression, but it is unclear whether functional impairment plays a causal role in depression or depression exacerbates functional impairment (Freedland and Carney, 2000).

There is also some evidence to suggest that pathophysiological factors may contribute to the development of CHF. Inflammatory cytokines seem to have a role in the progression of CHF, and there is evidence suggesting that elevated cytokine levels lead to cognitive disturbances including depression (Reichenberg et al., 2001).

No evidence currently exists as to whether exercise can reduce depression in patients with CHF; however, positive findings have been shown when exercise has been prescribed for older adults with depression (Mather et al., 2002). In a review of the psychological factors associated with CHF, MacMahon and Yip (2002) highlight the current paucity of work in this area. In total, only 12 studies (seven cross-sectional, five longitudinal) were identified which addressed CHF and psychological well-being. Eight of the studies examined depression in patients with CHF and the remaining four studies examined anxiety, social support, and/or coping styles in patients with CHF. No evidence is available from randomized controlled trials (RCTs), and the reported studies only included hospitalized patients or hospital outpatients, and often had few participants. From the evidence currently available it would appear that the prevalence of depression among the CHF population is relatively high and there appears to be a correlation between depression and repeated hospital admissions, independent of initial disease severity. Depression may also be an independent risk factor for mortality in CHF patients (Murberg *et al.*, 1999).

Anxiety frequently presents comorbidly with depression. Due to the poor prognosis associated with CHF, anxiety may be a factor present in many patients suffering from CHF. However, there is a paucity of research concerning anxiety among patients with CHF, and it is currently impossible to confirm or refute this hypothesis. Anxiety should be of concern to health care professionals as stress can cause an increase in heart rate, which has a negative effect on coronary artery perfusion through shorter diastole. Tachycardia reduces myocardial oxygen supply, while increasing myocardial oxygen demand. This can become cyclical for patients who are worried about their physical condition, and subsequently increases their anxiety which can result in even poorer cardiac output (MacMahon and Yip, 2002). Furthermore, anxiety and depression can have a major effect on health care utilization. For example, studies have shown that anxious and depressed patients accrue four times the hospitalization costs of non-depressed patients (Allison *et al.*, 1995), and medical costs are 41% higher in depressed cardiac patients (Frasure-Smith *et al.*, 2000).

METHOD

As research studies examining the role of exercise for patients with CHF are still in their infancy, it is important to consider not only the relationship between QOL/depression/ exercise and CHF, but to review all the relevant evidence for advocating exercise for this patient group. This review covers studies published in English between 1966 and August 2003, on the effect of exercise training with heart failure patients. The studies were identified by searching the following electronic databases: MedLine; Science citation index; Social Sciences citation index; BIDS; Bandolier; CINAHL, Cochrane Database of Systematic Reviews (CDSR); EMBASE; NHS; National Research Register (NRR); PSYCHLIT; and Current Research in Britain (CRIB), using the search terms: "*exercise training*," "*physical training*," "*aerobic*," "*anaerobic*," "*heart failure*," "*left ventricular failure*," "*cardiac failure*," "*quality of life*," "*depression*," and "*emotional*." The reference lists of identified articles were also scrutinized for additional studies that conformed to the specified inclusion criteria. Studies included had the effects of exercise training in terms of physical performance, QOL or health care utilization as the main outcome measures.

Due to the variations that existed in the study design, patient group, study setting, and outcome measures used in the studies, a qualitative review of the obtained studies was performed.

REVIEW OF EVIDENCE

Thirty-seven studies met the defined selection criteria (Table 5.1). Of these, 17 were RCTs, 8 were randomized crossover trials, 3 were non-RCTs and 9 were pretest/posttest studies. The provision of exercise training was, in the majority of cases, supervised and hospital-based, with data collection taking place in a hospital laboratory setting. Investigation of long-term effects was rare and 41% (15/37) of the training programs lasted eight weeks or less. Only 35% (6/17) of the RCTs outlined their method of

Table 5.1 Research studies examining the role of exercise for patients with CHF

AUTHOR	STUDY DESIGN	n	AGE (YRS) MEAN (RANGE)	GENDER	ACTIVITY	DURATION	FREQUENCY	INTENSITY AS PERCENTAGE OF HEART RATE	TRAINING PERIOD	TRAINING EFFECTS
Belardinelli et al. (Italy) 1999	Prospective RCT	99	C = 56, T = 53	M/F	B	40 m	3×/week, 2×/week	60% peak VO$_2$	52 weeks	Positive
Belardinelli et al. (Italy) 1995	Non-RCT	27	57	M/F	B	30 m	3×/week	40% peak VO$_2$ uptake	8 weeks	Positive
Cider et al. (Sweden) 1997	Prospective RCT	24	C = 65, T = 62	M/F	CT	15 m	3×/week	60% of 1 rep max HR	20 weeks	Positive
Coats et al. (UK) 1992	RCT	17	R = 61, T = 65	M	B (HB)	20 m	5×/week	70–80% peak HR	8 weeks	Positive
Conn et al. (USA) 1982	Pretest/posttest	10	44–71	M/F (F = 1)	B (HB)	NS	3–5×/week	70–80% max HR	8 weeks	Positive
Davey et al. (UK) 1992	RCT	22	64	M	B (HB)	20 m	5×/week	70–80% max HR	8 weeks	Positive
Delagardelle et al. (Luxembourg) 2002	Prospective RCT	20	ET = 60.4 (47–70), CT = 56.3 (35–70)	M	B/ST	40 m	3×/week	75% VO$_2$ peak	16 weeks	CT superior to ET alone
Delagardelle et al. (Luxembourg) 1999	Pretest/posttest	14	57	M/F	T, B	60 m	3×/week	75% peak VO$_2$	24 weeks	Positive
European Heart Failure Training Group (UK) 1998	RCT	134	60.5	M/F	B, C (HB)	20/12 m	4–5×/week	70–80% peak HR	6–16 weeks	Positive
Gordon et al. (Sweden) 1996	Prospective RCT	21	60	M	KE	15 m	NS	TG1 = 35% abs peak TG2 = 65–75% abs peak	8 weeks	Positive
Hambrecht et al. (Germany) 2000	Prospective RCT	73	C = 54, T = 55	M	B (HB)	10 m 20 m	4–6×/week, 1×/day	70% peak VO$_2$ max	2 weeks (hospital) 24 weeks (home)	Positive

Study	Design	N	Age	M/F	Type	Distance	Frequency	Intensity	Duration	Outcome
Houghton et al. (UK) 2002	Pretest/posttest	36	69 (48–80)	M/F	W, T (HB)	NS	NS	NS	NS	Mixed
Jette et al. (Germany) 1991	Prospective RCT	39	50.8	M	J, C, B, W	5 m/30 m/15 m/ 30–60 m	3–7×/week	70–80% peak HR	4 weeks	Inconclusive
Johnson et al. (UK) 1998	Prospective RCT	18	C = 63, T = 70	M/F	IM	15 m	2×/daily	15% max IMP	8 weeks	Positive
Kavanagh et al. (Canada) 1996	Non-RCT	30	C = 65, T = 62	M/F	W (HB)	NS	5×/week	50–60% VO_2 max	52 weeks	Positive
Keteyian et al. (USA) 1996	Prospective RCT	40	56	M	B, T, R, A	43 m	3×/week	60–80% of HR	24 weeks	Positive
Kiilavuori et al. (Finland) 1996	Prospective RCT	27	52	M/F (F = 1)	B, W, R, S (HB)	B = 30 m (supervised) HB = NS	B = 3×/week (supervised) HB = NS	50–60% peak VO_2 later acc to HR	24 weeks	Positive
Koch et al. (France) 1992	Prospective RCT	25	C = 64, T = 56	M/F	KB	90 m	3×/week	NS	12 weeks	Positive
Maiorana et al. (Australia) 2000	RCT	13	60	M	CT, B, T, IM	60 m	3×/week	70–85% peak HR	8 weeks	Positive
McConnell et al. (USA) 2003	Prospective Cohort	24	64	M/F	B/RE	60 m	3×/week	70–85% max HR	12 weeks	Positive
McKelvie et al. (Canada) 2002	Prospective RCT	181	C = 66, T = 65	M/F	B, IM (HB)	NS	3×/week	60–70% max HR	52 weeks	Mixed
Meyer et al. (Germany) 1996	RCT	18	52	NS	B, W, T, E	B = 15 m, W = 10 m, T and E = 20 m	5×/week, 3×/week, 3×/week,	50% max WR	6 weeks	Positive
Oka et al. (USA) 2000	Prospective RCT	40	Range = 30–76	M/F	T, RE (HB)	HB = 40–60 m	3×/week (T), 2×/week (RE)	70% peak HR	12 weeks	Positive
Owen and Croucher (UK) 2000	RCT	22	C = 81, T = 81, R = 82	M/F	CT	10 m warm up 4.5 m activity 10 m cool down	1×/week	70% max of age predicted max pulse rate	12 weeks	Inconclusive
Quitan et al. (Austria) 1999	Prospective RCT	25	C = 54, T = 57	M/F	B, SE	60 m	2×/week, 3×/week (from week five)	50% VO_2 max	12 weeks	Positive
Radzewitz et al. (Germany) 2002	Pretest/posttest	88	65.8 (39–79)	M/F	B, IM	20–25 m	1×/week	60–80% peak VO_2	4 weeks	Positive

(Table 5.1 continued)

Table 5.1 Continued

AUTHOR	STUDY DESIGN	n	AGE (YRS) MEAN (RANGE)	GENDER	ACTIVITY	DURATION	FREQUENCY	INTENSITY AS PERCENTAGE OF HEART RATE	TRAINING PERIOD	TRAINING EFFECTS
Scalvini et al. (Italy) 1992	Pretest/ posttest	12	55/57	M	B	10 m ↑ 2 m every 4th day	2×/daily	70% max workload	5 weeks	Positive
Shephard et al. (Canada) 1998	Pretest/ posttest	21	62	M/F	W	NS	5×/week	60–70%peak O_2 uptake	16 weeks	Positive
Silva et al. (Brazil) 2002	Prospective RCT	24	C = 56, T = 48	M/F	W, RE	30–60 m	3×/week	60–80% max HR	12 weeks	Positive
Sullivan et al. (USA) 1988	Pretest/ post test	16	54	NS	B, W, J	60 m	3–5×/week	75% of peak VO_2	16–24 weeks	Positive
Taylor (UK) 1999	RCT	8	61	M	B	30 m	3×/week	45–70% peak O_2	8 weeks	Inconclusive
Tyni-Lenne et al. (Sweden) 1996	Prospective RCT	21	60	M	KE	15 m	3×/week	70% peak performance	8 weeks	Positive
Tyni-Lenne et al. (Sweden) 1998	RCT	24	M:58/ F:60	M/F	KE	15 m	3×/week	65–75% peak WR	8 weeks	Positive
Tyni-Lenne et al. (Sweden) 1997	RCT	16	R = 63, T = 62	F	KE	15 m	3×/week	65–75% baseline WR	16 weeks	Positive
Tyni-Lenne et al. (Sweden) 1999	RCT	24	C = 62, B = 62 KE = 64	M/F	B, KE	B = 20 m, KE = 32–36 m	3×/week	60–75% peak WR	8 weeks	Positive
Wielenga et al. (Netherlands) 1999	Prospective RCT	80	C = 65, T = 63	M	W, B, BG	30 m	3×/week	Target HR	12 weeks	Inconclusive
Willenheimer et al. (Sweden) 1998	Prospective RCT	50	64	M/F	B	15 m/6 weeks, 45 m/10 weeks	2×/week	80% max HR	16 weeks	Positive

Notes: RCT = Randomized Controlled Trial; C = control group; T = training group; R = resting first group; M = Male/F = Female; J = jogging; C = calisthenics; B = cycle ergometer; W = walking; R = rowing; S = swimming; KE = knee extensor exercises; T = treadmill; KB = 'Koch bench'; CT = circuit training; IM = inspiratory muscle training; BG = ball games; RE = resistance exercises; SE = step exercises; E = exercises (not specified); HR = heart rate; WR = work rate; HB = home-based component; NS = not specified.

randomization and in many instances when descriptions were provided these were vague and incomplete (e.g., no mention of the method of allocation). While 75% (28/37) of the studies detailed their inclusion and, in some cases, exclusion criteria for patient recruitment, but only 40% (15/37) provided information about the recruitment procedure adopted. When the recruitment procedure was detailed, participants tended to represent convenience samples (e.g., patients attending a particular clinic) or volunteers. Patients with other illnesses that frequently coexist within the wider heart failure population were often excluded. For example, 22% (8/37) excluded patients with diabetes, while 51% (19/37) excluded individuals with chronic obstructive airways disease. Finally, the majority of these studies were small. Sample size: 25 participants or less 62% (23/37); 26–50 participants 22% (8/37); 51–150 participants 13% (5/37).

Age of study participants

The annual incidence of CHF increases exponentially with age, from a rate of two per thousand in the fifth decade of life to fifty per thousand in the eighth decade (Kannel, 1989). Even so, mean patient age was below 65 years in 73% (27/37) of the reported studies (see Table 5.1). Only two studies specifically examined age variation and how this might affect a patient's response to physical exercise (Owen and Croucher, 2000; Willenheimer et al., 1998). Both studies suggest that physical exercise is not only safe but also beneficial for "older" chronic heart failure patients. Nevertheless, the former study (Willenheimer et al., 1998) had a small sample, was short-term, and most participants were close to 70 years of age. Although the latter study (Owen and Croucher, 2000) included "older" patients (M = 81 years), they emphasized that further investigation was required regarding the benefits of exercise upon morbidity and mortality, on-going compliance, and safety for this age group.

Gender of study participants

The overall prevalence of heart failure is reported to be similar in men and women (Ho et al., 1993; McDonagh et al., 1997; Schocken et al., 1992) yet women were grossly under represented in the studies under review. Gender distribution was reported in all but two studies. While 12 studies included males only, only one study focused exclusively on females (see Table 5.1). In studies where both males and females were included there still existed a strong bias towards male participants (e.g., male/female ratios of 26 : 1, 9 : 1, 5 : 1). Of those studies that included both female and male patients with CHF, only two examined the differences that may exist between male and female CHF patients in their response to physical exercise (Tyni-Lenne et al., 1998; Willenheimer et al., 1998).

Nature and intensity of the exercise

The majority of studies used either a cycle ergometer, or combined exercise programs (i.e., cycle ergometer and/or walking and/or jogging and/or swimming, or circuit training). Five studies focused upon resistance exercise training in the form of knee-extensor or leg muscle training (see Table 5.1). Completion rates were not recorded for eight of the studies and compliance rates were not recorded for nineteen of the studies. Seventeen studies cited completion rates for the exercise programs as being between 90% and 100% with twelve ranging between 50% and 89%. Compliance rates were again quite favorable, with 14 studies reporting more than 80% compliance and 4 studies reporting between 50% and 80%. Unfortunately, none of the studies attempted to assess patients' acceptance and appropriateness of such regimes, and their ability to adopt such procedures on an individual long-term basis. A total of 10 studies incorporated a home-based exercise component focusing upon physical fitness levels (see Table 5.1). Eight provided patients with a cycle ergometer and/or treadmill or pedometer for use in their home over a relatively short time period, with two studies prescribing an individualized walking program over a 36 and 52-week-period respectively. While choosing to implement an exercise training program in patients' homes, none of the studies capitalized upon this approach by providing an account of the pros and cons of the procedure in comparison with hospital-based exercise training.

Outcome measures and health care utilization

The studies under review had diverse outcome measures (e.g., lactic acidosis threshold, respiratory quotient, ventilatory threshold, ejection fraction, mean pulmonary artery pressure, peak oxygen uptake, cardiac output, blood pressure, citrate synthetase, anaerobic threshold). The most common recorded positive effects on physiological physical performance indicators were oxygen uptake, resting heart rate, maximal heart rate, sub-maximal heart rate, systolic blood pressure, and ventilation.

Health care utilization issues and mortality were addressed in only one study (Belardinelli et al., 1999). This study found that mortality were lower in the training group (RR = 0.37, 95% CI, 0.17–0.84; $p = 0.01$) and hospital readmission rates were higher in the control group (RR = 0.29, 95% CI, 0.11–0.84; $p = 0.02$). No cost-effectiveness analyses have yet to be published.

QUALITY OF LIFE

As shown in Table 5.2, only 54% (20/37) of the reviewed studies also measured QOL. Studies incorporating a quality of life component varied widely in the approach and instrument used and in the results obtained. All but one of the studies (Willenheimer et al., 1998) reported QOL outcomes from the patients' perspective. Nineteen out of the twenty studies used self-administered questionnaires, two of these also used a researcher administered component and one study used semi-structured patient interviews. Three studies did not specify the instrument used (Coats et al., 1992; Houghton et al., 2002; Koch et al., 1992), with one study not specifying the implementation process (Houghton et al., 2002). Only 20% (4/20) of studies included a global QOL assessment, as part of an assessment battery (Kavanagh et al., 1996; Shephard et al., 1998; Wielenga et al., 1998a; Willenheimer et al., 1998). Generic QOL measures were included in seven studies (Cider *et al.*, 1997; Quittan *et al.*, 1999; Radzewitz *et al.*, 2002; Tyni-Lenne *et al.*, 1996, 1997, 1998, 1999). The MLWHFQ and CHFQ disease-specific questionnaires were adminsistered in five (Belardinelli *et al.*, 1999; McConnell *et al.*, 2003; McKelvie *et al.*, 2002; Owen and Croucher, 2000; Tyni-Lenne *et al.*, 1999) and four (Johnson *et al.*, 1998; Kavanagh *et al.*, 1996; Oka *et al.*, 2000; Shephard *et al.*, 1998) studies respectively. Ten studies (50%) employed a battery approach, using more than one questionnaire to evaluate different domains of QOL, for example, functional status, emotional health, and symptoms (Cider *et al.*, 1997; Kavanagh *et al.*, 1996; Radzewitz *et al.*, 2002; Shephard *et al.*, 1998; Tyni-Lenne *et al.*, 1996, 1997, 1998, 1999; Wielenga *et al.*, 1998a; Willenheimer *et al.*, 1998). None of the studies used a preference-based assessment. Positive effects on QOL were reported in 65% (13/20) of studies, but only six studies considered the relationship between QOL and physiological outcomes (Belardinelli *et al.*, 1995; Houghton *et al.*, 2002; Kavanagh *et al.*, 1996; Quittan *et al.*, 1999; Radzewitz *et al.*, 2002; Shephard *et al.*, 1998).

Only one study adopted the optimal method for assessing QOL in CHF trials as recommended by Berry and McMurray (1999); a combination of a generic and disease specific questionnaires, together with a patient's self-reported global health response. Tyni-Lenne *et al.* (1999) used the MLWHFQ (a CHF disease specific questionnaire), the SIP (a measurement of health or illness related QOL), and the SOC Scale (assessing the prerequisites for coping capacity and indicating general QOL). The findings relating to QOL were inconclusive, with cycle training showing only a significant improvement for the SIP management score, and knee-extensor training showing significant improvements, for certain categories of the MLWHFQ and SIP, but not for the Sense of Coherence (SOC) scale, with none of the intergroup differences being significant. However, the study was characterized by small patient numbers ($n = 24$), a short study duration (eight weeks), and a relatively young patient group ($M = 63 \pm 10$ years).

In terms of assessing the effect of exercise upon emotional well-being, only two studies used measurements that evaluated this specifically. Radzewitz *et al.* (2002) used the Hospital, Anxiety and Depression Scale (HADS) – a descriptive screening procedure employed to assess anxiety and depression as mental limitations, together with the SF-36 questionnaire. The intervention included cycle ergometer and inspiratory muscle training. Although they found significant improvements in the mental health dimension of the SF-36 ($p = 0.002$), no significant improvements were found for either the anxiety or depression dimensions of the HADS. Wielenga *et al.* (1998b) used the Heart Patients Psychological Questionnaire (HPPQ) – a measure of well-being, feelings of being disabled, displeasure, and social inhibition, together with patients' self-assessment of general well-being (SAGWB) – comprising a single question on a scale of one to five relating to health improvement. They implemented a combined exercise program including cycle ergometer, treadmill walking, and ball games. The HPPQ showed marginal significant improvements in the training group ($p = 0.06$), with significant group differences for the "feelings of being disabled" dimension ($p < 0.001$). The patients' SAGWB also showed significant improvements in the training group ($p < 0.001$).

Table 5.2 Summary of exercise and CHF studies including a quality of life measure

AUTHOR	QUALITY OF LIFE MEASUREMENT	IMPLEMENTATION	OUTCOME
Belardinelli et al., 1999	MLWHFQ	Baseline and 2, 14, 26 months	QOL score improved ($p < 0.001$) in 'T' group after 2 mths, remained stable at 12 months and follow up
Cider et al., 1997	NHP/QLQ-HF	Baseline and study completion (20 weeks)	NHP: significant improvement found in 'C' group in social life, hobbies and holidays. QLQ-HF: no significant differences (no p values or CIs reported)
Coats et al., 1992	Likert scale	End of each study phase (i.e., 8 weeks training/8 weeks restricted activity)	Improvement in 'T' group for breathlessness ($p < 0.001$) and fatigue ($p < 0.001$), daily activities ($p < 0.001$), ease of these activities ($p < 0.01$) (No CIs reported)
Houghton et al., 2002	NS	NS	Significant positive correlation for total score on QofL and pedometer score ($p = 0.04$) and calf blood flow ($p = 0.04$). No correlation between QofL and treadmill exercise ($p = 0.14$)
Johnson et al., 1998	CHFQ	Baseline and study completion (8 weeks)	No significant difference between group scores
Kavanagh et al., 1996	CHFQ/SG	Baseline and 16, 26, 52 weeks	CHFQ showed trends in improvement for 'T' group; fatigue ($p < 0.001$), dyspnoea ($p < 0.115$), emotional function ($p < 0.132$), mastery ($p < 0.149$). SG = 14% improvement sustained over 52 weeks (No CIs reported)
Koch et al., 1992	Visual scale	Baseline and study completion (12 weeks)	Improvement estimate: 63% in 'T' group, spontaneous variation only 4% in 'C' group (no p values or CIs reported)
McConnell et al., 2003	MLWHFQ	Baseline and study completion (12 weeks)	Improved perception from baseline to study completion ($p = 0.008$)
McKelvie et al., 2002	MLWHFQ	Baseline and 12, 52 weeks	Slight improvement in exercise group after 12 weeks – not significant. No significant difference between groups at 52 weeks
Oka et al., 2000	CHFQ	Baseline and study completion (12 weeks)	'T' group improvement in fatigue ($p = 0.02$), emotion ($p = 0.01$), sense of mastery (0.04) (no CIs reported)

Study	Instrument	Timing	Results
Owen and Croucher 2000	MLWHFQ	Baseline and study completion (12/26 weeks)	No change in scores for 'C' or 'T' groups (scores not reported)
Quittan et al., 1999	MOS SF-36	Baseline and study completion (12 weeks)	Improvement in 'T' group for vitality ($p < 0.0001$) physical role ($p < 0.001$), physical ($p = 0.02$) and social functioning ($p = 0.0002$)
Radzewitz et al., 2002	SF-36/HADS	Baseline and study completion (4 weeks)	SF-36 showed significant changes for physical functioning, role-physical, bodily pain, general health, vitality, role-emotional, mental health. HADS – no significant changes for anxiety and depression
Shephard et al., 1998	CHFQ/SG	Baseline and study completion (16 weeks)	Improvement in 'T' group CHFQ scores: fatigue ($p < 0.001$). SG showed 14% improvement ($p < 0.0035$) (no CIs reported)
Tyni-Lenne et al., 1996	SIP/SOC	Baseline and study completion (8 weeks)	SIP scores improved in 'T' group ($p = 0.03$–0.005). SOC scores did not differ
Tyni-Lenne et al., 1998	SIP/SOC	Baseline and study completion (8 weeks)	Overall SIP scores improved for men ($p < 0.002$) and women ($p < 0.005$). SOC scores showed slight improvement for women ($p < 0.03$) (no CIs reported)
Tyni-Lenne et al., 1997	SIP/SOC	Baseline and 8, 16 weeks	SIP physical scores improved in 'T' group ($p < 0.04$). No change in SOC score (no CIs reported)
Tyni-Lenne et al., 1999	MLWHFQ/ SIP/SOC	Baseline and study completion (8 weeks)	Significant improvement in some MLWHFQ and SIP scores (knee-extensor only). No significant improvement in intergroup differences for any measurement (no CIs reported)
Wielenga et al., 1999	HPPQ/SAGWB	Baseline and study completion (12 weeks)	HPPQ: Marginal significant difference between 'C' and 'T' group ($p = 0.06$). SAGWB: higher for 'T' group ($p < 0.0001$) (no CIs reported)
Willenheimer et al., 1998	D–F index/ Global QOL/PA score	Baseline and study completion (16 weeks)	Global QOL improved in 'T' group ($p < 0.01$). In 'T' group correlation found between D–F index and Global QOL ($r = 0.44$, $p < 0.05$)

Notes: SIP = Sickness Impact Profile; SOC = Sense of Coherence Scale; NHP = Nottingham Health Profile; QLQ–HF = Quality of Life Questionnaire–Heart Failure; D–F index = Dysponea–Fatigue Index; Global QOL = Global Quality of Life; PA score = Physical Activity Score; CHFQ = Chronic Heart Failure Questionnaire; HPPQ = Heart Patients Psychological Questionnaire; SAGWB = Self-Assessment of General Well-Being; MLWHFQ = Minnesota Living with Heart Failure Questionnaire; CHFQ = Chronic Heart Failure Questionnaire; SG = Standard Gamble Test; CI = confidence intervals.

REVIEW OF MECHANISMS

Exercise interventions for patients with CHF are still primarily focused upon the physical as opposed to the psychological benefits of such programs. As a review of the literature has shown, there remains many unanswered questions regarding the suitability of exercise programs for various groups of patients with CHF. For example, exercise training in elderly patients with CHF is made more difficult by the multiple comorbidities often present, such as obstructive lung disease, peripheral vascular disease, angina pectoris, arthritis, and neuromuscular disorders. Also, older patients may have problems in attending hospital-based exercise programs due to restricted mobility and transportation problems. Home-based or community-based programs may be more appealing to this patient group and should be considered when developing research protocols for older patients with CHF.

It is unclear whether the under representation of women is due to the selection process and/or inclusion criteria adopted for a study, or due to women not wishing to take part. With respect to the latter, it has been speculated that women may be reluctant to enter cardiac rehabilitation studies as exercise is not deemed to be an appropriate activity for them, or they experience transportation difficulties, or they are required to leave a sick spouse to attend hospital-based programs (Fleg, 2002). If this is the case, these factors need to be considered and addressed by researchers when developing research proposals to ensure studies are inclusive of both genders.

It is currently impossible to assess the effect of exercise on CHF patients' QOL as various instruments have been utilized, producing diverse outcomes. A review of studies that have included a QOL measurement would suggest that measuring patients' well-being is currently an adjunct as opposed to an integral component of assessing the success of an exercise intervention. None of the reviewed studies explained why they chose to utilize a particular instrument, and in the case of a battery assessment, why certain instruments were chosen to be used in combination.

Leidy et al. (1999) reviewed 41 randomized controlled trials to identify recent trends in the assessment of QOL outcomes in patients with CHF, although only 4 of the studies featured, evaluated the influence of exercise, the review suggested that an exercise intervention was effective in improving the QOL. However, the review was unable to identify a single instrument that was reliable and reproducible. Berry and McMurray (1999), in their assessment of QOL evaluations in patients with CHF, echo this opinion and call for improvements to the design of available instruments to enhance sensitivity to real treatment effects, and the method of their administration in clinical research.

There is still no definitive QOL questionnaire that will accurately assess the physical, emotional, and social benefits of exercise interventions for patients with CHF. However, based upon the evidence available to date, it is recommended that a battery approach, using both a generic and disease-specific QOL questionnaire, should be used to provide the most reliable and valid outcomes.

Debilitating physical symptoms, frequent hospitalizations, forced retirement, and financial stress can all lead to significant depression in patients with CHF (Freedland et al., 1991; MacMahon and Yip, 2002; Martensson et al., 2003; Skotzko et al., 2000; van Jaarsveld et al., 2001). The evidence suggests that a significant number of patients with CHF experience depression. MacMahon and Yip (2002) advocate addressing the reasons behind depression in CHF patients with either medication or cognitive behavior therapy, leading to possible improvements in patients' QOL, a reduction in hospital admissions and lowering the mortality rate. However, the majority of CHF patients are elderly with a number of other comorbidities requiring medication (most of the patients with CHF are taking an average of 6 medications, and it is not unusual for patients to be taking up to 15 medications (Mair *et al.*, 1999)). Therefore, the prescribing of further medications to treat depression may not be suitable. Likewise, cognitive behavior therapy may be inappropriate for an elderly population managing a range of comorbidites. Exercise, on the other hand, is an activity that can be incorporated into an individual's life, with both physiological and psychological well-being as possible outcomes.

Taking psychological factors into consideration appears to have considerable importance in evaluating the effectiveness of exercise programs for patients with CHF. Assuming that the short-term effects of exercise training are favorable, it is likely that patients will experience and thus report improvements in their QOL and symptoms of depression. However, at this time it is hard to say which type or intensity of exercise is best for improving QOL. Furthermore, none of the available studies allowed for the assessment of the long-term impact of such exercise training upon patients' QOL, including depression.

RCTs need to be encouraged, with depression being included as an endpoint. It is necessary for studies examining the effects of exercise upon patients with CHF, to include robust measures of depression. Studies need to assess the baseline psychological status of their patient population, and the subsequent effects of an exercise program upon psychological status. A validated measurement of depression in patients with CHF does not currently exist, however, the adoption of an instrument, such as the HADS, together with patients' self-assessment of their psychological status will lead to a greater understanding of the role of exercise for the psychological health of patients with CHF.

A major aspect overlooked in all the studies reported in the systematic review is the relationship between self-efficacy and exercise. A positive relationship has been found between self-efficacy and exercise behavior in cardiac populations (Vidmar and Rubinson, 1994), and self-efficacy has been found to be the strongest predictor of physical activity in patients with CHF (Oka *et al.*, 1996). Evangelista *et al.* (2001) examined the relationship between psychosocial variables and compliance in CHF patients, and found that exercise regimens caused the greatest adherence problems due to a lack of self-motivation, lack of energy, and presence of physical symptoms. Oka *et al.* (1999) found an association between physical fitness levels and self-efficacy, suggesting that self-efficacy may be an indicator for physical ability. Interestingly, there was a lack of association between perception of physical condition and actual physical ability, but self-reported physical condition was associated with emotional well-being. This suggests that physical condition may be influenced by a patients' emotional state and not represent their actual physical ability.

The evidence suggests a strong relationship between self-efficacy, emotional well-being, and exercise. In light of this, there is possibly a need for change in exercise interventions for CHF patients that focus upon enhancing self-efficacy and psychosocial improvements, as these factors may be more important outcome indicators for short-term and long-term physical improvements than fitness tests.

IMPLICATIONS FOR THE RESEARCHER

Although recommendations on exercise testing and training for patients with heart failure exist, there is still insufficient evidence to promote exercise training for all CHF patients. No data exists at the present time concerning the prognostic implications of different training approaches, intensities, or duration for patients with CHF, or the effect upon mortality. To date, reported studies provide evidence relating to selected patients, usually including small numbers, often excluding older patients and women and involving just one centre.

The European Heart Failure Training Group (1998) have highlighted many unanswered questions that require consideration:

- Is exercise training practical in different settings (i.e., are home-based exercise programs as safe as hospital-supervised exercise training)?
- Can training effects be maintained over the long term?
- Are mortality and morbidity affected by exercise training?
- Is exercise training for heart failure patients cost-effective?

It is noteworthy that a recent meta-analysis of 9 studies, involving 801 CHF patients with chronic heart failure (ExTraMATCH collaborative, 2004), found an overall reduction in mortality for those participating in properly supervised medical training programs, albeit participants within this meta-analysis were predominantly male and younger than the average CHF patient.

One of the main challenges in exercise trials is differentiating the outcomes of exercise training from other types of interventions, which participants may receive within their rehabilitation programs. Many medical settings where supervised training interventions take place include other lifestyle interventions, for example, nutrition and stress management classes. Furthermore, medical staff may be alerted to participants' worsening symptoms, which may lead to additional medical intervention (Whellan *et al.*, 2004). There is also the possibility that participants receive more pharmacotherapy (ExTraMATCH, 2004). Therefore, researchers need to track and record educational and medical interventions that may be provided to an exercise group.

Although some studies have demonstrated positive outcomes in some dimensions of QOL for patients with heart failure, the above limitations of study design apply. It is unclear which type of exercise is best for improving QOL or what is the minimum intensity required to improve QOL. When QOL measures are included in exercise interventions they tend to be an adjunct to physiological aspects of the study, as opposed to an integral component. None of the reviewed studies detailed their reasons for including a particular QOL measure, and where more than one measure was used, why they chose that particular combination. Future research studies should attempt to use a combination of a generic and disease-specific QOL measures together with a patient's self-reported global health response.

Most of the exercise programs have been delivered in groups and/or with health professional supervision. It is possible that the improvements in QOL demonstrated in many studies may be due to this social contact as opposed to the exercise regime per se. For example, the study by McKelvie *et al.* (2002) illustrates the possible superior role of psychosocial as opposed to biophysical mechanisms in improving QOL. The intervention comprised an initial three months of supervised exercise training in a medical setting, followed by nine months of training at home on an exercise cycle. A consistent finding of the study was the loss of training and QOL effect after the initial three months of supervised training. By the end of 12 months follow-up, there was no difference between patients in the intervention and control arms. Therefore, future investigations should examine the effect upon QOL when exercise is performed in "natural environments" (i.e., the patient's home), both with and without supervision. Larger studies are also required to explore the relationship between self-efficacy, emotional well-being, and exercise together with behavioral and physiological aspects of physical activity and physical fitness levels

Although depression has been shown to affect a substantial proportion of the CHF population, there is an overall paucity of research that has examined the effects of exercise upon the psychological status of patients with heart failure. Evidence from studies that have included a specific psychological measure have produced inconclusive findings. Further work is required to investigate whether exercise does have a positive effect upon psychological status, in terms of mode, intensity and duration, and whether variations exist between different patient groups with CHF (i.e., older patients, women, severity of condition).

IMPLICATIONS FOR THE HEALTH PROFESSIONAL AND HEALTH SERVICE DELIVERY

There remains a lack of information concerning two important points to practitioners:

1 whether particular groups of heart failure patients should be encouraged to adopt a program of exercise and;
2 if exercise training is deemed appropriate, what should be the nature, duration, frequency, and intensity of the program.

Health care providers need validated research findings, which will enable the prescription of appropriate exercise regimens for patients with CHF. At present there remains a paucity of high quality evidence to support the further development of guidelines for health care providers or patients regarding the subject of exercise and heart failure. For all grades of heart failure, the goals of therapy are to decrease symptoms, decrease morbidity, and prolong life. Although the initial work is extremely promising, whether exercise can help achieve these aims remains uncertain.

Based upon the current available evidence, recommendations for exercise training for patients with CHF need to consider the individual patient in terms of the severity of their CHF, comorbidities, and their general well-being.

In order to assist the health professional, the Working Group on Cardiac Rehabilitation and Exercise Physiology and Working Group on Heart Failure of the European Society of Cardiology (2001) has published the following recommendations: An exercise training program should be started only with patients who are clinically stable for at least four weeks. Clinical stability is defined by stable symptoms, as identified by the New York Heart Association (NYHA) class, and stable fluid balance. Caution should be taken when systolic blood pressure is below 80 mmHg at rest, resting heart rate is below 50 beats/min or above 100 beats/min. A cardiopulmonary exercise test should be performed before starting a training program and relative and absolute contraindications to exercise training should be considered (include: stable chronic CHF, minimal peak VO_2 of 10 mL/kg/min; optimal medical treatment. Exclude: active viral or autoimmune myocarditis; obstructive disease; serious arrhythmias).

Additionally, the American Association of Cardiovascular and Pulmonary Rehabilitation (1999) recommends: Exercise training in CHF should consider the pathology of the patient, the patient's individual response to exercise, and the gas exchange data obtained during cardiopulmonary exercise testing prior to training. Although both aerobic and strength training are recommended, the latter should focus only on low resistance, high repetition exercises, and are not appropriate for all chronic heart failure patients.

Emerging evidence indicates self-reported components of physical condition may be influenced by a patient's current emotional state and may not represent their actual physical ability. Therefore, diminished emotional well-being should be considered when exercise and physical activity recommendations are given based on self-reported physical ability (Oka *et al.*, 1999). Furthermore, if improvements in self-perceptions can be accomplished, changes in exercise behavior should be more sustainable. Therefore, practitioners should aim to enhance self-efficacy by encouraging patients to evaluate their physical progress and tailor exercise programs/physical activities to a patient's own needs and capabilities.

WHAT WE KNOW SUMMARY

- Patients with CHF show evidence of anxiety and depression and experience a dramatic reduction in their QOL.
- Significant improvements in exercise capacity have been demonstrated in CHF patients included in clinical trials.
- The evidence suggests that exercise can play an important role in improving the function and QOL of patients with CHF.

WHAT WE NEED TO KNOW SUMMARY

- Studies are required to examine the effect of exercise on psychological status in CHF. We need to know if different modes, intensities, and durations of exercise have an effect upon the psychological status of patients with CHF.
- There is currently no validated and reliable instrument for measuring the psychological and emotional effects of exercise upon patients with CHF, within clinical practice.
- We need to know what people with CHF think about participating in exercise programs, if training effects (both physical and psychological) are maintained

without supervision, and if an exercise regime can be maintained independently in the long-term.

- We need to know more about adherence to exercise programs (facility and home-based) and effectiveness of interventions, which are driven by accepted behavior change strategies.

- Studies have been characterized by statistically small numbers of participants, diverse study design and inclusion criteria, limited numbers of older patients and women, strict exclusion criteria, various training methods, and short training periods. There is a requirement for randomized controlled long-term trials, with adequate sample sizes, and longer follow-up, and patients whose characteristics are different to those already included in studies (i.e. more patients who are 65 years plus, female and with comorbidities).

- Studies have excluded patients (particularly the elderly) with significant comorbidities, such as obstructive lung disease, peripheral vascular disease, arthritis, angina pectoris, and neuromuscular disorders, and are therefore atypical of patients seen in every day clinical practice. It is not known which type of exercise training is practical in patients with comorbidities or whether these patients can improve their functional capacity.

- The reliability and validity of QOL questionnaires for use with CHF patients in exercise studies requires further development in order to establish the physical, social, and emotional benefits of different exercise activities.

- The cost-effectiveness of exercise training for reducing morbidity and mortality in patients with heart failure has not been examined.

REFERENCES

Albanese, M. C., Plewka, M., Gregori, D., Fresco, C., Avon, G., Caliandro, D. *et al.* (1999). Use of medical resources and quality of life patients with chronic heart failure: a prospective survey in a large Italian community hospital. *The European Journal of Heart Failure, 1*, 411–417.

Allison, T. G., Williams, D. E., Miller, T. D., Patten, C. A., Bailey, K. R., Squires, R. W. *et al.* (1995). Medical and economic costs of psychological distress in patients with coronary artery disease. *Mayo Clinic Proceedings, 70*, 809–810.

American Association of Cardiovascular and Pulmonary Rehabilitation (1999). *Guidelines for Cardiac Rehabilitation Programs* (3rd edn). Champaign, IL: Human Kinetics Publishers.

Andrews, F. and Withey, S. (1974). Developing measures of perceived life quality: results from several national surveys. *Social Indicators Research, 1*, 1–26.

Belardinelli, R., Georgiou, D., Scocco, V., Barstow, T. J., and Purcarco, A. (1995). Low intensity exercise training in patients with chronic heart failure. *Journal of the American College of Cardiology, 26*, 975–982.

Belardinelli, R., Georgiou, D., Cianci, G., and Purcaro, A. (1999). Randomized controlled trial of long-term moderate exercise training in chronic heart failure: effects on functional capacity, quality of life, and clinical outcome. *Circulation, 99*, 1173–1182.

Berry, C. and McMurray, J. (1999). A review of quality-of-life evaluations in patients with congestive heart failure. *Pharmacoeconomics, 16*, 247–271.

Bonneux, L., Barendregt, J. J., and Meeter, K. (1994). Estimating clinical morbidity due to ischaemic heart disease and congestive heart failure: the future rise of heart failure. *American Journal of Public Health, 84*, 20–28.

Braunwald, E. (1988). *Heart Disease: A Textbook of Cardiovascular Medicine* (4th edn). Philadelphia, PA: WB Saunders.

Buselli, E. F. and Stuart, E. M. (1999). Influence of psychosocial factors and biopsychosocial interventions on outcomes after myocardial infarction. *Journal of Cardiovascular Nursing, 13*, 60–72.

Canadian Cardiovascular Society (1994). Diagnosis and management of heart failure: Canadian Cardiovascular Society – Consensus Development Conference Guidelines. *Canadian Journal of Cardiology, 10*, 613–654.

Carels, R. (2004). The association between disease severity, functional status, depression and daily quality of life in congestive heart failure patients. *Quality of Life Research, 13*, 63–72.

Cider, A., Tygesson, H., Hedberg, M., Seligman, L., Wennerblom, B., and Sunnerhagen K. S. (1997). Peripheral muscle training in patients with clinical signs of heart failure. *Scandinavian Journal of Rehabilitation Medicine, 29*, 121–127.

Clarke, S. P., Frasure-Smith, N., Lesperance, F., and Bourassa, M. G. (2000). Psychosocial factors as predictors of functional status at 1 year in patients with left ventricular dysfunction. *Research in Nursing and Health, 23*, 290–300.

Coats, A. J., Adamopoulos, S., Radaelli, A., McCance, A., Meyer, T. E., Bernardi, L. *et al.* (1992). Controlled trial of physical training in chronic heart failure: exercise performance, hemodynamics, ventilation, and automatic function. *Circulation, 85*, 2119–2131.

Conn, E. H., Williams, R. S., and Wallace, A. G. (1982). Exercise responses before and after physical conditioning in patients with severely depressed left ventricular function. *American Journal of Cardiology, 49*, 296–300.

Davey, P., Meyer, T., Coats, A., Adamopoulos, S., Casadei, B., Conway, J. *et al.* (1992). Ventilation in chronic heart failure: effects of physical training. *British Heart Journal, 68*, 473–477.

Davies, M. K., Hobbs, F. D. R., Davis, R. C., Kenkre, J. E., Roalfe, A. K., Hare, R. *et al.* (2001). Prevalence of left-ventricular systolic dysfunction and heart failure in the Echocardiographic Heart of England Screening study: a population based study. *The Lancet, 358*, 439–444.

Delagardelle, C., Feiereisen, P., Krecke, R., Essamri, B., and Beissel, J. (1999). Objective effects of a 6 months' endurance and strength training program in outpatients with congestive heart failure. *Medicine and Science in Sports Exercise, 31*, 1102–1107.

Delagardelle, C., Feiereisen, P., Autier, P., Shita, R., Krecke, R., and Beissel, J. (2002). Strength/endurance training versus endurance training in congestive heart failure. *Medicine and Science in Sports Exercise, 34*, 1868–1872.

Deyo, R. A., Inui, T. S., Leininger, J., and Overman, S. (1982). Physical and psychosocial function in rheumatoid arthritis: clinical use of a self-administered health status instrument. *Archives of Internal Medicine, 142*, 879–882.

Dracup, K., Walden, J. A., Stevenson, L. W., and Brecht, M. L. (1992). Quality of life in patients with advanced heart failure. *Journal of Heart and Lung Transplantation, 11*, 273–279.

Dugmore, L. D., Tipson, R. J., Phillips, M. H., Flint, E. J., Stentiford, N. H., Bone, M. F. *et al.* (1999). Changes in cardiorespiratory fitness, psychological well-being, quality of life, and vocational status following a 12 month cardiac exercise rehabilitation programme. *Heart, 81*, 359–366.

Dupuy, H. J. (1984). The psychological general well-being (PGWB) index. In N. K. Wenger, M. E. Mattson, and C. D. Furberg (Eds). *Assessment of Quality of Life in Clinical Trials of Cardiovascular Therapies* (pp. 170–184). New York: Le Jacq.

Eaker, E. D., Sullivan, L. M., Kelly-Hayes, M., D'Agostino, R. B., Sr, and Benjamin, E. J. (2004). Anger and hostility predict the development of atrial fibrillation in men in the Framingham Offspring Study. *Circulation, 109*, 1267–1271.

European Heart Failure Training Group (1998). Experience from controlled trials of physical training in chronic heart failure. *European Heart Journal, 19*, 466–475.

EuroQoL Group (1990). EuroQol-a new facility for the measurement of health related quality of life. *Health Policy*, *16*, 199–208.

Evangelista, L. S., Berg, J., and Dracup, K. (2001). Relationship between psychosocial variables and compliance in patients with heart failure. *Heart and Lung*, *30*, 294–301.

ExTraMATCH collaborative (2004). Exercise training meta-analysis of trials in patients with chronic heart failure. *British Medical Journal*, *328*, 189.

Fleg, J. L. (2002). Can exercise conditioning be effective in older heart failure patients? *Heart Failure Reviews*, *7*, 99–103.

Frasure-Smith, N., Lesperance, F., Gravel, G., Masson, A., Juneau, M., Talajic, M. *et al.* (2000). Depression and health-care costs during the first year following myocardial infarction. *Journal of Psychosomatic Research*, *48*, 471–478.

Freedland, K. E. and Carney, R. M. (2000). Psychosocial considerations in elderly patients with heart failure. *Clinical Geriatric Medicine*, *16*, 649–661.

Freedland, K. E., Carney, R. M., Rich, M. W., Krone, R. J., and Smith, L. J. (1991). Depression in elderly patients with congestive heart failure. *Journal of Geriatric Psychiatry and Neurology*, *24*, 59–71.

Gordon, A., Tyni-Lenne, R., Persson, H., Kaijser, L., Hultman, E., and Sylven, C. (1996). Markedly improved skeletal function with local muscle training in patients with chronic heart failure. *Clinical Cardiology*, *19*, 568–574.

Gorkin, L., Norvell, N. K., and Rosen, R. C. (1993). Assessment of quality of life as observed from the baseline data of the Studies of Left Ventricular Dysfunction (SOLVD) trial quality-of-life substudy. *American Journal of Cardiology*, *71*, 1069–1073.

Grady, K. L., Jalowiec, A., and White-Williams, C. (1995). Predictors of quality of life in patients with advanced heart failure awaiting transplantation. *Journal of Heart and Lung Transplantation*, *14*, 2–10.

Hambrecht, R., Gielen, S., Linke, A., Fiehn, E., Yu, J., Walther, C. *et al.* (2000). Effects of exercise training on left ventricular function and peripheral resistance in patients with chronic heart failure: a randomized trial. *Journal of the American Medical Association*, *283*, 3095–3101.

Havranek, E. P., Ware, M. G., and Lowes, B. D. (1999). Prevalence of depression in congestive heart failure. *American Journal of Cardiology*, *84*, 348–350.

Ho, K. K., Pinsky, J. L., Kannel, W. B., and Levy, D. (1993). The epidemiology of heart failure: the Framingham Study. *Journal of the American College of Cardiology*, *22*(Suppl. 4), 6A–13A.

Hobbs, F. D. R., Kenkre, J. E., Roalfe, A. K., Davis, R. C., Hare, R., and Davies, M. K. (2002). Impact of heart failure and left ventricular systolic dysfunction on quality of life: a cross-sectional study comparing common chronic cardiac and medical disorders and a representative adult population. *European Heart Journal*, *23*, 1867–1876.

Houghton, A. R., Harrison, M., Cowley, A. J., and Hampton, J. R. (2002). Assessing exercise capacity, quality of life and haemodynamics in heart failure: do the tests tell us the same thing? *European Journal of Heart Failure*, *4*, 289–295.

Hunt, S. M. (1986) Measuring health in clinical care and clinical trials. In G. Teeling-Smith (Ed.). *Measuring Health: A Practical Approach* (pp. 7–21). Chichester, West Sussex, UK: John Wiley.

Jaarsma, T., Halfens, R., Abu-Saad, H. H., Dracup, K., Stappers, J., and van Ree, J. (1999). Quality of life in older patients with systolic and diastolic heart failure. *European Journal of Heart Failure*, *1*, 151–160.

Jette, M., Heller, R., Landry, F., and Blumchen, G. (1991). Randomized 4-week exercise program in patients with impaired left ventricular function. *Circulation*, *84*, 1561–1567.

Jiang, W., Alexander, J., Christopher, E., Kuchibhatla, M., Gaulden, L. H., Cuffe, M. S. *et al.* (2001). Relationship of depression to increased risk of mortality and rehospitalization in patients with congestive heart failure. *Archives of Internal Medicine*, *161*, 1849–1856.

Johnson, P. H., Cowley, A. J., and Kinnear, W. J. M. (1998). A randomized controlled trial of inspiratory muscle training in stable chronic heart failure. *European Heart Journal*, *19*, 1249–1253.

Kannel, W. B. (1989). Epidemiological aspects of heart failure. *Cardiology Clinics*, *7*, 1–9.

Kavanagh, T., Myers, M. G., Baigrie, R. S., Mertens, D. J., Sawyer, P., and Shephard, R. J. (1996). Quality of life and cardiorespiratory function in chronic heart failure: effects of 12 months' aerobic training. *Heart*, *76*, 42–49.

Keteyian, S. J., Levine, A. B., Brawner, C. A., Kataoka, T., Rogers, F. J., Schairer, J. R. *et al.* (1996). Exercise training in patients with heart failure: a randomized controlled trial. *Annals of Internal Medicine*, *124*, 1051–1057.

Kiilavuori, K., Sovijarvi, A., Naveri, H., Ikonen, T., and Leinonen, H. (1996). Effect of physical training on exercise capacity and gas exchange in patients with chronic heart failure. *Chest*, *110*, 985–991.

Koch, M., Douard, H., and Broustet, J. P. (1992). The benefit of graded physical exercise in chronic heart failure. *Chest*, *101* (Suppl. 5), 231S–235S.

Konstam, M., Dracup, K., Baker, D., Bottorff, M. B., Brooks, N. H., Dacey, R. A. *et al.* (1994). *Heart Failure: Evaluation and Care of Patients with Left Ventricular Systolic Dysfunction*. Clinical Practice Guideline No. 11. AHCPR Publication No. 94–0612. Agency for Health Care Policy and Research, Public Health Service. Rockville, MD: US Department of Health and Human Services.

Lavie, C. J. and Milani, R. V. (1995). Effects of cardiac rehabilitation programs on exercise capacity, coronary risk factors, behavioral characteristics, and quality of life in a large elderly cohort. *American Journal of Cardiology*, *15*, 177–179.

Lavie, C. J. and Milani, R. V. (1997). Effects of cardiac rehabilitation, exercise training, and weight reduction on exercise capacity, coronary risk factors, behavioral characteristics, and quality of life in obese coronary patients. *American Journal of Cardiology*, *79*, 397–401.

Leidy, N. K., Rentz, A. M., and Zyczynski, T. M. (1999). Evaluating health-related quality-of-life outcomes in patients with congestive heart failure: a review of recent randomised controlled trials. *Pharmacoeconomics*, *15*, 19–46.

Linden, W., Stossel, C., and Maurice, J. (1996). Psychosocial interventions for patients with coronary artery disease: a meta-analysis. *Archives of Internal Medicine*, *156*, 745–752.

McConnell, T. R., Mandak, J. S., Sykes, J. S., Fesniak, H., and Dasgupta, H. (2003). Exercise training for heart failure patients improves respiratory muscle endurance, exercise tolerance, breathlessness, and quality of life. *Journal of Cardiopulmonary Rehabilitation*, *23*, 10–16.

McDonagh, T. A., Morrison, C. E., Lawrence, A., Ford, I., Tunstall-Pedoe, H., McMurray, J. J. *et al.* (1997). Symptomatic and asymptomatic left-ventricular systolic dysfunction in an urban population. *Lancet*, *350*, 829–833.

McKelvie, R. S., Teo, K. K., Roberts, R., McCartney, N., Humen, D., Montague, T. *et al.* (2002). Effects of exercise training in patients with heart failure: the Exercise Rehabilitation Trial (EXERT). *American Heart Journal*, *144*, 23–30.

MacMahon, K. M. and Yip, G. Y. (2002). Psychological factors in heart failure: a review of the literature. *Archives of Internal Medicine*, *162*, 509–516.

McMurray, J. and Dargie, H. J. (1992). Trends in hospitalisation for chronic heart failure in the United Kingdom. *European Heart Journal*, *13*, 350.

McMurray, J. and Davie, A. P. (1996). The pharmacoeconomics of ACE inhibitors in chronic heart failure. *Pharmacoeconomics*, *9*, 188–197.

Maiorana, A., O'Driscoll, G., Cheetham, C., Collis, J., Goodman, C., Rankin, S. *et al.* (2000). Combined aerobic and resistance exercise training improves functional capacity and strength in CHF. *Journal of Applied Physiology*, *88*, 1565–1570.

Mair, F. S., Crowley, T. S., and Bundred, P. E. (1996). Prevalence, aetiology and management of heart failure in general practice. *British Journal of General Practice*, 46, 77–79.

Mair, F. S., Ling, M., and Lloyd-Williams, F. (1999). *A Study of Patient Perceptions of Heart Failure*. Report submitted to North West Regional Health Authority, UK. RDO/18/71.

Martensson, J., Dracup, K., Canary, C., and Fridlund, B. (2003). Living with heart failure: depression and quality of life in patients and spouses. *Journal of Heart and Lung Transplantation*, 22, 460–467.

Mather, A. S., Rodriguez, C., Guthrie, M., McHarg, A. M., Reid, I. C., and McMurdo, M. E. (2002). The effects of exercise on depressive symptoms in older adults with poorly responsive depressive disorder: a randomised controlled trial. *British Journal of Psychology*, 180, 411–415.

Meyer, K., Schwaibold, M., Westbrook, S., Beneke, R., Hajric, R., Gornandt, L. *et al.* (1996). Effects of short-term exercise training and activity restriction on functional capacity in patients with severe chronic congestive heart failure. *American Journal of Cardiology*, 78, 1017–1022.

Miller, A. B. (2002). Heart failure and depression. *European Journal of Heart Failure*, 4, 401–402.

Moser, D. K. (2002). Psychosocial factors and their association with clinical outcomes in patients with heart failure: why clinicians do not seem to care. *European Journal of Cardiovasular Nursing*, 1, 183–188.

Moser, D. K. and Worster, P. L. (2000). Effect of psychosocial factors on physiologic outcomes in patients with heart failure. *Journal of Cardiovascular Nursing*, 14, 106–115.

Murberg, T. A., Bru, E., Svebak, S., Tveteras, R., and Aarsland, T. (1999). Depressed mood and subjective health symptoms as predictors of mortality in patients with congestive heart failure: a two-years follow-up study. *International Journal of Psychiatric Medicine*, 9, 311–326.

O'Connor, G. T., Buring, J. E., Yusuf, S., Goldhaber, S. Z., Olmstead, E. M., Paffenbarger, R. S., Jr *et al.* (1989). An overview of randomized trials of rehabilitation with exercise after myocardial infarction. *Circulation*, 80, 234–244.

Oka, R. K., Gortner, S. R., Stotts, N. A., and Haskell, W. L. (1996). Predictors of physical activity in patients with chronic heart failure secondary to either ischemic or idiopathic dilated cardiomyopathy. *American Journal of Cardiology*, 77, 159–163.

Oka, R. K., DeMarco, T., and Haskell, W. L. (1999). Perceptions of physical fitness in patients with heart failure. *Progress in Cardiovascular Nursing*, 14, 97–102.

Oka, R. K., DeMarco, T., Haskell, W. L., Botvinick, E., Dae, M. W., Bolen, K. *et al.* (2000). Impact of a home-based walking and resistance training program on quality of life in patients with heart failure. *American Journal of Cardiology*, 85, 365–369.

Oldridge, N. B., Guyatt, G. H., Fischer, M. E., and Rimm, A. A. (1988). Cardiac rehabilitation after myocardial infarction: combined experience of randomized clinical trials. *Journal of the American Medical Association*, 260, 945–950.

Oldridge, N., Perkins, A., Marchionni, N., Fumagalli, S., Fattirolli, F., and Guyatt, G. (2002). Number needed to treat in cardiac rehabilitation. *Journal of Cardiopulmonary Rehabilitation*, 22, 22–30.

Owen, A. and Croucher, L. (2000). Effect of an exercise programme for elderly patients with heart failure. *European Journal of Heart Failure*, 2, 65–70.

Patrick Green, C., Porter, C. B., Bresnahan, D. R., and Spertus, J. A. (2000). Development and evaluation of the Kansas city cardiomyopathy questionnaire: a new health status measure for heart failure. *Journal of the American College of Cardiology*, 35, 1245–1255.

Quittan, M., Sturm, B., Wiesinger, G., Pacher, R., and Fialka-Moser, V. (1999). Quality of life in patients with chronic heart failure: a randomized controlled trial of changes induced by a regular exercise program. *Scandinavian Journal of Rehabilitation Medicine*, 31, 223–228.

Radzewitz, A., Miche, E., Herrmann, G., Nowak, M., Montanus, U., Adam, U. *et al.* (2002). Exercise and muscle strength training and their effect on quality of life in patients with chronic heart failure. *European Journal of Heart Failure, 4,* 627–634.

Reichenberg, A., Yirmiya, R., Schuld, A., Kraus, T., Haack, M., Morag, A. *et al.* (2001). Cytokine-associated emotional and cognitive disturbances in humans. *Archives of General Psychiatry, 58,* 445–452.

Report of the American College of Cardiology/American Heart Association Task Force on Practice Guidelines (1995). Guidelines for the evaluation and management of heart failure. *Circulation, 92,* 2764–2784.

Rodriguez-Artalejo, F., Guallar-Castillon, P., Banegas, J. R., and del Rey Calero, J. (1997). Trends in hospitalisation and mortality for heart failure in Spain. *European Heart Journal, 18,* 1771–1779.

Rogers, W. J., Johnstone, D. E., Yusuf, S., Weiner, D. H., Gallagher, P., Bittner, V. A. *et al.* (1994). Quality of life among 5,025 patients with left ventricular dysfunction randomized between placebo and enalapril: the Studies of Left Ventricular Dysfunction, The SOLVD Investigators. *Journal of the American College of Cardiology, 23,* 393–400.

Rumsfeld, J. S., Havranek, E., Masoudi, F. A., Peterson, E. D., Jones, P., Tooley, J. F. *et al.* (2003). Cardiovascular outcomes research consortium depressive symptoms are the strongest predictors of short-term declines in health status in patients with heart failure. *Journal of the American College of Cardiology, 42,* 811–817.

Scalvini, S., Marangoni, S., Volterrani, M., Schena, M., Quadri, A., and Levi, G. F. (1992). Physical rehabilitation in coronary patients who have suffered from episodes of cardiac failure. *Cardiology, 80,* 417–423.

Schocken, D. D., Arrieta, M. I., Leaverton, P. E., and Ross, E. A. (1992). Prevalence and mortality rate of congestive heart failure in the United States. *Journal of the American College of Cardiology, 20,* 301–306.

Schwarz, K. A. and Elman, C. S. (2003). Identification of factors predictive of hospital readmissions for patients with heart failure. *Heart and Lung, 32,* 88–99.

Shephard, R. J., Kavanagh, T., and Mertens, D. J. (1998). On the prediction of physiological and psychological responses to aerobic training in patients with congestive heart failure. *Journal of Cardiopulmonary Rehabilitation, 18,* 45–51.

Silva, M. S., Bocchi, E. A., Guimaraes, G. V., Padovani, C. R., Silva, M. H., Pereira, S. F. *et al.* (2002). Benefits of exercise training in the treatment of heart failure: study with a control group. *Arquivos Brasileiros de Cardiologia, 79,* 351–362.

Skotzko, C. E., Krichten, C., Zietowski, G., Alves, L., Freudenberger, R., Robinson, S. *et al.* (2000). Depression is common and precludes accurate assessment of functional status in elderly patients with congestive heart failure. *Journal of Cardiac Failure, 6,* 300–305.

Steptoe, A., Mohabir, A., Mahon, N. G., and McKenna, W. J. (2000). Health related quality of life and psychological well being in patients with dilated cardiomyopathy. *Heart, 83,* 645–650.

Stewart, A. L. and Ware, J. E. (Eds). (1992). *Measuring Functioning and Well-being: The Medical Outcomes Study Approach.* Durham, NC: Duke University Press.

Stewart, A. L., Greenfield, S., Hays, R. D., Wells, K., Rogers, W. H., Berry, S. D. *et al.* (1989). Functional status and well-being of patients with chronic conditions: results from the Medical Outcomes Study. *Journal of the American Medical Association, 262,* 907–913.

Stewart, K. J., McFarland, L. D., Weinhofer, J. J., and Brown C. S. (1999). Safety and efficacy of weight training soon after myocardial infarction. *Journal of Cardiopulmonary Rehabilitation, 18,* 37–44.

Stewart, S., MacIntyre, K., Hole, D. J., Capewell, S., and McMurray, J. J. (2001) More "malignant" than cancer? Five-year survival following a first admission for heart failure. *European Journal of Heart Failure*, 3, 315–322.

Stewart, S., Jenkins, A., Buchan, S., McGuire, A., Capewell, S., and McMurray, J. J. V. (2002). The current cost of heart failure to the National Health Service in the UK. *European Journal of Heart Failure*, 4, 361–371.

Sullivan, M. J., Higginbotham, M. B., and Cobb, F. R. (1988). Exercise training in patients with severe left ventricular dysfunction. *Circulation*, 78, 506–515.

Taylor, A. (1999). Physiological response to a short period of exercise training in patients with chronic heart failure. *Physiotherapy Research International*, 4, 237–249.

The National Heart Foundation of New Zealand, Cardiac Society of Australia and New Zealand, and the Royal New Zealand College of General Practitioners Working Party (1997). New Zealand guidelines for the management of chronic heart failure. *New Zealand Medical Journal*, 110, 99–107.

The Task Force of the Working Group on Heart Failure of the European Society of Cardiology (1997). The treatment of heart failure. *European Heart Journal*, 18, 736–753.

The Task Force on Heart Failure of the European Society of Cardiology (1995). Guidelines for the diagnosis of heart failure. *European Heart Journal*, 16, 741–751.

Tyni-Lenne, R., Gordon, A., and Sylven, C. (1996). Improved quality of life in chronic heart failure patients following local endurance training with leg muscles. *Journal of Cardiac Failure*, 2, 111–117.

Tyni-Lenne, R., Gordon, A., Jansson, E., Bermann, G., and Sylven, C. (1997). Skeletal muscle endurance training improves peripheral oxidative capacity, exercise tolerance, and health-related quality of life in women with chronic congestive heart failure secondary to either ischemic cardiomyopathy or idiopathic dilated cardiomyopathy. *American Journal of Cardiology*, 80, 1025–1029.

Tyni-Lenne, R., Gordon, A., Europe, E., Jansson, E., and Sylven, C. (1998). Exercise based rehabilitation improves skeletal muscle capacity exercise tolerance, and quality of life in both women and men with chronic heart failure. *Journal of Cardiac Failure*, 4, 9–17.

Tyni-Lenne, R., Gordon, A., Jensen-Urstad, M., Dencker K., Jansson, E., and Sylven, C. (1999). Aerobic training involving a minor muscle mass shows greater efficiency than training involving a major muscle mass in chronic heart failure patients. *Journal of Cardiac Failure*, 5, 300–307.

van Jaarsveld, C. H., Sanderman, R., Miedema, I., Ranchor, A. V., and Kempen, G. I. (2001). Changes in health-related quality of life in older patients with acute myocardial infarction or congestive heart failure: a prospective study. *Journal of the American Geriatric Society*, 49, 1052–1058.

Vidmar, P. M. and Rubinson, L. (1994). The relationship between self-efficacy and exercise compliance in a cardiac population. *Journal of Cardiopulmonary Rehabilitation*, 14, 246–254.

Walden, J. A., Stevenson, L. W., Dracup, K., Hook, J. F., Moser, D. K., Hamilton, M. *et al.* (1994). Extended comparison of quality of life between stable heart failure patients and heart transplant recipients. *Journal of Heart and Lung Transplantation*, 13, 1109–1118.

Wenger, N. K., Froelicher, E. S., Smith, L. K., Ades, P. A., Berra, K., Blumenthal, J. A. *et al.* (1995). Cardiac rehabilitation as secondary prevention: Agency for Health Care Policy and Research and the National Heart, Lung and Blood Institute. *Clinical Practice Guideline: Quick Reference Guide for Clinicians*, 17, 1–23.

Whellan, D. J., O'Connor, C. M., and Pina, I. (2004). Training trials in heart failure: time to exercise restraint? *American Heart Journal*, 147, 190–192.

Wielenga, R. P., Erdman, R. A. M., Huisveld, I. A., Bol, E., Dunselman, P. H., Baselier, M. R. *et al.* (1998a). Effect of exercise training on quality of life in patients with chronic heart failure. *Journal of Psychosomatic Research*, 45, 459–464.

Wielenga, R. P., Huisveld, I. A., Bol, E., Dunselman, P. H. J. M., Erdman, R. A., Baselier, M. R. *et al.* (1998b). Exercise training in elderly patients with chronic heart failure. *Coronary Artery Disease*, *9*, 765–770.

Wielenga, R. P., Huisveld, I. A., Bol, E., Dunselman, P. H. J. M., Erdman, R. A., Baselier, M. R. *et al.* (1999). Safety and effects of physical training in chronic heart failure. *European Heart Journal*, *20*, 872–879.

Willenheimer, R., Erhardt, L., Cline, C., Rydberg, E., and Israelsson, B. (1998). Exercise training in heart failure improves quality of life and exercise capacity. *European Heart Journal*, *19*, 774–781.

Working Group on Cardiac Rehabilitation and Exercise Physiology and Working Group on Heart Failure of the European Society of Cardiology (2001). Recommendations for exercise training in chronic heart failure patients. *European Heart Journal*, *22*, 125–135.

Zellweger, M. J., Osterwalder, R. H., Langewitz, W., and Pfisterer, M. E. (2004). Coronary artery disease and depression. *European Heart Journal*, *25*, 3–9.

Exercise and psychological well-being for individuals with Human Immunodeficiency Virus and Acquired Immunodeficiency Syndrome

WILLIAM W. STRINGER

HIV AND AIDS

HIV and AIDS are global health problems. The Center for Disease Control (CDC) and the Joint United Nations Programme on HIV/AIDS predicted that worldwide in 2003, over 40 million people would be living with HIV/AIDS, an estimated 5 million people will have acquired HIV, and 3 million people would have died of AIDS. In the United States alone, it is estimated that 1 in 200 people are HIV positive (Center for Disease Control, 2004).

HIV is primarily transmitted via sexual contact with blood, semen, and vaginal secretions. One of the primary targets of the HIV virus is the $CD4^+$ T helper cell. Once the virus is inside the body, it binds to the $CD4^+$ receptor on the surface of the cell and is internalized. This eventually can result in the death of the cell. Attack on $CD4^+$ lymphocytes results in a marked depletion of these cells and a reduction in the ability of the immune system to respond to common infectious agents. This immune suppression increases a person's vulnerability to opportunistic infections, malignancies, as well as loss of lean body mass. Progression from HIV^+ to AIDS is a metric of the current status of the host's immune system. The average time from initial infection with HIV to AIDS is 8–10 years, and $CD4^+$ cell counts (an excellent marker of immune status and prognosis) decrease by approximately 50–75 cells/mm³/year (Vergis, 2000). When $CD4^+$ cell counts decrease below 200 cells/ mm³ the patient is defined as having AIDS (Castro et al., 1992).

The stage of HIV disease can also be defined as mild (early or asymptomatic, >500 $CD4^+$ cells/mm³), moderate (mid-stage, early symptomatic, or pre-AIDS, 200–500 $CD4^+$ cells/mm³), and severe (advanced or AIDS, <200 $CD4^+$ cells/mm³). Patients with less than 50 $CD4^+$ cells/mm³ are considered to have an end stage immunodeficiency. Another commonly used marker of immune system function and prognosis is the HIV polymerase chain reaction (PCR) assessment of viral load. An undetectable viral load is optimal, and the number increases (e.g., increased viral particles circulating) when the disease progresses or is poorly controlled. Medical therapy for HIV is indicated when the $CD4^+$ cell counts are in the range of 200–350 cells/mm³. $CD4^+$ cell counts can markedly increase and viral loads can markedly decrease (immune reconstitution) when patients are placed on highly active anti-retroviral therapy (e.g., HAART). HAART is a combination of medications from the nucleoside reverse transcriptase inhibitor (NRTIs), non-nucleoside reverse transcriptase inhibitor (NNRTIs), and protease inhibitor (PIs), families.

NEUROPSYCHOIMMUNOLOGY MODEL

Early epidemiologic studies which focused on coping with HIV demonstrated that active strategies (i.e., fighting spirit, planning a course of action, exercise) resulted in less depression and higher self-esteem compared to HIV negative controls (Namir et al., 1987). The perceived epidemiological association of exercise with a decrease in psychological symptoms in HIV^+ individuals led to the conceptualization of the effects of stress on psychosocial, neuroendocrine, and immunologic function (psychoneuroimmunology) in HIV^+ individuals (Antoni et al., 1990; LaPerriere et al., 1994b) (see Figure 6.1).

The proposed mechanism behind psychoneuroimmunology is that stressors (with a decreased sense of control) can cause increased anxiety, depression, diminished coping skills, and loss of sleep. This in turn, increases the activation of the sympathetic nervous system, increasing levels of epinephrine, norepineprine, and cortisol. These hormones can act to suppress the function of the immune system, for example, T cells (cells that are involved with cellular immunity – $CD4^+$ cells are included here), B cells (cells that are involved with humoral immunity and antibody production), and natural killer cells (cells that are capable of killing other cells), thereby resulting in more rapid progression of HIV. Consequently, interventions that decrease stress or increase control

Figure 6.1 Effect of stressors on immune system function and possible mitigation by aerobic exercise.

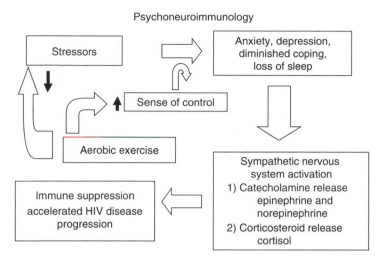

Source: Adapted from Antoni *et al.* (1990).

(i.e., coping mechanisms) of stress, for example, moderate exercise (see Taylor, 2000), may improve psychological, neuroendocrine, and immunological functional parameters and overall health in HIV$^+$ individuals.

METHOD

This chapter reviews the existing literature, focusing on the use of exercise training (e.g., aerobic exercise, progressive resistance exercise (PRE), or both) to improve the psychological well-being of HIV positive (HIV$^+$) individuals across the disease spectrum from asymptomatic HIV$^+$ individuals to AIDS. The review does not focus on AIDS patients with extensive lean body mass reduction (>10%) or studies that have used anabolic agents (e.g., testosterone, growth hormone) as the primary intervention, even when exercise was a component of the study, as these agents may affect psychological well-being in ways that confound the effects of exercise training. An extensive search of several reference databases (Medline, CKNAHL, Cochrane, EMBASE, and PsychLit) was performed using the time window of 1981 to present and the search terms: HIV, aerobic exercise training, strength training, quality of life (QOL), depression, well-being, anxiety, and coping. Eight primary studies were appropriate for this review (see Table 6.1) although all suffered from methodological problems that included either a lack of control group (1), small sample size (6), or very short (<3 months) duration of study (6). Recent reviews were also examined to integrate the HIV medical literature, HIV medical therapy, and the aerobic and strength effects of exercise in HIV.

Table 6.1 Studies on the effect of exercise on psychological well-being in HIV

AUTHOR	NUMBER OF PARTICIPANTS/ CONCURRENT CONTROL GROUP	TYPE OF EXERCISE/ DURATION/ RESISTANCE	HIV STAGE	RESULTS/FITNESS CHANGE?	STUDY LIMITATIONS	COMMENTS/ DROP OUT RATE	INSTRUMENT
LaPerriere et al. (1991)	39 (39M), 22 performed exercise, no data on ethnicity. A non-exercising concurrent HIV$^+$ control group present	Cycle ergometer training/ 10 weeks/ no resistance	Mean CD4$^+$ count >900 cells/μL – no AIDS defining diagnosis	POMS – Tension– anxiety and depression–dejection in exercising seropositive subjects remained stable when compared to non-exercising seropositive controls (who worsened)/there was no change in calculated (not measured) VO$_2$ max	Small sample size, short study (10 weeks), no documentation of drop out rate, all male participants, no data on ethnicity, aerobic fitness (VO$_2$ max) changes with exercise program calculated, not measured	Very similar population and results in reference (LaPerriere et al., 1990), a 5 week program with 50 participants. Drop out rate not documented	Profile of Mood States (POMS, McNair et al., 1981)
MacArthur et al. (1993)	25 (24M, 1F), no data on ethnicity/no concurrent HIV$^+$ control group	Treadmill/ 24 weeks, 2 different aerobic training intensities (Low vs High)	Mean CD4$^+$ count in the 6 who completed the study was 209 ± 115 cells/μL	Improved anxiety and depression scores with exercise training at either intensity; however, the scores on the General Health Questionnaire-28 (GHQ-28, Goldberg and Hilliar, 1979)	Small sample size, short study (24 weeks), large drop out rate (76%), 96% male participants, no data on ethnicity, no analysis of subjects by intention to treat,	Drop out rate, 76% (6 completed the study and were labeled "compliant"	GHQ-28

(Table 6.1 continued)

Study	Participants	Intervention	CD4 count	Results	Limitations	Outcome measures
Lox et al. (1995)	33 (33M), no data on ethnicity/ concurrent non-exercising HIV+ control group present	Cycle ergometer/ 12 weeks/ yes (12 subjects)	Mean CD4+ count ~302 ± 350 cells/μL, aerobic 403 ± 392, resistance training 149 ± 240, control 311 ± 341, all participants on antiretrovirals	did not correlate with exercise compliance/ the 6/25 compliant study participants had an increase in VO₂ max of 24%. Both aerobic and resistance exercise groups demonstrated improvements in positive and negative mood and satisfaction with life compared to the control group. The changes in the aerobic group compared to the resistance training group were greater/ aerobic fitness was not measured, however exercise heart rate for isotask did decrease 12% without changes in the weight training or control groups	Small sample size, short study (12 weeks), all male participants, no data on ethnicity, poor randomization into subgroups (markedly different CD4 counts). Randomization poor with markedly different CD4 counts and AIDS status/ drop out rate 3%. no control group	Positive and Negative Affect Schedule (PANAS, Watson et al., 1998) and Satisfaction with Life Scale (SWLS, Diener et al., 1985)
Stringer et al. (1998)	26 (24M, 2F), 29% Hispanic, 20% African American/	Cycle ergometer training/ 6 weeks/no resistance	Mean CD4+ count 266 ± 128 cells/μL (all participants on Zidovudine	Overall QOL, hope, and desire to continue living improved significantly in the both exercising	Small sample size, very short study (6 weeks), 93% male participants, non-standardized. Drop out rate 23%	HIV specific QOL questionnaire (Ertl et al., 1996)

Table 6.1 Continued

AUTHOR	NUMBER OF PARTICIPANTS/ CONCURRENT CONTROL GROUP	TYPE OF EXERCISE/ DURATION/ RESISTANCE	HIV STAGE	RESULTS/FITNESS CHANGE?	STUDY LIMITATIONS	COMMENTS/ DROP OUT RATE	INSTRUMENT
	concurrent non-exercising HIV$^+$ control group present	exercise	or Zidovudine + didanosine)	groups, relative to non-exercising controls. Exercising groups improved the LAT 10–25 % and VO$_2$max in the heavy group improved 13%. There was no change in the moderate intensity exercise VO$_2$ max	psychological well-being/QOL questionnaire		
Smith et al. (2001)	60 (52M, 8F), 26% Hispanic or African–American/ concurrent non-exercising HIV$^+$ control group present	Walking – treadmill or track/ 12 weeks/ none	Mean CD4$^+$ count 328 ± 69 cells/µL (most subjects on 2 or fewer antiretroviral medications, 7 subjects (29%) were on protease inhibitor therapy)	No change in rating of perceived exertion/VO$_2$ max increased 7% in the exercising group	Small sample size, short study (12 weeks), 86% male participants, Borg scale (a perceived exertion scale) is equated in this study to changes in QOL/psycho-gical well-being, exercising group	Drop out rate 18%	Borg (Borg, 1982)

Study	Subjects	Exercise/duration	CD4 count	Results	Limitations	Drop out	Measures
Rojas et al. (2003)	33 (23M, 10F), 100% Caucasians/ concurrent non-exercising HIV+ control group was present	Mixture of stretching, aerobic, (circuit training, running, walking or obstacle course), and resistance training in each session/ 16 week	Mean CD4+ count 425 ± 215 cells/μL	Psychological well-being improved in both exercising and control groups; therefore, no statistically significant effect. VO_2 max increased 9% in the exercising group	had the greatest attrition Small sample size, short study (16 weeks), 69% male participants, poor randomization of males/females in exercising group relative to the control, non-standardized, variegated exercise	Drop out/ non-compliance rate 15%	Medical Outcomes Study in HIV (MOS-HIV; Zander et al., 1994)
Neidig et al. (2003)	60 (52M, 8F), 36% African–American/ concurrent non-exercising HIV+ control group was present	Cycle, treadmill or walking/ 12 weeks	Mean CD4+ count 347 ± 87 cells/μL (75% on antiretrovirals)	Exercise participants showed a reduction in depressive symptoms on all indices Center for Epidemiological Studies–Depression (CES–D), Beck Depression Inventory (BDI), and POMS. Results on all depression scales were well correlated with each other/fitness change not specifically reported	Small sample size, short study (12 weeks), 86% male participants	Drop out rate 20%	CES–D (Radloff, 1977), BDI (Beck and Steer, 1993), and POMS (Mc Nair et al., 1981)

(Table 6.1 continued)

Table 6.1 Continued							
AUTHOR	NUMBER OF PARTICIPANTS/ CONCURRENT CONTROL GROUP	TYPE OF EXERCISE/ DURATION/ RESISTANCE	HIV STAGE	RESULTS/FITNESS CHANGE?	STUDY LIMITATIONS	COMMENTS/ DROP OUT RATE	INSTRUMENT
Baigis et al. (2004)	99 (79M, 20F), 55% African–American, 32% Caucasian, 10% Hispanic, 2% other. Concurrent non-exercising HIV$^+$ control group was present	Exercise group received a 20 minute workout on a ski machine 3 × per week/ 15 weeks/ controls received a 1 nurse visit per week	Mean CD4$^+$ count 350–365 ± 90 cells/µL (75% on antiretrovirals)	No difference between exercise and control group at week 15 on any Health Related Quality of Life (HR-QOL), except MOS-HIV overall subscale (67.5 vs 55.4, $p = 0.02$). There were non-significant trends on the other scales favoring exercise/ there was no improvement in aerobic fitness in the exercising group	Small sample size, short study (15 weeks), 93% male participants, no change in aerobic fitness in the exercising group, therefore the "dose" of exercise may not have been adequate	20 % overall drop out rate 24% in exercise group, 14% in control)	MOS-HIV

THE CASE FOR PHYSICAL ACTIVITY/EXERCISE IN HIV

Improvements in aerobic and strength parameter with exercise in HIV

Several recent reviews have summarized the impact of aerobic and strength exercise training in a broad spectrum of HIV^+ disease (from asymptomatic individuals to patients clinically ill with AIDS and reduced lean body mass (Dudgeon *et al.*, 2004; Mars, 2003; Nixon *et al.*, 2003; Stringer, 1999, 2001)). From the preponderance of evidence in these primary studies (Johnson *et al.*, 1990; MacArthur *et al.*, 1993; Perna *et al.*, 1999; Pothoff *et al.*, 1994; Rigsby *et al.*, 1992; Roubenoff *et al.*, 1999; Smith *et al.*, 2001; Stringer *et al.*, 1998), it is clear that 6–12 weeks of moderate aerobic exercise sessions (3 times per week for 1 hr) significantly improves (15–30%) aerobic capacity (maximal oxygen uptake, VO_2 max) and lactic acidosis threshold (LAT).

PRE alone has been demonstrated (9 studies) to improve strength (10–60%) and lean body mass (1–4%) in HIV/AIDS patients, using 6–16 weeks of three, 1 hr PRE training sessions per week. These studies are summarized in detail elsewhere (Dudgeon *et al.*, 2004; Stringer, 2003). Interestingly, the addition of androgenic therapy (e.g., testosterone, nandrolone, oxandrolone) did not contribute more to strength than the PRE alone, although weight and fat free mass did increase in the groups given androgen therapy.

The combination of strength and aerobic exercise training has also been studied, and appears to have similar beneficial effects on aerobic capacity and lean body mass (Grinspoon *et al.*, 2000; Lox *et al.*, 1995; Rigsby *et al.*, 1992; Strawford *et al.*, 1999); however, the conclusions are limited by the small sample sizes utilized in these studies.

Improvements in CD4+ cell counts and viral loads with exercise in HIV

Not even a single study has demonstrated a statistically significant improvement in either viral load or $CD4^+$ cell counts with 6–16 weeks of aerobic or PRE training, although many small studies have been performed (LaPerriere *et al.*, 1991, 1994a; Perna *et al.*, 1999; Rigsby *et al.*, 1992; Smith *et al.*, 2001; Stringer *et al.*, 1998). The lack of statistically significant improvements in $CD4^+$ counts is likely due, in part, to study size and variability of $CD4^+$ counts superimposed on the perceived or actual (small) exercise effect (Stringer *et al.*, 1998). The converse of this argument is important, in that no study has demonstrated a statistically significant fall in $CD4^+$ counts, despite exercise levels that were designed as moderate and heavy intensities (Stringer *et al.*, 1998). This suggests that moderate and even heavy exercise intensities do not appear to have adverse effects on $CD4^+$ counts.

Improvements in psychological well-being with exercise in HIV

The return of a positive HIV test result often results in feelings of hopelessness, sadness, depression, loneliness, detachment, fearfulness, and suicidal ideation (Ciesla and Roberts, 2001). Pretest and posttest counseling, availability of effective medical and pharmacological care, and continued asymptomatic state appear to reduce these symptoms;

however, asymptomatic HIV$^+$ subjects have approximately twice the risk of depression compared to non-HIV$^+$ controls (Ciesla and Roberts, 2001). Also, as Chesney and Folkman (1994) have demonstrated, psychological symptoms can return with increased intensity when physical health related issues of AIDS appear (e.g., skin changes, weight loss, dyspnea, diarrhea, reduction in mental functioning, etc.). When defining symptoms of AIDS manifest, there is additional risk of depression (approximately 2X) compared to asymptomatic HIV$^+$ individuals (Ostrow et al., 1989). Physical and psychological disability are clearly additive, and combine to markedly reduce global quality of life in individuals with HIV.

Aerobic exercise training to improve the psychological manifestations of HIV/AIDS has been less well examined; however, several studies have focused on improving QOL, anxiety, and depression using aerobic exercise alone, or in combination with resistance exercise (see Table 6.1). One of the early attempts to mitigate psychological stress, related to HIV notification, used moderate exercise as part of a controlled pre/posttest counseling intervention (LaPerriere et al., 1990, 1991). In these studies, LaPerriere et al., utilized 39 subjects from a homogeneous AIDS risk group (asymptomatic gay males, mean CD4$^+$ count >900 cells/μL, between 18 and 40 years old), and administered a 5–10 week aerobic exercise training program (stationary bike, 45 min 3 times per week). The control group did only the pre/posttest counseling. Improvement in the subjects' aerobic capacity was demonstrated with no significant effects on CD4$^+$ cell counts. They also found that there were no significant changes in the Profile of Mood States (POMS; McNair et al., 1981) scores in the exercising group (relative to initial assessments) between weeks 5 and 7 of the study, whereas the control group worsened (i.e., POMS scores worsened in the tension–anxiety and/or depression–dejection categories).

MacArthur et al. (1993) studied 25 HIV$^+$ subjects with a mean CD4$^+$ count of 209 $\pm$ 115 cells/μL using an uncontrolled 24 week treadmill aerobic exercise program. Although the drop out rate was 76%, making the interpretation of results difficult (these results were likely heavily biased by the lack of intention to treat analysis), they did document improved anxiety and depression scores with exercise training using the 28 question General Health Questionnaire (GHQ-28; Goldberg, 1978) instrument.

More recently, Lox et al. (1995) studied 33 subjects with a mean CD4$^+$ count of 302 $\pm$ 350 cells/μL using groups that performed either aerobic or resistance exercise training for 12 weeks. There was a non-exercising (stretching and flexibility) control group. They found that both groups (aerobic and resistance) demonstrated improvements in positive and negative mood scores (Positive and Negative Affect Schedule, PANAS; Watson et al., 1998), as well as improved satisfaction with life (Satisfaction with Life Scale, SWLS; Diener et al., 1985) compared to the control group. They also noted that the improvements were more substantial in the aerobic group, compared to the resistance group, possibly due to the larger intervention effect (or stimulus) of aerobic exercise relative to resistance exercise.

Stringer et al. (1998) published a controlled study involving 26 HIV$^+$ subjects with a mean CD4$^+$ count of 266 $\pm$ 128 cells/μL. These subjects performed a 6 week aerobic exercise program at two different work intensities (moderate and heavy). Overall QOL, as assessed by a 23 question HIV specific QOL of life questionnaire, improved significantly in both exercising groups relative to the non-exercising control group. This QOL instrument broadly documented their increased satisfaction with aerobic exercise relative to non-exercising controls; however, the psychological well-being/QOL instrument was not as well standardized as other HIV QOL instruments (e.g., the MOS-HIV; Zander et al., 1994).

Smith et al. (2001) reported on 60 HIV$^+$ subjects, with a mean CD4$^+$ count of 328 ± 69 cells/μL, who participated in a 12 week walking program. They utilized the Borg (1982) scale to evaluate relative perceived exertion (RPE) and reported no difference in the rating of perceived exertion in the exercising group, relative to the controls. However, RPE may not reflect QOL as measured by other more standardized psychological well-being instruments.

Rojas et al. (2003) studied 33 HIV$^+$ subjects, with a mean CD4$^+$ count of 425 ± 215 cells/μL, during a 16 week aerobic exercise training program (combined with resistance training in each session). They found that psychological well-being, as measured by the MOS-HIV instrument, improved in both the exercising and control groups, leading to a lack of statistically significant difference between the groups in their study. It is not clear if the control group may have significantly benefited from their self-help group involvement (78.5% were involved), during the intervention, resulting in improvements in all arms of the study (exercise and control), thereby resulting in a lack of a statistically significant difference.

Neidig et al. (2003), in an extension of their 2001 study, reported on 60 HIV$^+$ individuals, with mean CD4$^+$ count of 347 ± 87 cells/μL, who underwent 12 weeks of aerobic exercise training (e.g., cycle, treadmill, or walking). They demonstrated a reduction in depressive symptoms using three separate instruments: CES–D (Radloff, 1977), BDI (Beck and Steer, 1993), and POMS. The results on these three instruments were highly correlated with each other.

Finally, Baigis et al. (2004) studied the effectiveness of a supervised, home-based exercise intervention in HIV individuals relative to a control, non-exercising group. Ninety-nine subjects were enrolled (mean CD4$^+$ cell count 360 ± 90 cells/μL) and the intervention group underwent a 15 week, 20 min, 3 times per week home-based moderate intensity exercise program. A 15 weeks there was no difference in physical fitness, Health Related Quality of Life (HR-QOL) on an HIV specific instrument (MOS-HIV, only statistically significant difference was on the overall health subscale), or changes in CD4$^+$ counts relative to the control group. The results of this study may have suffered from an inadequate exercise dosage or frequency, as well as a markedly different drop out rate in the exercising versus control groups (see Table 6.1).

Dudgeon et al. (2004) in an excellent review of the physiological and psychological effects of exercise interventions in HIV disease concluded that:

1 The physiologic parameters of aerobic fitness (e.g., strength, endurance, time to fatigue, and body composition) in HIV$^+$ individuals improve with aerobic exercise.
2 The immunologic effects of exercise training are conflicting and non-uniform.
3 Exercise training has been effectively used to treat depression and anxiety in non-HIV$^+$ individuals, and depression and anxiety are very common in HIV$^+$ individuals.
4 Only minimal data is currently available regarding the effects of exercise on psychological well being, including the dose, duration, and frequency which is not determined at this time.

From the recent review by Dudgeon *et al.* (2004) and the studies reviewed in this chapter, it is suggested, but not proven (due to methodological problems) that aerobic exercise interventions may result in improved psychological well-being for people suffering with HIV/AIDS. Unfortunately, the minimum "dose" of exercise required to observe an effect (if present) is not known.

If exercise can improve psychological well-being, what is the likely mechanism? It may be mediated by the effect of aerobic exercise on improving coping mechanisms (especially positive mental attitude or optimism), decreasing the deleterious effects of stressors, as postulated by the psychoneuroimmunology theory (see Figure 6.1). However, definitive proof is not provided in the studies reviewed in this chapter as cortisol, epinephrine, and norepinephrine levels were not measured in any of these studies, and changes in immunologic function (e.g., $CD4^+$ cells, viral loads) have been small, variable, conflicting, and not statistically significant. Further, the direct effect (and minimal "dose") of exercise on psychological well-being in this population remains relatively unexplored. All of these studies suffer from methodological problems, including small sample sizes, short studies, suboptimal research design (i.e., not blinded), lack of intention to treat analysis, lack of a "placebo" intervention, and/or true randomization (see Table 6.1).

How best to measure psychological well-being or QOL in studies of HIV and exercise?

An enormous number of scales to evaluate psychological well-being have been developed and utilized with respect to the effect of aerobic exercise on psychological well-being in HIV, although they have not been uniformly applied. Essentially each study has utilized a different instrument. These include the POMS, the GHQ-28, the PANAS, the SWLS, an HIV specific QOL Questionnaire, the Borg scale, the MOS–HIV scale, the CES–D, and the BDI, see Table 6.1 for references. All of these instruments have reported very similar and positive results when exercise has been used as the stimulus, and when compared head to head (Neidig *et al.*, 2003), and appear to provide reproducible, reliable, disease specific indicators of improvements in psychological well-being. None of these instruments have been utilized longitudinally to assess psychological well-being or health related QOL. Instruments that broadly measure QOL appear to be most effective in detecting differences in the exercise intervention; however, more specific scales for anxiety, depression, or mood appear to document benefits as well.

SUMMARY OF FINDINGS FROM EXERCISE STUDIES

A 6–12-week program of aerobic exercise alone, or in combination with resistance exercise, three times per week for 45 min, has been demonstrated to improve aerobic fitness. However the effects on psychological well-being are less well understood. There is some modest evidence that mood and QOL may improve while decreasing symptoms of depression and anxiety in HIV^+ individuals given an exercise intervention; however, methodological problems noted in the individual studies (see Table 6.1) make the resulting evidence only modest at best. In addition, the majority of the research has focused primarily on Caucasian males, making the generalizability of the data to other races or genders difficult. As the current recommendations surrounding HIV exercise programs are not significantly different from the recommendations by the American College of Sports Medicine (ACSM) for adults (ACSM, 2000), for other health benefits, it is not unreasonable to provide these recommendations to patients for their potential psychological well-being effects. However, the exercise dose (length × frequency × intensity) to obtain psychological well-being effects (if it exists) may indeed differ from these ACSM recommendations. It has also been suggested that aerobic exercise may be more effective than resistance exercise alone in improving psychological well-being, although no specific hypothesis, as to why, has been advanced (Rojas *et al.*, 2003). Despite the lack of convincing evidence that aerobic exercise affects psychological well-being in HIV$^+$ individuals, it should be considered as a readily available, non-drug therapy intervention to improve physical fitness, as well as possibly psychological well-being.

IMPLICATIONS FOR THE RESEARCHER

Longer-term studies of the effects of aerobic exercise training on QOL (i.e., >12 weeks) should be undertaken to better understand the sustained relationship between HIV and exercise. A more reasonable event horizon for long-term follow-up would be 3–5 years, which would be more similar to studies of heart failure and cancer. This would allow life table and survival analysis to proceed to determine the long-term effects of aerobic exercise on mortality. In addition, due to the high rate of "drop outs" from all of the exercise training studies, future investigations should focus on the characteristics of the "drop outs" from the exercise program, as well as utilize an intention to treat analysis to better understand the true overall value of an exercise program. An important question would be "Are the 'drop outs' in the intervention group (and the control) primarily related to physical, psychological, or both factors?" and researchers should clearly document why drop outs occur. Researchers should attempt to standardize instruments aimed at assessing psychological well-being in HIV, or at least compare the internal validity of these several instruments with each other during the study, similar to the study conducted by Neidig *et al.* (2003). Finally, as the medical therapy of HIV becomes increasingly complex with multiple medications, toxicities, and side effects, appropriate randomization of subjects with much larger numbers in each arm of the study must be achieved to prevent both Type I and Type II statistical errors.

IMPLICATIONS FOR THE EXERCISE PRACTITIONER

Since studies have documented the effectiveness of exercise in improving physical fitness across the span of HIV disease; from asymptomatic HIV$^+$ to full blown AIDS with reduction in lean body mass, the exercise recommendations should mirror the ACSM guidelines for adults. However, the evidence for psychological well-being improvements with exercise are less clear from the available studies and the exercise level recommendations for patients with depression and/or mood disorders, may not be equivalent to the ACSM guidelines. In any event, an exercise program for

HIV$^+$ patients should be a sustained program combining aerobic exercise (i.e., cycling, walking, running, hiking) with a smaller component of resistance training to maximize fitness gains; however, the "dose" of exercise to achieve psychological well-being benefits is not known. With evidence of high drop out among many of the reported studies, there may be scope for recommending a range of exercise doses that are tailored to the needs of this population to maximize adherence.

In any event, the program should be scaled to the current physical status of the patient. A cardiopulmonary exercise test (CPET) should be considered prior to an exercise prescription to identify subtle signs of cardiac or pulmonary disease that could portend early infection, especially in patients above 40 years of age (Stringer, 2000). In addition, regular follow-up CPET (at least annually, and earlier if significant changes occur in physical status or disease state) should occur to allow early detection of systemic disease. Finally, exclusions to this exercise recommendation (e.g., uncontrolled hypertension, peripheral vascular disease, diabetics with severe autonomic neuropathy) should likely follow ACSM recommendations.

IMPLICATIONS FOR THE HEALTH ANALYST AND POLICY MAKER

The implications for health policy are related to the fact that exercise has enormous potential, is widely available, and is an inexpensive non-drug therapy. Improvements in physical and psychological well-being may be achieved in the HIV$^+$ population through this important therapy. Safe and easy-to-use environments for exercise are important for HIV$^-$, as well as HIV$^+$ populations, and must be made increasingly available by policy makers and urban designers. All HIV$^+$ patients should be able to avail themselves of expertise in exercise physiology, exercise prescriptions, resistance exercise training equipment, and trained staff that are aware of proper precautions (i.e., gloves, sterilization strategies) in case of accidental blood loss (American Academy of Pediatrics, 1999). Other precautionary measures are not necessary due to the very low risk of HIV transmission during sporting events as calculated by the American Medical Society for Sports Medicine (AMSSM) and the American Academy of Sports Medicine (AASM) (AMSSM and AASM, 1995).

 ## WHAT WE KNOW SUMMARY

- HIV and AIDS markedly increase the incidence and prevalence of depressive symptoms.
- In the studies reviewed here, aerobic exercise training was associated with quantifiable improvements in aerobic fitness; however, the effects on psychological well-being are less certain. The studies reviewed here have observed a decrease in the rate of depressive symptoms and improved QOL/psychological well-being in HIV$^+$ subjects (regardless of disease stage) using a very wide variety of QOL instruments.
- The exercise program (e.g., dose) to improve fitness should consist of 45 min, three times per week of aerobic exercise combined with a smaller component of resistance training.

- The "dose" (length × duration × intensity) for changes in psychological well-being have not been determined from existing studies.
- "Drop outs" are a significant problem with exercise programs in HIV/AIDS patients and should engender adequate preplanning to prospectively identify barriers to continued participation.
- Aerobic exercise appears to provide greater improvements in psychological well-being when compared to resistance exercises in some studies.

WHAT WE NEED TO KNOW SUMMARY

- The long-term effects of aerobic exercise program (i.e., >12 weeks) on psychological well-being.
- The long-term effects of an aerobic exercise program on mortality, physical, and psychological morbidity.
- The effect that complicated drug regimens (HAART) will have on the importance of aerobic exercise training on psychological well-being in HIV.
- The mechanism of improvements in QOL and psychological well-being with exercise.
- What is the minimum exercise stimulus ("dose") required to generate improvements in psychological well-being.

REFERENCES

American Academy of Pediatrics (1999). Issues related to human immunodeficiency virus transmission in schools, child care, medical settings, the home, and community. *Pediatrics, 104*, 318–324.

American College of Sports Medicine (2000). *ACSM's Guidelines for Exercise Testing and Prescription* (6th edn). Hagerstown, MD: Lippincott, Williams & Wilkins.

AMSSM and AASM (1995). Human immunodeficiency virus and other blood-borne pathogens in sports: the American Medical Society for Sports Medicine (AMSSM) and the American Academy of Sports Medicine (AASM) Joint Position Statement. *Clinical Journal of Sports Medicine, 5*, 199–204.

Antoni, M. H., Schneiderman, H., Fletcher, M. A., Goldstein, D., Ironson, G., and LaPerriere, A. (1990). Psychoneuroimmunology and HIV-1. *Journal of Consulting and Clinical Psychology, 58*, 38–49.

Baigis, J., Korniewicz, D. M., Chase, G., Butz, A., Jacobson, D., and Wu, A. W. (2004). Effectiveness of a home-based exercise intervention for HIV infected adults: a randomized trial. *Journal of the Association of Nurses in AIDS Care, 13*, 33–45.

Beck, A. T. and Steer, R. A. (1993). *Beck Depression Inventory Manual* (6th edn). Philadelphia, PA: Lippincott, Williams & Wilkins.

Borg, S. A. (1982). Psychological basis of perceived exertion. *Medicine, Science, Sports, and Exercise, 14*, 377–381.

Castro, K. G., Ward, J. W., and Slutsker, J. W. (1992). 1993 Revised classification system for HIV infection and expanded surveillance case definition for AIDS among adolescents and adults. *Morbidity and Mortality Weekly Report, 41*, 961–962.

Center for Disease Control (n.d.). *Quick facts: Rapid testing April 2003–April 2004.* Retrieved October 23, 2004, from http://www.cdc.gov

Chesney, M. A. and Folkman, S. (1994). Psychological impact of HIV disease and implications for intervention. *Psychiatry Clinics of North America, 17*, 163–182.

Ciesla, J. A. and Roberts, J. E. (2001). Meta-analysis of the relationship between HIV infection and risk for depressive disorders. *American Journal of Psychiatry, 158*, 725–730.

Diener, E., Larsen, R. J., and Griffin, S. (1985). The satisfaction with life scale. *Journal of Personality Assessment, 49*, 71–75.

Dudgeon, W. D., Phillips, K. D., Bott, C. M., and Hand, G. A. (2004). Physiological and psychological effects of exercise interventions in HIV disease. *AIDS Patient Care and STDs, 18*, 81–98.

Ettl, M., Hays, R. D., Cunningham, W., Shapiro, M. F., and Beck, C. K. (1996). Assessing health-related quality of life in disadvantaged populations. In B. Spiker (Ed.). *Quality of Life and PharmacoEconomics in Clinical Trials* (2nd edn, pp. 595–604). New York: Lippencott Raven Publishers.

Goldberg, D. P. and Hilliar, V. F. (1979). A scaled version of the general health questionnaire. *Psychological Medicine, 9*, 139–145.

Grinspoon, S., Corcoran, C., Parlman, K., Costello, M., Rosenthal, D., Anderson, E. *et al.* (2000). Effects of testosterone and progressive training in eugonadal men with AIDS wasting. *Annals of Internal Medicine, 133*, 348–355.

Johnson, J., Anders, G., Blanton, H., Hawkes, C., Bush, B., McAllister, K. *et al.* (1990). Exercise dysfunction in patients seropositive for the human immunodeficiency virus-1. *American Review of Respiratory Diseases, 141*, 618–622.

LaPerriere, A., Antoni, M. H., Schneiderman, N., Ironson, G., Klimas, N. G., Caralis, P. *et al.* (1990). Exercise intervention attenuates emotional distress and natural killer cell decrements following notification of positive serologic status for HIV-1. *Biofeedback and Self-Regulation, 15*, 229–242.

LaPerriere, A., Fletcher, M. A., Antoni, M. H., Klimas, N. G., Ironson, G., and Schneiderman, H. (1991). Aerobic exercise training in an AIDS risk group. *International Journal of Sports Medicine, 12*, S53–S57.

LaPerriere, A., Antoni, M. H., Ironson, G., Perry, A., McCabe, A., Klimas, N. G. *et al.* (1994a). Effects of aerobic exercise training on lymphocyte subpopulations. *International Journal of Sports Medicine, 15*, S127–S130.

LaPerriere, A., Ironson, G., Antoni, M. H., Schneiderman, N., Klimas, N. G., and Fletcher, M. A. (1994b). Exercise and psychoneuroimmunology. *Medicine, Science, Sports, and Exercise, 26*, 182–190.

Lox, C. L., McAuley, E., and Tucker, R. S. (1995). Exercise as an intervention for enhancing subjective well-being in an HIV-1 population. *Journal of Sports and Exercise Psychology, 17*, 345–362.

MacArthur, R. D., Levine, S. D., and Berk, T. J. (1993). Supervised exercise training improves cardiopulmonary fitness in HIV-infected persons. *Medicine, Science, Sports, and Exercise, 25*, 684–688.

McNair, D. M., Lorr, M., and Dropplemen, L. F. (1981). *EITS Manual of the Profile of Mood States (POMS)*. San Diego, CA: Educational and Industrial Testing Service.

Mars, M. (2003). What limits exercise in HIV positive individuals? *International Sports Medicine Journal, 4*, 1–15.

Namir, S., Wolcott, D., and Fawzy, F. (1987). Coping with AIDS: psychological and health implications. *Journal of Applied Social Psychology, 17*, 309–328.

Neidig, J., Smith, B. A., and Brasher, D. E. (2003). Aerobic exercise training for depressive symptom management in adults living with HIV infection. *Journal of the Association of Nurses in AIDS Care, 14*, 30–40.

Nixon, S., O'Brien, K., Glazier, R. H., and Tynan, A. M. (2003). *Aerobic Exercise Interventions for People with HIV/AIDS (Cochrane Review)*. The Cochrane Library, Issue 4. Oxford: Update Software.

Ostrow, D., Monjan, A., and Joseph, J. (1989). HIV-related symptoms and psychological function in a cohort of homosexual men. *American Journal of Psychiatry*, *146*, 737–742.

Perna, F. M., LaPerriere, A., Klimas, N. G., Makemson, D., Perry, A., Goldstein, A. *et al.* (1999). Cardiopulmonary and CD4 changes in response to exercise training in early symptomatic HIV infection. *Medicine, Science, Sports, and Exercise*, *31*, 973–979.

Pothoff, G., Wasserman, K., and Ostmann, H. (1994). Impairment of exercise capacity in various groups of HIV-infected patients. *Respiration*, *61*, 80–85.

Radloff, L. S. (1977). The CES–D scale: a self report depression scale for research in the general population. *Applied Psychological Measurement*, *1*, 385–401.

Rigsby, L. W., Dishman, R. K., Jackson, A. W., Baclean, G. S., and Raven, P. B. (1992). Effects of exercise training on men seropositive for the human immunodeficiency virus-1. *Medicine, Science, Sports, and Exercise*, *24*, 6–12.

Rojas, R., Schlicht, W., and Hautzinger, M. (2003). Effects of exercise training on quality of life, psychological well-being, immune status, and cardiopulmonary fitness in an HIV-1 positive population. *Journal of Sports and Exercise Psychology*, *25*, 440–455.

Roubenoff, R., Weiss, L., McDermott, A., Heflin, T., Cloutier, G. J., Wood, M. *et al.* (1999). A pilot study of exercise training to reduce trunk fat in adults with HIV associated fat redistribution. *AIDS*, *13*, 1373–1375.

Smith, B. A., Neidig, J., Nickel, J., Mitchell, G. L., Para, M., and Fass, R. (2001). Aerobic exercise: effects on parameters related to fatigue, dyspnea, weight and body composition in HIV-infected adults. *AIDS*, *15*, 693–701.

Strawford, A., Barbieri, T., Van Loan, M., Parks, E., Catlin, D., Barton, N. *et al.* (1999). Resistance exercise and supraphysiologic androgen therapy in eugonadal men with HIV-related weight loss: a randomized controlled trial. *Journal of the American Medical Association*, *281*, 1282–1290.

Stringer, W. W. (1999). HIV and aerobic exercise: current recommendations. *Sports Medicine*, *28*, 387–393.

Stringer, W. W. (2000). Mechanisms of exercise limitation in HIV$^+$ individuals. *Medicine, Science, Sports, and Exercise*, *32*, S412–S421.

Stringer, W. W. (2001). The role of aerobic exercise for HIV$^+$/AIDS patients. *International Sports Medicine Journal*, *1*, 1–5.

Stringer, W. W. (2003). HIV, AIDS, and exercise. In L. Lemura and S. Von Duvillard (Eds). *Medicine and Exercise Science: Clinical Application and Physiological Principals* (1st edn, pp. 455–481). Philadelphia, PA: Lippincott, Williams, & Wilkins.

Stringer, W. W., Berezovskaya, M., O'Brien, W. A., Beck, C. K., and Casaburi, R. (1998). The effect of exercise training on aerobic fitness, immune indices, and quality of life in HIV$^+$ patients. *Medicine, Science, Sports, and Exercise*, *30*, 11–16.

Taylor, A. H. (2000). Physical activity, anxiety, and stress. In S. J. H. Biddle, K. R. Fox, and S. H. Boutcher (Eds). *Physical Activity and Psychological Well-being* (pp. 10–45). London: Routledge.

Vergis, E. N. (2000). Natural history of HIV-1 infection. *Infectious Disease Clinics of North America*, *14*, 809–825.

Watson, D., Clark, L. A., and Tellegen, A. (1998). Development and validation of brief measures of positive and negative affect: the PANAS scales. *Journal of Personality and Social Psychology*, *54*, 1063–1070.

Zander, K., Palitzsch, M., Kirchberger, I., Jagel-Guedes, E., Jager, H., von Steinbuchel, N. *et al.* (1994). The medical outcome study in HIV-infection (MOS-HIV). *AIDS-Forschung (AIFO)*, *5*, 241–246.

CHAPTER 7

Exercise and quality of life in cancer survivors

KERRY S. COURNEYA

In this chapter, the evidence regarding the effects of exercise on quality of life (QOL) in cancer survivors is summarized. Brief overviews of the pathophysiology and epidemiology of cancer is provided before reviewing the major medical treatments for this disease and their implications for QOL. Next, the concept of QOL is discussed and how it has been defined and measured in the cancer field. A brief review of the QOL interventions that are currently available to cancer survivors is offered. After that, the published research on exercise and QOL in cancer survivors up to 2001 is summarized and then a more detailed review of studies published in 2002 and 2003 is included. Subsequently, the possible mechanisms that may account for the generally positive effects of exercise on QOL in cancer survivors are described. Lastly, future research directions for this field and the practical implications of the research are discussed.

PATHOPHYSIOLOGY OF CANCER

Unlike normal cells, cancer cells undergo a series of genetic mutations that allow them to grow and divide indefinitely (Gribbon and Loescher, 2000). As cancer cells accumulate, they often adhere together and develop into a mass called a tumor or neoplasm. There are benign tumors that grow and enlarge only at the site where they began. Malignant or cancerous tumors, however, have the potential to compress, invade, and destroy the normal tissue that surrounds them. Moreover, they are able to spread (i.e., metastasize) throughout the body via the bloodstream or lymph system and form "colony" tumors at new sites. As the cancer continues to spread, it typically invades and destroys the healthy tissue of vital organs (e.g., brain, lung, liver), which ultimately results in death. The term cancer actually represents over 100 diseases that can virtually occur in any tissue or organ in the body. Most cancers however, fall into four major classifications based on the type of cell from which they arise. Carcinomas are cancers that develop from epithelial cells that line the surfaces of the body, glands, and internal organs. They comprise 80–90% of all cancers and include the most common types of cancer such as prostate, colon, lung, cervical, and breast. Cancers can also arise from the cells of the blood (i.e., leukemias), the immune system (i.e., lymphomas), and connective tissues such as bones, tendons, cartilage, fat, and muscle (i.e., sarcomas).

EPIDEMIOLOGY OF CANCER

Cancer is a major public health burden worldwide (Parkin *et al.*, 2001). In the United States alone, over 1.35 million new cases of cancer are expected to be diagnosed in 2004 (American Cancer Society, 2004). The lifetime probability of being diagnosed with cancer in the United States is about 41%. This means that approximately two out of every five Americans will be diagnosed with cancer at some point in their lifetime. Moreover, cancer is the second leading cause of death in America behind heart disease, with over 560,000 deaths from cancer expected in 2004. The four most common cancers – prostate, breast, colorectal, and lung – account for over 50% of all new diagnoses and deaths (see Table 7.1). In terms of demographics, men are slightly more likely to develop and die from cancer than women, but cancer incidence and mortality increases dramatically with age (see Table 7.2). More specifically, about 76% of all cancers are diagnosed in persons aged 55 and older.

Despite the relatively high mortality rates for various cancers, the prospects for surviving the disease have improved significantly over the past few decades due to earlier

Table 7.1 Estimated new cancer cases and deaths for the major cancer sites by sex, United States, 2004

SITE	ESTIMATED NEW CASES			ESTIMATED NEW DEATHS		
	TOTAL	MALE	FEMALE	TOTAL	MALE	FEMALE
All sites	1,368,030	699,560	668,470	563,700	290,890	272,810
Breast	217,440	1,450	215,990	40,580	470	40,110
Prostate	230,110	230,110	—	29,900	29,900	—
Lung	173,770	93,110	80,660	160,440	91,930	68,510
Colorectal	14,694	73,620	73,320	56,730	28,320	28,410

Source: Adapted from the American Cancer Society, 2004.
Note: Excludes basal and squamous cell skin cancers and in situ carcinomas except urinary bladder.

Table 7.2 Percentage of the population developing the most common invasive cancers over selected age intervals by sex, United States, 1998–2000

SITE	GENDER	BIRTH TO 39	40–59	60–79	BIRTH TO DEATH
All sites	Male	1.36	8.03	33.92	44.77
	Female	1.92	9.01	22.61	38.03
Prostate	Male	0.01	2.28	14.20	17.15
Breast	Female	0.44	4.14	7.53	13.36
Lung	Male	0.03	1.02	5.80	7.69
	Female	0.03	0.79	3.93	5.73
Colorectal	Male	0.06	0.86	3.94	5.88
	Female	0.06	0.67	3.05	5.49

Source: Adapted from the American Cancer Society, 2004.
Note: Excludes basal and squamous cell skin cancers and in situ carcinomas except urinary bladder.

detection and better treatments. The most recent estimate of the five year relative survival rate across all cancers and disease stages is 63% (American Cancer Society, 2004). This figure climbs to over 90% for some of the most common cancers (e.g., prostate, breast, and colorectal) if they are detected early (see Table 7.3). The high incidence rates and good survival rates have resulted in almost 10 million cancer survivors currently alive in the United States. Parenthetically, throughout this chapter the term cancer survivor – as suggested by the National Coalition for Cancer Survivorship – is used to refer to any individual diagnosed with cancer, from the time of discovery and for the rest of life.

MEDICAL TREATMENTS FOR CANCER

Although the prognosis for surviving cancer is often very good, it almost always requires medical intervention. The most common treatment modalities for cancer are surgery,

Table 7.3 Five-year relative survival rates for the most common cancers by stage at diagnosis, United States, 1992–1999				
SITE	ALL STAGES (%)	LOCAL (%)	REGIONAL (%)	DISTANT (%)
Prostate	97.5	100.0	100.0	34.0
Breast	86.6	97.0	78.7	23.3
Colorectal	62.3	90.1	65.5	9.2
Lung	14.9	48.7	16.0	2.1

Source: Adapted from the American Cancer Society, 2004.
Note: Rates are adjusted for normal life expectancy and are based on cases diagnosed from 1992–1999 followed through 2000.

radiation therapy, and systemic (i.e., drug) therapy. These medical interventions have documented survival advantages but they can also negatively affect the QOL. Surgery is the oldest and most common cancer therapy that is still in use today (Frogge and Cunning, 2000). More individuals are cured by surgery than by any other cancer therapy. Unfortunately, surgery is only successful if the cancer is localized to a small area. There can be significant morbidity associated with surgery depending on the location and extent of the operation (e.g., wound complications, infections, loss of function, decreased range of motion, diarrhea, dyspnea, pain, numbness, lymphedema, fatigue, anxiety).

Radiation therapy has been used to treat cancer since the early 1900s (Hilderley, 2000). Approximately 60% of cancer survivors will receive radiation therapy at some point during their treatments (Maher, 2000). Radiation therapy can cure some cancers if they are localized and it can also provide palliative relief if the cancer is incurable. External beam radiation therapy, the most common method of delivering radiation, is typically delivered in repeated small doses (i.e., fractions) over a 5–8 week period in order to maximize the killing of cancer cells and minimize the damage to normal cells. Nevertheless, toxicity to healthy tissues does occur, and it is dependent on the dose and site that is irradiated (Maher, 2000). Radiation therapy can cause both acute toxicities and late effects including pain, blistering, reduced elasticity, decreased range of motion, nausea, fatigue, dry mouth, diarrhea, lung fibrosis, and cardiomyopathy (Maher, 2000).

Unfortunately, up to 60% of cancer survivors have micrometastatic disease at the time of diagnosis (Frogge and Cunning, 2000). That is, the disease has already spread from the original site but it is undetectable by standard diagnostic methods. Consequently, systemic therapy (i.e., drugs) is prescribed to many cancer survivors. The three major types of systemic therapy are chemotherapy, endocrine or hormone therapy, and biologic or immunotherapy. Chemotherapy is usually administered intravenously or orally and is given in repeated courses or cycles of 2–4 weeks apart over a 3–6 month period. Chemotherapy may cause significant side effects including fatigue, anorexia, nausea, anemia, neutropenia, thrombocytopenia, peripheral neuropathies, ataxia, alopecia, and cardiotoxicity (Camp-Sorrell, 2000). The incidence and severity of these side effects depends on the type of drugs, mechanisms of action, drug dosage, administration schedule, presence of other comorbidities, and the use of supportive care interventions (Camp-Sorrell, 2000). The side effects from chemotherapy can appear immediately, within a few weeks or months, or even years after treatment has been completed (i.e., late effects). Moreover, the side effects that occur during treatments can either dissipate quickly after treatment (i.e., acute) or linger long after treatments (i.e., chronic).

Hormone therapy is usually administered orally (continuously or intermittently) for many years and can have significant side effects such as weight gain, muscle loss, proximal muscle weakness, fat accumulation in the trunk and face, osteoporosis, fatigue, hot flashes, and increased susceptibility to infection. Lastly, biologic therapies are the newest treatments and influence the body's own defense mechanisms to act against cancer cells or potentiate the effects of other drugs (Battiato and Wheeler, 2000). These treatments tend to be better tolerated than chemotherapy but can still produce significant side effects similar to chemotherapy.

More commonly, combinations of cancer therapies (i.e., surgery, radiotherapy, and systemic therapy) are used to treat cancer. The timing and sequence of the treatments varies depending on the cancer and its stage. It is possible that some cancer survivors may be treated on multiple occasions with multiple modalities, either concurrently or sequentially, for many months or years. Consequently, it is easy to see that such prolonged and intensive medical treatments may take a heavy toll on QOL.

QOL IN CANCER SURVIVORS

The concept of QOL has significant meaning for cancer survivors and has risen to prominence in the cancer field over the past two decades. QOL has become a legitimate and important endpoint in clinical trials of cancer survivors and in cancer care practice itself (Ferrans, 2000). Unfortunately, QOL is a difficult concept to characterize and there is no universal agreement on its definition. Farquhar (1995) has noted that many QOL definitions can be placed into two broad categories: global definitions and component definitions. Global definitions focus on overall happiness and satisfaction with life without making reference to any particular component of life. Most cancer researchers have not adopted this broad and overarching definition of QOL. On the other hand, component definitions break down QOL into a series of component parts that are thought to be essential to QOL. Most cancer researchers have adopted this definition of QOL (Ferrans, 2000), although there is no consensus on the number and nature of QOL components that are relevant for cancer survivors. The most commonly mentioned components of QOL in the cancer field include physical, functional, emotional, cognitive, spiritual, and social. Farquhar (1995) has noted that such component definitions are likely to contribute to the global evaluations of QOL. Figure 7.1 depicts how this notion might be conceptualized in the exercise domain.

There is also agreement among practitioners that QOL is both personal and subjective (Ferrans, 2000). Consequently, QOL is primarily measured by self-report. Although some cancer researchers have used generic QOL measures such as the Short-Form Health Survey (SF-36; Ware and Sherbourne, 1992), most have adopted one of the many cancer-specific QOL measures that have been developed over the past two

Figure 7.1 Schematic representation of the associations between exercise, QOL components, and global QOL.

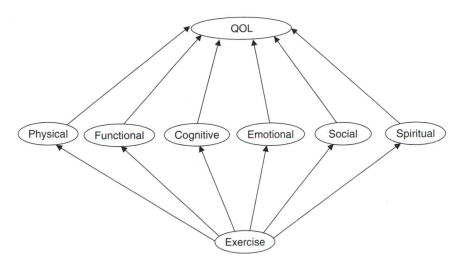

decades. Although too numerous to mention each by name, the most common cancer-specific QOL measures include the Cancer Rehabilitation Evaluation System (CARES, Schag and Heinrich, 1990), the European Organization for Research and Treatment of Cancer Quality of Life Questionnaire (EORTC QLQ-C30; Aaronson *et al.*, 1993), the Functional Living Index – Cancer (FLIC; Schipper *et al.*, 1984), and the Functional Assessment of Cancer Therapy scale (FACT; Cella *et al.*, 1993). All these scales assess multidimensional components of QOL (e.g., physical, functional, emotional, and social well-being) with items that are specifically relevant to cancer survivors. The FACT scale appears to be the most popular for exercise researchers.

CURRENT INTERVENTIONS TO ENHANCE QOL IN CANCER SURVIVORS

The acceptance of QOL as an important endpoint in cancer care has spurred a major research effort into strategies to maintain and enhance QOL in cancer survivors both during and after treatments. In attempting to delineate the potential role of exercise in this regard, it is important to be aware of other QOL interventions that are currently offered to cancer survivors. This knowledge will allow exercise researchers to address the issue of how exercise might complement existing QOL interventions. Here, a brief overview of some of the currently accepted QOL interventions for cancer survivors is provided.

The most common psychosocial QOL interventions for cancer survivors include cognitive-behavioral therapies (e.g., relaxation training, meditation, hypnotherapy), informational and educational strategies (e.g., procedural, medical), counselling or psychotherapy (e.g., psychodynamic, existential), peer and professional support groups, and other alternative treatments (e.g., music therapy, aromatherapy, art therapy). An early meta-analysis of 45 randomized controlled trials (RCTs) found little ($ds = 0.19–0.28$) but significant effects on emotional well-being, functional well-being, symptoms, and global QOL (Meyer and Mark, 1995). There were, however, no significant differences among the different categories of interventions (e.g., cognitive-behavioral, informational/educational, psychotherapy). A more recent meta-analysis used a different analytical technique and included 37 RCTs (Rehse and Pukrop, 2003). This meta-analysis found an overall moderate-to-large effect ($d = 0.65$) of these interventions on QOL. In additional moderator analyses, the researchers reported that the effects were larger for men – informational/educational interventions, longer interventions, self-report measures of QOL, functional versus emotional adjustment, and better quality studies (Rehse and Pukrop, 2003). However, in a subsequent multivariate analysis, only length of the intervention was predictive of a larger effect.

In terms of specific psychosocial interventions, Luebbert *et al.* (2001) conducted a meta-analysis of 15 RCTs focusing exclusively on relaxation training in cancer survivors. Their analysis showed significant moderate effects ($ds = 0.34–0.55$) on blood pressure, pulse rate, nausea, pain, depression, tension, anxiety, mood, and hostility, but not fatigue, confusion, or vigor. Moreover, a qualitative review of group psychotherapy concluded that there is compelling evidence that this intervention improves the QOL of cancer survivors (Blake-Mortimer *et al.*, 1999). Clearly, there is good data to support the utility of psychosocial interventions in enhancing QOL in cancer survivors. One limitation of this genre of QOL interventions, however, is that they are largely psychosocial in nature and less likely to address the physical and functional problems encountered by cancer survivors (Courneya and Friedenreich, 1997a,b).

The primary intervention available to address the physical and functional problems of cancer survivors is physical therapy. Physical therapy is a mainstay of supportive care interventions for cancer survivors and has been shown to enhance physical and functional outcomes (Gerber *et al.*, 2001). The main limitation of physical therapy is that it has tended to focus on rehabilitating specific impairments, such as range of motion, chewing and swallowing, and lymphedema, rather than general physical conditioning. Lastly, medical treatments also play an important role as QOL interventions. For example, drugs have been developed to address QOL issues in cancer survivors, such as pain, nausea and vomiting, depression, and anemia/fatigue. The main limitation with drugs and other medical interventions is that they often have side effects of their own that cause problems. To address some of the limitations of current QOL interventions for cancer survivors, researchers have begun to examine the utility of exercise in this population.

EXERCISE AND QOL IN CANCER SURVIVORS

There have been many recent reviews on the topic of exercise and QOL in cancer survivors and the reader is directed to these reviews for a detailed analysis of studies published prior to 2002 (e.g., Courneya, 2003; Courneya *et al.*, 2002, 2004). Here, a summary of that literature is provided before a more detailed review of the studies published in 2002 and 2003. The initial summary of the earlier research is based on the review by Courneya (2003). Following Courneya (2003), the review is divided into breast versus "other" cancer survivors, and into two time periods – during versus posttreatment.

Breast cancer survivors during treatment

Courneya (2003) located 14 studies that examined the effects of exercise in breast cancer survivors during treatment. Twelve of the studies tested exercise interventions and all but one of the interventions was conducted during chemotherapy or combined adjuvant therapy. The intervention designs were equally divided between RCTs and uncontrolled trials (i.e., pre-post) and the sample sizes ranged from 10 to 99. The studies were equally divided between supervised and home-based exercise programs. Almost all studies tested an aerobic exercise intervention based on traditional exercise prescription guidelines. The length of the exercise interventions ranged from 6 to 26 weeks. The studies examined a wide range of biopsychosocial outcomes including functional capacity, body composition, mood states (e.g., anxiety, depression), symptoms (e.g., nausea, fatigue, sleep disturbances, body dissatisfaction), and general QOL. The specific QOL benefits that were demonstrated included fatigue, nausea, physical well-being, functional well-being, satisfaction with life, and overall QOL.

Courneya (2003) noted that these studies were generally of good quality, consisting of RCT design with appropriate controls, supervised exercise sessions, an appropriate exercise stimulus, objective fitness indicators, and validated psychometric scales. The primary methodological limitations he noted were: (a) the RCT methodology was not well described (e.g., enrollment, randomization, blinding, analytical plan), (b) the samples were small and convenient, and (c) the exercise interventions did not coincide with the medical treatment in its entirety. This last point means that we do not have definitive data on the effects of an exercise intervention during an entire treatment protocol.

Breast cancer survivors after treatment

Courneya (2003) reported on 14 studies that examined exercise in breast cancer survivors after treatment although only 7 actually tested an exercise intervention. Moreover, most of the intervention studies were uncontrolled trials. The sample sizes ranged from 12 to 28 and most of the exercise interventions were supervised. Most studies tested aerobic exercise although two examined a combined aerobic and resistance training program. Most studies followed traditional exercise prescription guidelines with one study examining the effects of an acute bout of exercise. The most common outcomes studied were biologic (e.g., immune system, physical fitness, lymphedema) with lesser attention paid to psychosocial variables (e.g., anxiety, depression, satisfaction with life). In terms of the QOL results, the studies demonstrated improvements with exercise in depression, anxiety, mood, self-esteem, physical well-being, satisfaction with life, and overall QOL.

Compared to the studies during breast cancer treatment, Courneya (2003) characterized the studies after breast cancer treatment as generally less methodologically rigorous. Only 2 of the 14 studies had controls and 8 of the studies relied on self-reports of exercise. Other limitations of the intervention studies include small convenience samples, relatively short exercise interventions, heterogeneous participants that spanned the survivor continuum from several months to many years postdiagnosis, and limited follow-up. Finally, the observational studies were mostly cross-sectional.

Other cancer survivors during treatments

Courneya (2003) reviewed 10 studies that examined the effects of exercise in other cancer survivor groups during treatments. Six studies examined mixed cancer survivors (e.g., breast, testicular, non-Hodgkin's lymphoma, multiple myeloma) immediately after high dose chemotherapy and stem cell transplantation; and one study each examined adolescents with mixed cancers (e.g., leukemia) on chemotherapy, adults with mixed cancers (e.g., Hodgkin's and non-Hodgkin's lymphoma) on mixed treatments, postsurgical stomach cancer survivors, and postsurgical colorectal cancer survivors on chemotherapy. Seven studies tested interventions and five of those used an RCT design. The sample sizes ranged from 5 to 70 and most interventions tested supervised exercise. Six studies tested an aerobic exercise intervention while one focused on resistance exercise. The length of the exercise programs ranged from 2 to 16 weeks. The studies examined a wide range of biopsychosocial outcomes including functional capacity, body composition, natural killer cell cytotoxic activity, mood states (e.g., anxiety and depression), symptoms (e.g., nausea, fatigue, pain), and general QOL. The reported QOL benefits included improvements in pain, anxiety, depression, vigor, anger, fatigue/energy, physical well-being, functional well-being, emotional well-being, social well-being, and satisfaction with life. Courneya (2003) noted similar strengths and weaknesses of these studies as the studies on exercise during breast cancer treatment.

Other cancer survivors after treatments

Courneya (2003) reported on nine studies that examined exercise in other cancer survivors after treatments. Four studies examined mixed cancer survivors (e.g., breast, non-Hodgkin's lymphoma, leukemia, prostate), two studies examined mixed childhood/adolescent cancer survivors (e.g., Hodgkin's, lymphoma, leukemia), and one study each examined prostate cancer survivors, head/neck cancer survivors, and colorectal cancer survivors. Six studies tested interventions but none were RCTs. The sample sizes ranged from 6 to 32 and most of the studies reported a supervised aerobic exercise intervention following a traditional exercise prescription. The interventions examined biopsychosocial outcomes including functional capacity, body composition, hemoglobin levels, and general QOL. In terms of QOL results, exercise resulted in improvements in fatigue, depression, anxiety, physical appearance, and overall QOL. As a group, the studies on exercise after treatments in other cancer survivors were not as methodologically rigorous as the studies during treatment.

RECENT RESEARCH

A literature search was conducted in February 2004 to locate more recent research published in 2002 and 2003. The CD-ROM databases of CancerLit, CINAHL, HERA-CLES, MEDLINE, PsycINFO, and SPORT Discus were searched using key words that related to cancer (i.e., cancer, oncology, tumor, neoplasm, carcinoma), the postdiagnosis time period (i.e., rehabilitation, therapy, adjuvant therapy, treatment, intervention, palliation), and exercise (i.e., exercise, physical activity, physical therapy, sport, weight training). To be included in the review, a study had to be published in a peer-reviewed journal in 2002 or 2003 and examine aerobic or resistance exercise training. Sixteen studies were located that examined the effects of exercise on QOL in cancer survivors (see Table 7.4).

The 16 recent studies have examined breast, prostate, colorectal, and mixed (i.e., more than one cancer) cancer survivors. The ages of participants ranged from the early 20s to 80s but most participants were between 40 and 69 years old. Most of the studies included cancer survivors at various stages of the cancer experience (e.g., during treatments, soon after treatments, long-term survivors). Study designs consisted of nine RCTs with usual care controls, two non-RCTs with usual care controls, and four pre-post designs with no controls. The sample sizes ranged from 9 to 135. In 13 studies the exercise program was supervised whereas in three it was home-based.

Nine studies tested an aerobic exercise training program, six tested a combined aerobic and resistance training program, and one tested resistance training alone. The majority of studies followed traditional exercise prescription guidelines in terms of frequency, intensity, and duration. The length of the exercise interventions ranged from 3 to 24 weeks. The studies examined a wide range of biopsychosocial outcomes including functional outcomes (e.g., aerobic capacity, body composition, flexibility, strength, energy expenditure), QOL, mood states (e.g., anxiety, depression), sleep patterns, and biologic outcomes (e.g., hemoglobin, immune function). In terms of results, almost all studies showed some statistically significant improvements after completion of the exercise program including improvements in exercise capacity, body composition, overall QOL, QOL subdomains, mood states, metabolic hormones, and fatigue.

Overall, the quantity and quality of research on exercise in cancer survivors has increased significantly over the past two years. The majority of recent studies have tested supervised exercise interventions and have employed RCT methodology. Moreover, almost all studies have obtained objective fitness assessments and used well-validated QOL measures. Nevertheless, there are still significant limitations in these studies including poorly described RCT methodologies, small convenience samples, relatively short exercise interventions, exercise interventions that did not coincide with the treatment in its entirety, heterogeneous participants that spanned the survivor continuum from several months to many years posttreatment, and limited follow-up.

MECHANISMS OF ENHANCED QOL FROM EXERCISE IN CANCER SURVIVORS

Overall, the results of almost 70 studies to date suggest that exercise can improve QOL in cancer survivors both during and after treatments. Several biopsychosocial

Table 7.4 Studies of exercise in cancer survivors (January 2002–December 2003)

AUTHOR	SAMPLE	DESIGN	EXERCISE PROGRAM	OUTCOME VARIABLES	RESULTS
Observational studies					
Pinto *et al.* (2002)	69 breast cancer survivors, % on treatment not reported	Prospective Cohort	Self-reported over 12 months	Mood states, symptoms, social support, QOL, coping, exercise participation	Exercising at or below recommended levels versus no exercise associated with higher levels of physical functioning
Intervention studies					
Burnham and Wilcox (2002)	18 posttreatment breast/colon patients	RCT	Supervised low intensity (25–35% HRR) or moderate intensity (40–50% HRR) aerobic exercise program, 3×/week, for 10 weeks	Aerobic capacity, body fat, flexibility, QOL, symptoms	Exercise groups ↑ aerobic capacity, flexibility, ↓ body fat, ↑ QOL compared with control. No differences between exercise groups
Kolden *et al.* (2002)	40 postsurgical breast cancer survivors, 65% were receiving chemotherapy	Pre-post test	Supervised group exercise training including aerobic and resistance training, 3×/week for 16 weeks	Aerobic capacity, QOL, body fat, anxiety, depression, strength, flexibility	Exercise training ↑ flexibility, aerobic capacity, strength and multiple QOL subscales
Coleman *et al.* (2003)	16 Multiple Myeloma cancer survivors receiving HDC and BMT	RCT	Combined aerobic and strength training program, 3×/week for 30–60 min for 6 months	Mood states, sleep, body composition, aerobic capacity and strength	Exercise training ↑ lean body composition versus control. Trends towards a difference for multiple QOL outcomes
Courneya *et al.* (2003a)	93 postsurgical colorectal cancer survivors, 66% were receiving adjuvant therapy	RCT	Home-based exercise program, 3–5×/week, moderate intensity for 20–30 mins	QOL, SWL, depression, anxiety, aerobic fitness, fatigue, body composition, flexibility	Primary analysis revealed no significant differences. Ancillary analyses (↑ versus ↓ fitness) differences on overall QOL and multiple subdomains

Study	Design	Population	Intervention	Outcomes	Results
Courneya et al. (2003b)	RCT	96 mixed cancer survivors attending group therapy, 44% were receiving radiation or chemotherapy	Home-based aerobic exercise program, 3–5×/week, moderate intensity for 20–30 mins	QOL, SWL, depression, anxiety, aerobic fitness, fatigue, body composition, flexibility	Exercise group showed ↑ in FWB, ↓ fatigue, body composition compared with control
Courneya et al. (2003c)	RCT	52 postmenopausal breast cancer survivors, 46% on hormone therapy	Supervised moderate intensity (70–75%) aerobic exercise program, 3×/week for 15 weeks	Aerobic capacity, QOL, body composition	Exercise group showed ↑ in VO_{2peak}, QOL and multiple QOL subdomains versus control
Dimeo et al. (2003)	Pre-post test	66 mixed cancer survivors receiving conventional or HDC	Daily supervised moderate intensity aerobic exercise program during hospitalization (30 ± 10 days)	Physical performance (walking speed, RPE), hemoglobin concentration	Physical performance remained unchanged during hospitalization, hbg ↓ during this time
Fairey et al. (2003)	RCT	52 postmenopausal breast cancer survivors, 46% on hormone therapy	Supervised moderate intensity (70–75%) aerobic exercise program, 3×/week for 15 weeks	Fasting insulin, glucose, IGF-1, 2, IGFBP-1, 3 and molar ratio	Exercise group showed ↓ IGF-1, ↑ IGFBP-3 and molar ratio versus control
Hayes et al. (2003a)	Non-RCT	12 mixed cancer patients receiving HDC	Combined supervised moderate aerobic and resistance training program, 3×/week for 12 weeks. Controls performed stretching	Energy expenditure – singly and doubly labeled water technique and body composition	Exercise led to ↑ in TEE, FFM versus control
Hayes et al. (2003b)	Non-RCT	12 mixed cancer patients receiving HDC	Combined supervised moderate aerobic and resistance training program, 3×/week for 12 weeks. Controls performed stretching	White blood cell count, lymphocyte function, CD3+, CD4+, CD8+	No significant effects of exercise on any immunologic outcome versus control

(Table 7.4 continued)

Table 7.4 Continued

AUTHOR	SAMPLE	DESIGN	EXERCISE PROGRAM	OUTCOME VARIABLES	RESULTS
McKenzie and Kalda (2003)	14 posttreatment breast cancer survivors with unilateral upper extremity lymphedema	RCT	Supervised progressive 8-week upper body resistance and aerobic exercise training program	Lymphedema and QOL	Exercise resulted in no changes in arm circumference or arm volume. Exercise ↑ in 4 SF-36 subdomains versus control
Oldervoll et al. (2003)	9 posttreatment fatigued Hodgkins cancer survivors	Pre-post test	Home-based aerobic exercise training program 3×/week, 40–60 min for 20 weeks	Aerobic capacity, lung function, fatigue, QOL	Exercise led to ↑ in aerobic capacity, physical functioning and ↓ in fatigue
Pinto et al. (2003)	21 posttreatment breast cancer survivors, % receiving treatment not reported	RCT	Supervised moderate intensity aerobic exercise program, 3×/week for 12 weeks	Aerobic capacity, mood states, affect, body esteem	Exercise led to ↑ in body image, and trends for fitness and distress versus control at posttreatment
Segal et al. (2003)	155 prostate cancer survivors on Androgen Deprivation Therapy	RCT	Supervised progressive, moderate intensity resistance training program, 3×/week for 12 weeks	Fatigue, QOL, strength, body composition	Resistance training led to ↓ fatigue, ↑ QOL and upper and lower body strength versus control
Young-McCaughan et al. (2003)	46 mixed cancer survivors, 24% were undergoing treatment	Pre-post test	Combined aerobic and strength training program, 2×/week for 12 weeks	Aerobic capacity, sleep patterns and QOL	Exercise led to ↑ in aerobic capacity, sleep patterns and QOL

Notes: HRR = heart rate reserve; SWL = satisfaction with life; FWB = functional well-being; RPE = rating of perceived exertion; IGF = insulin-like growth factor; IGFBP = IGF binding protein; TEE = total energy expenditure; FFM = fat free mass; HDC = high dose chemotherapy; CD = cluster designation.

Figure 7.2 Model of exercise and QOL in cancer survivors during treatment.

QOL	General (i.e., noncontent-specific) happiness and satisfaction with life
↑	
Symptom distress	Psychological/emotional well-being (e.g., anxiety, depression, anger, hope, pride)
↑	
Symptom interference	Functional well-being (e.g., activities of daily living, leisure activities, work), social well-being (i.e., interaction with others), spiritual well-being (e.g., meaning, purpose)
↑	
Symptom occurrence	Physical well-being (e.g., nausea, pain, fatigue, dyspnea, insomnia, poor appetite, constipation, diarrhea, weight change, asthenia, cachexia), cognitive well-being (e.g., attention, confusion)
↑	
Mechanisms	Biologic (e.g., hemoglobin, physical fitness), psychologic (e.g., self-efficacy, distraction), Social (e.g., interaction, support)
↑	
Exercise	Type, amount (frequency, intensity, duration), progression, context (i.e., physical and social environment)

Source: Reprinted with permission from Courneya, 2001.

mechanisms may explain the QOL improvements in cancer survivors that result from exercise training. Courneya (2001) has proposed a simple organizational model on how exercise might enhance QOL during cancer treatment (see Figure 7.2). First, exercise may alter one of the many hypothesized biopsychosocial mechanisms thought to underlie improved coping and adjustment to cancer (e.g., fitness, self-efficacy, social interaction). In turn, changes in these biopsychosocial mechanisms may alleviate or prevent the occurrence of many of the common symptoms and side effects associated with cancer and its treatments (e.g., fatigue, insomnia, pain, anorexia). Amelioration of these effects may then positively impact a patient's ability to perform activities of daily living, leisure activities, interactions with others, and so on. Finally, enhanced physical and social activities may improve psychological distress/well-being (e.g., anxiety, depression) thereby improving overall QOL.

Only two studies have examined the potential mechanisms of change between exercise and QOL in cancer survivors. Schwartz (1999) examined the associations among exercise, fatigue, and QOL in 27 breast cancer survivors who participated in an 8 week home-based exercise program during their chemotherapy treatments. The exercise program consisted of aerobic activities performed at low-to-moderate intensity for 15–30 min, 3–4 days per week. Exercise behavior was measured by a functional fitness test (i.e., the 12 min walk test). To examine mediation, QOL was regressed on exercise (i.e., fitness) and fatigue using a stepwise regression analysis. Results showed that only fatigue entered the regression equation. While this analytical technique is not consistent with the recommendations for testing mediation by Baron and Kenny (1986), and a functional fitness test is not an ideal exercise measure, the results do suggest that the

Figure 7.3 Mediation of QOL by peak oxygen consumption from the REHAB Trial.

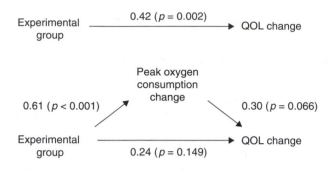

Source: Adapted from Courneya *et al.* (2003c).

effects of exercise/fitness on QOL may be mediated by fatigue. The small sample and observational design, however, preclude any definitive conclusions from being drawn.

More recently, Courneya *et al.* (2003c) conducted a RCT to determine the effects of a 15 week exercise training program on cardiovascular fitness and QOL in 53 post-menopausal breast cancer survivors who had completed adjuvant therapy with or without current hormone therapy use. They reported significant effects of the intervention on various fitness indices including peak oxygen consumption and peak power output, and various psychosocial measures including QOL, fatigue, happiness, and self-esteem. Multiple regression analyses were used to provide a statistical test of the possible mediating role of fitness following the guidelines of Baron and Kenny (1986).

For change in peak oxygen consumption as the mediator, there was evidence of statistical mediation for changes in QOL (see Figure 7.3) and the trial outcome index (not presented), and evidence of failed mediation for self-esteem (see Figure 7.4). For change in peak power output as the mediator, there was evidence of statistical mediation for change in fatigue (see Figure 7.5) and the trial outcome index (not presented), and evidence of failed mediation for self-esteem (see Figure 7.6). Results for the other psychosocial outcomes were inconclusive. These data suggest that fitness changes may mediate the effects of exercise on fatigue and QOL in cancer survivors. The self-esteem changes, however, were independent of fitness changes and may have resulted from increased social interaction or a sense of accomplishment in completing the exercise program. Taken together, the studies by Schwartz (1999) and Courneya *et al.* (2003c) support one possible mechanism for how exercise may enhance QOL in cancer survivors, namely, by increasing fitness and reducing fatigue (i.e., exercise → fitness → fatigue → QOL).

FUTURE RESEARCH DIRECTIONS

There is a growing interest in the possible role of exercise in enhancing QOL in cancer survivors. Preliminary research suggests that exercise may be an effective QOL intervention, particularly for breast cancer survivors and for the posttreatment time period

Figure 7.4 Failed mediation of self-esteem by peak oxygen consumption from the REHAB Trial.

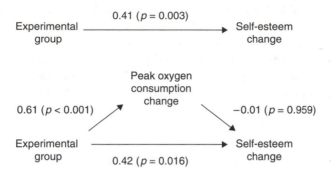

Source: Adapted from Courneya *et al.* (2003c).

Figure 7.5 Mediation of fatigue by peak power output from the REHAB Trial.

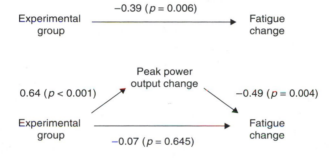

Source: Adapted from Courneya *et al.* (2003c).

Figure 7.6 Failed mediation of self-esteem by peak power output from the REHAB Trial.

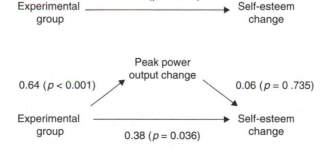

Source: Adapted from Courneya *et al.* (2003c).

in general. Moreover, the beneficial effects of exercise may extend beyond those provided by group psychotherapy alone (Courneya *et al.*, 2003b). It also seems that at least part of the beneficial effects of exercise on QOL are due to improvements in fitness and reductions in fatigue. Unfortunately, the studies are few in number and of limited quality. Encouragingly, more recent research has increased in both quantity and quality.

Future research is needed using rigorous RCT methodology to definitively answer questions concerning the role of exercise in enhancing QOL in cancer survivors both during and after treatment. Research should be extended beyond breast cancer survivors to many other cancer groups who may benefit from exercise. For breast cancer survivors, there is sufficient evidence to warrant second generation studies focusing on more specific questions, such as the optimal timing, type, volume, progression, and context for exercise. Research should also be extended beyond high-dose treatments with stem cell support to many other therapies that cancer survivors endure (e.g., radiation therapy, hormone therapy, biologic therapy). Lastly, studies are needed to further elucidate the mechanisms of change in QOL and to compare and integrate exercise with other currently accepted QOL interventions.

IMPLICATIONS FOR PRACTITIONERS

Based on the current evidence, the American Cancer Society has recommended regular exercise to all cancer survivors (Brown *et al.*, 2003). There are several special precautions for cancer survivors; therefore, the reader is referred to previous published guidelines for these safety issues (Courneya *et al.*, 2000, 2002). In general, exercise during adjuvant therapy is a major struggle for cancer survivors (e.g., Courneya and Friedenreich, 1997a,b) but it is still likely that benefits can be realized (Courneya, 2003). We have recommended low-to-moderate intensity exercise performed 3–5 days per week for 20–30 min each time, depending on baseline fitness levels and treatment toxicities (Courneya *et al.*, 2000, 2002). The exercise should be of moderate intensity in the range of 55–75% of maximal heart rate. Unfortunately, many cancer survivors receiving chemotherapy experience tachycardia, which makes heart rate alone an unreliable indicator of exercise intensity. Consequently, it may be also useful to monitor intensity with a rating of perceived exertion scale using the range of "somewhat hard" to "hard." The preferred exercise choice in cancer survivors is walking (Jones and Courneya, 2002) and this activity will likely be sufficient to meet the recommended intensity for most of the cancer survivors on adjuvant therapy. Exercise progression in cancer survivors during adjuvant therapy is unpredictable and does not always follow a linear course given the accumulating side effects of most cancer therapies. Cancer survivors should exercise to tolerance during adjuvant therapy, including reducing intensity and performing exercise in shorter durations (e.g., 10 min) if needed.

After treatments have been completed and many acute toxicities have dissipated, most of the cancer survivors can probably be recommended the public health guidelines from the American College of Sports Medicine and the United States Centers for Disease Control (American College of Sports Medicine, 1998). These organizations propose two different prescriptions for achieving health through physical activity. The more traditional prescription is to perform at least 20 min of continuous vigorous intensity exercise (i.e., ≥80% of maximal heart rate) on at least 3 days per week. The alternative prescription is to accumulate at least 30 min of moderate intensity exercise (i.e., 60–80% of maximal heart rate) in durations of at least 10 min on most (i.e., at least 5), preferably all, days of the week. Exercise trials in cancer survivors have generally followed the traditional prescription and there is some evidence that QOL benefits may be enhanced if cardiovascular adaptations occur (Courneya *et al.*, 2003c). Nevertheless, in the absence of clinical trials comparing the two prescriptions in cancer survivors, it seems reasonable to expect both the exercise prescriptions to yield health benefits.

WHAT WE KNOW SUMMARY

- The number of cancer survivors will continue to increase in the coming decades.
- Cancer and its treatments often have negative effects on QOL.
- Exercise has been shown to improve QOL, especially in breast cancer survivors, and especially after treatments have been completed.
- Exercise may improve QOL in cancer survivors beyond the benefits of group psychotherapy.
- Reduced fatigue may be one of the key factors explaining why exercise enhances QOL in cancer survivors.
- Exercise interventions that increase physical fitness may result in even greater improvements in QOL.

WHAT WE NEED TO KNOW SUMMARY

- What is the effect of exercise on QOL in cancer survivor groups other than breast (e.g., prostate, colorectal, lung, endometrial)?
- What is the effect of exercise on QOL during cancer treatments other than dose-intensive chemotherapy with stem cell support (e.g., external beam radiation therapy, brachytherapy, conventional chemotherapy, hormone therapy, biologic therapy)?
- What is the safety, feasibility, and efficacy of exercise for cancer survivors with advanced disease receiving palliative care?
- What is the optimal time course for initiating exercise in cancer survivors (e.g., before treatment, during treatment, immediately after treatment, 3–6 months posttreatment)?
- What is the optimal type, volume, progression, and context of exercise for optimizing QOL in cancer survivors?
- Which cancer survivors are likely to benefit the most from exercise (e.g., early disease stage, previous exercisers, younger age)?
- How does exercise compare to other interventions known to enhance QOL in cancer survivors (e.g., group psychotherapy, relaxation training, drugs)? Are the effects of exercise redundant or complementary (additive) to these interventions?

- What are the major determinants of exercise in cancer survivors (e.g., demographic, medical, social cognitive, environmental)?
- What interventions will be most effective in increasing exercise in cancer survivors (e.g., persuasive communications, environmental supports, oncologist recommendation, behavior modification strategies)?

REFERENCES

Aaronson, N. K., Ahmedzai, S., Bergman, B., Bullinger, M., Cull, A., Duez, N. J. *et al.* (1993). The European Organization for Research and Treatment of Cancer QLQ-C30: a quality-of life instrument for use in international clinical trials in oncology. *Journal of the National Cancer Institute*, *85*, 365–376.

American Cancer Society (2004). *Cancer Facts and Figures 2004*. Atlanta, GA: American Cancer Society.

American College of Sports Medicine Position Stand (1998). The recommended quantity and quality of exercise for developing and maintaining cardiorespiratory and muscular fitness, and flexibility in healthy adults. *Medicine and Science in Sports and Exercise*, *30*, 975–991.

Baron, R. M. and Kenny, D. A. (1986). The moderator-mediator variable distinction in social psychological research: conceptual, strategic, and statistical considerations. *Journal of Personality and Social Psychology*, *51*, 1173–1182.

Battiato, L. A. and Wheeler, V. S. (2000). Biotherapy. In C. H. Yarbro, M. Goodman, M. H. Frogge, and S. L. Groenwald (Eds). *Cancer Nursing: Principles and Practice* (pp. 543–579). Sudbury, MA: Jones & Bartlett Publishers.

Blake-Mortimer, C., Gore-Felton, R., Kimerling, J. M., Turner-Cobb, K., and Spiegel, D. (1999). Improving the quality and quantity of life among patients with cancer: a review of the effectiveness of group psychotherapy. *European Journal of Cancer*, *35*, 1581–1586.

Brown, J. K., Byers, T., Doyle, C., Courneya, K. S., Demark-Wahnefried, W., Kushi, L. H. *et al.* (2003). Nutrition and physical activity during and after cancer treatment: an American Cancer Society guide for informed choices. *CA: A Cancer Journal for Clinicians*, *53*, 268–291.

Burnham, T. R. and Wilcox, A. (2002). Effects of exercise on physiological and psychological variables in cancer survivors. *Medicine and Science in Sports and Exercise*, *34*, 1863–1867.

Camp-Sorrell, D. (2000). Chemotherapy: toxicity management. In C. H. Yarbro, M. Goodman, M. H. Frogge, and S. L. Groenwald (Eds). *Cancer Nursing: Principles and Practice* (pp. 444–486). Sudbury, MA: Jones & Bartlett Publishers.

Cella, D. F., Tulsky, D. S., Gray, G., Sarafian, B., Linn, E., Bonomi, A. *et al.* (1993). The functional assessment of cancer therapy scale: development and validation of the general measure. *Journal of Clinical Oncology*, *11*, 570–579.

Coleman, E. A., Coon, S., Hall-Barrow, J., Richards, K., Gaylor, D., and Stewart, B. (2003). Feasibility of exercise during treatment for multiple myeloma. *Cancer Nursing*, *26*, 410–419.

Courneya, K. S. (2001). Exercise interventions during cancer treatment: biopsychosocial outcomes. *Exercise and Sport Sciences Reviews*, *29*, 60–64.

Courneya, K. S. (2003). Exercise in cancer survivors: an overview of research. *Medicine and Science in Sports and Exercise*, *35*, 1846–1852.

Courneya, K. S. and Friedenreich, C. M. (1997a). Relationship between exercise during cancer treatment and current quality of life in survivors of breast cancer. *Journal of Psychosocial Oncology*, *5*, 120–127.

Courneya, K. S. and Friedenreich, C. M. (1997b). Relationship between exercise pattern across the cancer experience and current quality of life in colorectal cancer survivors. *Journal of Alternative and Complementary Medicine*, 3, 215–226.

Courneya, K. S., Mackey, J. R., and Jones, L. W. (2000). Coping with cancer: can exercise help? *The Physician and Sports Medicine*, 28, 49–73.

Courneya, K. S., Mackey, J. R., and McKenzie, D. C. (2002). Exercise for breast cancer survivors: research evidence and clinical guidelines. *The Physician and Sports Medicine*, 30, 33–42.

Courneya, K. S., Friedenreich, C. M., Quinney, H. A., Fields, A. L. A., Jones, L. W., and Fairey, A. S. (2003a). A randomized trial of exercise and quality of life in colorectal cancer survivors. *European Journal of Cancer Care*, 12, 347–357.

Courneya, K. S., Friedenreich, C. M., Sela, R. A., Quinney, H. A., Rhodes, R. E., and Handman, M. (2003b). The group psychotherapy and home-based physical exercise (group-hope) trial in cancer survivors: physical fitness and quality of life outcomes. *Psycho-Oncology*, 12, 357–374.

Courneya, K. S., Mackey, J. R., Bell, G. J., Jones, L. W., Field, C. J., and Fairey, A. S. (2003c). Randomized controlled trial of exercise training in postmenopausal breast cancer survivors: cardiopulmonary and quality of life outcomes. *Journal of Clinical Oncology*, 21, 1660–1668.

Courneya, K. S., Mackey, J. R., and Rhodes, R. E. (2004). Cancer. In L. M. LeMura and S. P. von Duvillard (Eds). *Clinical Exercise Physiology: Application and Physiological Principles* (pp. 387–404). Baltimore, MD: Lippincott Williams and Wilkins.

Dimeo, F., Schwartz, S., Fietz, T., Wanjura, T., Boning, D., and Thiel, E. (2003). Effects of endurance training on the physical performance of patients with hematological malignancies during chemotherapy. *Supportive Care in Cancer*, 11, 623–628.

Fairey, A. S., Courneya, K. S., Field, C. J., Bell, G. J., Jones, L. W., and Mackey, J. R. (2003). Effects of exercise training on fasting insulin, insulin resistance, insulin-like growth factors, and insulin-like growth factor binding proteins in postmenopausal breast cancer survivors: a randomized controlled trial. *Cancer Epidemiology, Biomarkers and Prevention*, 12, 721–727.

Farquhar, M. (1995). Definitions of quality of life: a taxonomy. *Journal of Advanced Nursing*, 22, 502–508.

Ferrans, C. E. (2000). Quality of life as an outcome of cancer care. In C. H. Yarbro, M. Goodman, M. H. Frogge, and S. L. Groenwald (Eds). *Cancer Nursing: Principles and Practice* (5th edn, pp. 243–258). Sudbury, MA: Jones & Bartlett Publishers.

Frogge, M. H. and Cunning, S. M. (2000). Surgical therapy. In C. H. Yarbro, M. Goodman, M. H. Frogge, and S. L. Groenwald (Eds). *Cancer Nursing: Principles and Practice* (pp. 272–285). Sudbury, MA: Jones & Bartlett Publishers.

Gerber, L., Hicks, J., and Shah, J. (2001). Rehabilitation of the cancer patient. In V. T. DeVita Jr, S. Hellman, and S. A. Rosenberg (Eds). *Cancer: Principles and Practice of Oncology* (6th edn, pp. 3089–3100). Philadelphia, PA: Lippincott Williams and Wilkins.

Gribbon, J. and Loescher, L. J. (2000). Cancer Biology. In C. H. Yarbro, M. Goodman, M. H. Frogge, and S. L. Groenwald (Eds). *Cancer Nursing: Principles and Practice* (5th edn, pp. 17–34). Boston, MA: Jones & Bartlett Publishers.

Hayes, S., Davies, P. S., Parker, T., and Bashford, J. (2003a). Total energy expenditure and body composition changes following peripheral blood stem cell transplantation and participation in an exercise programme. *Bone Marrow Transplantation*, 31, 331–338.

Hayes, S. C., Rowbottom, D., Davies, P. S., Parker, T. W., and Bashford, J. (2003b). Immunological changes after cancer treatment and participation in an exercise program. *Medicine and Science in Sports and Exercise*, 35, 2–9.

Hilderley, L. J. (2000). Principles of radiation therapy. In C. H. Yarbro, M. Goodman, M. H. Frogge, and S. L. Groenwald (Eds). *Cancer Nursing: Principles and Practice* (pp. 286–299). Sudbury, MA: Jones & Bartlett Publishers.

Jones, L. W. and Courneya, K. S. (2002). Exercise counseling and programming preferences of cancer survivors. *Cancer Practice, 10*, 208–215.

Kolden, G. G., Strauman, T. J., Ward, A., Kuta, J., Woods, T. E., Schneider, K. L. *et al.* (2002). A pilot study of group exercise training (GET) for women with primary breast cancer: Feasibility and health benefits. *Psycho-Oncology, 11*, 447–456.

Luebbert, K., Dahme, B., and Hasenbring, M. (2001). The effectiveness of relaxation training in reducing treatment-related symptoms and improving emotional adjustment in acute non-surgical cancer treatment: a meta-analytical review. *Psycho-Oncology, 10*, 490–502.

McKenzie, D. C. and Kalda, A. L. (2003). Effect of upper extremity exercise on secondary lymphedema in breast cancer patients: a pilot study. *Journal of Clinical Oncology, 21*, 463–466.

Maher, K. E. (2000). Radiation therapy: toxicities and management. In C. H. Yarbro, M. Goodman, M. H. Frogge, and S. L. Groenwald (Eds). *Cancer Nursing: Principles and Practice* (pp. 323–351). Sudbury, MA: Jones & Bartlett Publishers.

Meyer, T. J. and Mark, M. M. (1995). Effects of psychosocial interventions with adult cancer patients: a meta-analysis of randomized experiments. *Health Psychology, 14*, 101–108.

Oldervoll, L. M., Kaasa, S., Knobel, H., and Loge, J. H. (2003). Exercise reduces fatigue in chronic fatigued Hodgkins disease survivors – results from a pilot study. *European Journal of Cancer, 39*, 57–63.

Parkin, D. M., Bray, F., Ferlay, J., and Pisani, P. (2001). Estimating the world cancer burden: Globocan 2000. *International Journal of Cancer, 94*, 153–156.

Pinto, B. M., Trunzo, J. J., Reiss, P., and Shiu, S. Y. (2002). Exercise participation after diagnosis of breast cancer: trends and effects on mood and quality of life. *Psycho-Oncology, 11*, 389–400.

Pinto, B. M., Clark, M. M., Maruyama, N. C., and Feder, S. I. (2003). Psychological and fitness changes associated with exercise participation among women with breast cancer. *Psycho-Oncology, 12*, 118–126.

Rehse, B. and Pukrop, R. (2003). Effects of psychosocial interventions on quality of life in adult cancer patients: meta analysis of 37 published controlled outcome studies. *Patient Education and Counseling, 50*, 179–186.

Schag, C. A. and Heinrich, R. L. (1990). Development of a comprehensive quality of life measurement tool: CARES. *Oncology, 4*, 135–138.

Schipper, H., Clinch, J., McMurray, A., and Levitt, M. (1984). Measuring the quality of life of cancer patients: the Functional Living Index–Cancer: development and validation. *Journal of Clinical Oncology, 2*, 472–483.

Schwartz, A. L. (1999). Fatigue mediates the effects of exercise on quality of life. *Quality of Life Research, 8*, 529–538.

Segal, R., Reid, R. D., Courneya, K. S., Malone, S. C., Parliament, M. B., Scott, C. G. *et al.* (2003). Resistance exercise in men receiving androgen deprivation therapy for prostate cancer. *Journal of Clinical Oncology, 21*, 1653–1659.

Ware, J. J. and Sherbourne, C. D. (1992). The MOS 36-Item Short-form Health survey (SF-36): 1. Conceptual framework and item selection. *Medical Care, 30*, 473–483.

Young-McCaughan, S., Mays, M. Z., Arzola, S. M., Yoder, L. H., Dramiga, S. A., Leclerc, K. M. *et al.* (2003). Research and commentary: change in exercise tolerance, activity and sleep patterns, and quality of life in patients with cancer participating in a structured exercise program. *Oncology Nursing Forum, 30*, 441–454.

Effects of exercise on smoking cessation and coping with withdrawal symptoms and nicotine cravings

ADRIAN H. TAYLOR AND MICHAEL H. USSHER

The health risks associated with cigarette smoking are well established (Doll *et al.*, 1994; USDHHS, 1990), as is the fact that stopping smoking prolongs life and reduces morbidity (USDHHS, 1996). Unaided attempts to quit smoking have a success rate (>12-month continuous abstinence) of around 2–4% (Hughes *et al.*, 1992), while aided quit attempts, particularly through a combination of behavioral counseling and nicotine replacement therapy (NRT) or antidepressants (e.g., bupropion), can improve success rates to up to 30% (Hughes *et al.*, 2004; Silagy *et al.*, 2004). Nevertheless, more effective smoking cessation interventions are needed, including behavioral techniques, that are suitable for those who are unable or unwilling to use pharmacological products (e.g., pregnant smokers) or as an adjunct to commonly prescribed methods.

This chapter primarily focuses on the evidence for the role of exercise as a therapy in increasing the likelihood of successful quitting. However, another critical issue is whether involvement in sport and exercise can attenuate the likelihood of progression to becoming a regular smoker. This latter question will be dealt with at the end of the chapter, but it is important to note that cross-sectional studies have consistently shown that adolescents and adults who participate in greater levels of physical activity are less likely to smoke or smoke fewer cigarettes (Aarnio *et al.*, 1997; Aaron *et al.*, 1995; Abrams *et al.*, 1999; Baumert *et al.*, 1998; Boutelle *et al.*, 2000; Boyle *et al.*, 2000; Coulson *et al.*, 1997; Davis *et al.*, 1997; Melnick *et al.*, 2001; Pate *et al.*, 1996, 2002; Rainey *et al.*, 1996). It is also worth noting that smokers who are more physically active have reduced risk of disease (Hedblad *et al.*, 1997).

Exercise has been proposed as an aid for smoking cessation (Hill, 1981), but until recently there has been no systematic approach to understanding how any benefits occur. Understanding the mechanisms is important because it enables more precise guidance for the practitioner and quitter. For example, if exercise has little effect on psychological withdrawal symptoms but enables quitters to avoid weight gain, which is often a fear reported by potential quitters and a cause of relapse among quitters (Glasgow *et al.*, 1999; Levine *et al.*, 2001), then increasing overall energy expenditure during cessation will be the most important thing. However, if single sessions of exercise reduce cigarette cravings, help to manage mood and affect (Thayer *et al.*, 1994) and help prevent relapse then we need to know what duration, intensity, and type of exercise is most beneficial to enhance coping with withdrawal symptoms and possibly buffer the effects of cues or triggers to smoke.

Encouragingly, smokers trying to quit may be more receptive to initiating an active lifestyle than smokers in general (Doherty *et al.*, 1998; King *et al.*, 1996). Also, becoming more active has been positively associated with both confidence to maintain smoking abstinence (King *et al.*, 1996) and success at stopping smoking (Derby *et al.*, 1994; Paavola *et al.*, 2001; Sedgwick *et al.*, 1988). Exercise has been routinely recommended as an aid to smoking cessation by specialist smoking clinics (Hurt *et al.*, 1992), by pharmaceutical companies (Boots Company PLC, 1998), in self help guides (Ashelman, 2000; Marcus *et al.*, 2004), and in national guidelines (Raw *et al.*, 1998). However, evidence from surveys would suggest that exercise is not routinely recommended by physicians (Taylor, 2003). Also, exercise practitioners may have limited understanding of the issues associated with smoking cessation interventions and their effectiveness. Unrealistic expectations for success in quitting may provide a frustrating experience for both quitter and practitioner.

This chapter builds on previous reviews of exercise and smoking cessation (Fiore *et al.*, 1996; Nishi *et al.*, 1998; Ussher, 2005; Ussher *et al.*, 2000) but also presents the first review of a growing number of studies designed to assess whether single sessions of exercise have an acute effect on reducing tobacco cravings and withdrawal. Exploration of the characteristics (i.e., type, intensity, and duration) of single sessions of exercise may provide a more precise understanding of the potential beneficial role of exercise as a therapy for helping smokers to successfully quit.

In summary, the review seeks to address five main questions:

1 Do exercise interventions increase the likelihood of successful quit attempts?
2 How may the characteristics of studies and interventions have influenced the findings?
3 How may exercise interventions work?
4 Does a single session of exercise reduce urges to smoke and tobacco withdrawal symptoms during temporary abstinence?
5 Does involvement in sport and exercise reduce the likelihood of progression to smoking in adolescence?

CHAPTER 8

QUESTION 1: DO EXERCISE INTERVENTIONS INCREASE THE LIKELIHOOD OF SUCCESSFUL QUIT ATTEMPTS?

Search strategy and inclusion criteria

The specialized register of the Cochrane Tobacco Addiction group was searched for studies including "exercise" or "physical activity," together with electronic searches of Medline, PsychInfo, Dissertation Abstracts, CINAHL, EMBASE, and SPORTDiscus using the terms smoking, smoking cessation, exercise, and physical activity and intervention up to October 2004. Also a manual review of reference lists and additional searches on key authors was conducted.

In order to specifically address the effects of exercise, the only studies that were included considered programs of supervised or unsupervised exercise, as an adjunct to a smoking cessation intervention, compared to a smoking cessation program alone. Studies were selected that included an equivalent comparison group at baseline (i.e., randomly assigned). Interventions which included exercise in a multiple component smoking cessation program were excluded since the specific effects of exercise on smoking abstinence could not be addressed (e.g., Jonsdottir and Jonsdottir, 2001). Multiple risk factor interventions where smoking cessation was one of a number of health related outcomes were excluded for the same reason (e.g., Taylor *et al.*, 1998). Exercise interventions alone, without a concurrent smoking cessation program were excluded since none of these studies recorded the number of smokers who where trying to quit at the outset (e.g., McMurdo and Burnett, 1992).

Data was extracted from each study on research design (including setting); recruitment and randomization method; subject characteristics including age, gender, smoking behavior; sample size; description of exercise and smoking cessation programs (including number of sessions and duration); rates of exercise adherence; control conditions; length of follow-up; definition of cessation; and method of validation. The primary outcome was quitting at the longest follow-up using the strictest definition of abstinence reported in the study (e.g., continuous abstinence rather than point prevalence at the longest follow-up, since being a non-smoker at a particular follow-up time, may not be as a result of the intervention if relapse has already occurred and this is a new quit attempt).

Findings

The literature search identified ten studies which met the inclusion criteria, as shown in Table 8.1. Four studies showed significant differences in abstinence between a physically active group and a control group immediately at the end of treatment or at a later point in time (Marcus *et al.*, 1991, 1999, 2003a; Martin *et al.*, 1997). The most enduring positive effects for exercise on abstinence were at both the 3-month and 12-month follow-up points (Marcus *et al.*, 1999). The latter study showed a difference in abstinence rates for the exercise condition compared to the control of 11.9% versus 5.4% ($p = 0.05$, OR = 2.36, 95% CI, 0.97–5.70) at the 12-month follow-up. The other studies showed no significant effect for exercise on abstinence at the most distal measure of abstinence. It was apparent though that most studies showed positive effects in the interim period, with the effects usually greatest during or at the end of the treatment; reported net differences in favor of the exercise group were 23% (Hill, 1985), 50% (Marcus *et al.*, 1991), and 20% (Marcus *et al.*, 1995), at the end of the exercise program, and 7.3% (Marcus *et al.*, 2003a) after three months. In the study by Ussher *et al.* (2003), in which only those people who attended the quit day were considered (rather than all those being randomized and providing baseline data prior to the quit day), the exercise intervention (compared with the control group) led to significantly better abstinence two weeks after quitting (81% versus 64%).

A summary of study and intervention characteristics

Six of the studies had fewer than 25 people in each treatment arm. Five trials were limited to women (Marcus *et al.*, 1991, 1995, 1999, 2003b; Russell *et al.*, 1988), and one to men (Taylor *et al.*, 1988). In all but one of the studies a multi-session cognitive behavioral smoking cessation program was provided for intervention and control conditions. In five studies this began prior to quit day (Hill *et al.*, 1993; Marcus *et al.*, 1991, 1999, 2003b; Ussher *et al.*, 2003). All the studies recruiting current smokers set a quit date. The exercise program began before the quit date in six studies (Hill *et al.*, 1993; Marcus *et al.*, 1991, 1995, 1999, 2003b; Ussher *et al.*, 2003), on it in two (Hill, 1985; Martin *et al.*, 1997) and after the quit date in one (Russell *et al.*, 1988). Two studies entailed exercise program lasting for less than six weeks (Hill, 1985; Martin *et al.*, 1997). Most of the trials employed a supervised group-based exercise program, supplemented by a home-based program. Three studies (Marcus *et al.*, 1991, 1995, 1999) did not provide a home program. The strictest measure of abstinence was continuous in three studies (Marcus *et al.*, 1999, 2003a; Ussher *et al.*, 2003), point prevalence in six, and not specified in two (Russell *et al.*, 1988; Taylor *et al.*, 1988). Post-randomization dropouts were excluded from the denominator in two studies (Hill *et al.*, 1993; Taylor *et al.*, 1988).

QUESTION 2: HOW MAY THE STUDY AND INTERVENTION CHARACTERISTICS HAVE INFLUENCED THE FINDINGS?

Effects of research design on abstinence rates

A comparison of the studies was complicated by differences in study design and intervention, and by the relative paucity of research in this field. There were marked variations between studies in the length, type, and timing of the exercise intervention, in the design of the control condition and cessation program, and in the demographic factors recorded. In addition, there was a general absence of data relating to the physical activity levels of the control groups, and of either group during the follow-up period. Together, these factors restricted meaningful comparisons of results between studies.

Only four studies (Marcus *et al.*, 1997, 1999, 2003b; Martin *et al.*, 1997; Ussher *et al.*, 2003) had a sufficiently large sample size to have a good prospect of detecting a significant difference between the treatment and control conditions. One of the studies did not provide separate abstinence data for the experimental and control groups, although it was reported that no significant difference was found between the groups (Russell *et al.*, 1988). In addition to comparing the exercise condition with a control group, two of the studies examined the effectiveness of exercise versus nicotine gum (Hill *et al.*, 1993; Martin *et al.*, 1997). No significant differences were reported.

The study by Taylor *et al.* (1988) differed from the others in that the interventions were not intended to initiate smoking abstinence, but rather to maintain abstinence in smokers following acute myocardial infarction (AMI). Thus, the results, which did not show any evidence of benefit from exercise, cannot easily be generalized beyond the context of abstaining post-AMI smokers. This trial also compared the combined effect on smoking abstinence of four different exercise interventions with the combined effect of two different control interventions, so that it was not possible to relate outcomes for smoking cessation to specific interventions. This study is further limited by providing smoking cessation counseling for only one of the two control conditions.

The results of one of the studies showing a positive effect for exercise on smoking abstinence may have been confounded by the exercise group receiving a different cessation program than the control group (Martin *et al.*, 1997). In four of the studies the exercise condition received more staff contact time than the control (Hill, 1985; Marcus *et al.*, 1991; Martin *et al.*, 1997; Taylor *et al.*, 1988) leading to the question of whether the outcomes for abstinence were due to exercise alone or due to additional professional support.

Effects of exercise intervention characteristics on abstinence rates

It has been recommended that an exercise program should start before the quit date and continue into the period of abstinence (Raw *et al.*, 1998); yet, there was wide variation in the timing of the exercise program in the studies under review. For those beginning exercise either on or after the quit date (Hill, 1985; Martin *et al.*, 1997; Russell *et al.*, 1988) success rates may have been hampered by the demand to cope simultaneously

Table 8.1 A summary of randomized trials to investigate the effects of exercise interventions on smoking abstinence

AUTHOR	METHODS	PARTICIPANTS	INTERVENTIONS (GROUPS)	OUTCOMES	NOTES	RESULTS (% ABSTINENT)
Hill (1985)	Randomized to 2 groups	26 Canadian women and 10 men, mean age group = 40 yrs, mean cig/day = 32, smoking ≥10 cig/day	(a) CV activity: various, facility, 30 min, [2, 5] + home activity + [2,5] + CP [2,5] (b) Control, CP alone Exercise began on quit date	7-day PPA Validation: CO (ET, 1, 3, 6 months)	Contact time not balanced Control group advised to limit physical activity to pre-treatment levels	(a) 67, 55, 40, 41 (b) 44, 34, 29, 30 NS
Hill et al. (1993)	Randomized in blocks of 8 to 12, to 4 groups	43 US women and 39 men, mean age = 59 yrs (only 50+), mean cig/day = 28, (excludes 4 treatment dropouts and 8 non-attenders) Smoking for ≥30 yrs, not currently walking for exercise	(a) Walk: group/individual, facility/home, 15–35 min, 60–70% HR reserve, [1–3, 12]; (b) as (a) + CP [1–4, 12]; (c) CP as (b) + nicotine gum; (d) CP alone. Exercise began 1 week before quit date	5-day PPA Validation: CO <10 ppm (ET, 1, 4, 9 months)	(b) compared to (d) for effect of exercise program	(a) 25, 10, 20, 10 (b) 33, 33, 22, 28 (c) 45, 41, 50, 37 (d) 45, 32, 27, 32 NS
Marcus et al. (1991)	Recruitment: method not specified, Randomization method: not stated	20 US women, mean age = 39, mean cig/day = 28 Smoking ≥10 cig/day for ≥3yrs, exercise ≤ × 1 week	(a) CV equipment: group, facility 30–45 min, 70–85% HR maximum, [3, 15] + CP [2, 4] (b) CP only [2, 4]; Exercise began 3 wk before quit date	7-day PPA Validation: saliva cotinine <10 ng/ml (ET, 1, 3, 12 months)	Contact time not balanced	(a) 50, 40, 30, 20 (b) 0, 0, 0, 0 NS

(Table 8.1 continued)

Study	Recruitment/Randomization	Participants	Intervention	Outcome/Validation	Notes	Results
Marcus et al. (1995)	Recruitment: method not stated, Randomization method: not stated	20 US women, mean age 38, mean cig/day = 23. Exercise ≤ × 1 week	(a) CV equipment: group, facility, 30–45 min, 70–85% HR maximum [3, 15] + CP [1, 12] (b) CP as (a) + HE [3, 15]. Exercise began 3 wk before quit date	7-day PPA Validation: saliva cotinine <10 ng/ml (ET, 1, 3, 12 months)	Contact time balanced between (a) and (b)	(a) 30, 30, 30, 30 (b) 10, 10, 10, 10 (a) versus (b) at ET ($p < 0.05$)
Marcus et al. (1997, 1999)	Randomized to 2 groups	281 sedentary US women, mean age = 40 (18–65 yrs), mean cig/day = 22, smoked ≥10 cig/day for ≥3 yrs	(a) CV equipment: group, facility, 30–40 min, 60–85% HRR, [3, 12] + CP [1, 22] (b) CP as (a) [1, 12] + HE [3, 12]. Exercise began 3 wk before quit date	CA Validation: saliva cotinine <10 ng/ml, CO <8 ppm (ET, 3, 12 months)	Contact time matched. Less weight gain for (a) at 12 months	7-day PPA (a) 31, 25, 19 (b) 22, 14, 14 (a) versus (b) at 3 months ($p = 0.02$) CA (a) 19, 16, 12 (b) 10, 8, 5 (a) versus (b) at ET and 3 months ($p = 0.03$); at 12 months ($p = 0.05$)
Marcus et al. (2003a,b)	Randomized to 2 groups	217 sedentary US women, mean age = 43 years, mean cig/day = 21. Exercise <90 min/wk	(a) CBT + NRT + mod. ex. (45–59% HRR). CV equipment: group, facility [1, 8] + home-target of	7-day PPA + CA Validation: saliva cotinine <10 ng/ml, CO <8 ppm (ET, 3 and 12 months)	Contact time matched (a) 3.8% increase (up to ET) in VO₂ peak (ml/kg/min)	7-day PPA (a) 20, 12, 7 (b) 19, 5, 8 (a) versus (b) at 3 months ($p = 0.04$)

Table 8.1 Continued

AUTHOR	METHODS	PARTICIPANTS	INTERVENTIONS (GROUPS)	OUTCOMES	NOTES	RESULTS (% ABSTINENT)
			165 mins/week (b) CBT + NRT + wellness program [1, 8]. Exercise began 3 wk before quit day		(from intent to treat analysis). No weight gain differences	CA (a) 15, 7, 1 (b) 11, 4, 1 (no differences)
Martin et al. (1997)	Randomized to 3 groups	92 US women and 113 men, mean age = 42 yrs, mean cig/day = 27, exercise < × 1/wk ≥18 yrs, problem drinkers, alcohol/drug abstinence ≥3 months, smoking ≥10 cig/day	(a) CV activity: various, group/individual, facility/home, 15–45 min, 60–75% HR max, [1, 4] + CP [1, 12] (b) + CP as + nicotine gum (c) Different CP [1, 8] and Nicotine Anonymous meetings [3, 4]. Exercise began on quit date	7-day PPA for 7-day follow-up (i.e., ET), 24 hr PP for ET, 6 and 12 months. (a) Validation: CO <10 ppm 7 days, 6, 12 months	Contact time not matched, different cessation programs	(a) 60, 29, 27 (b) 52, 27, 27 (c) 31, 21, 26 (a) versus (c) at 7 days (ET) ($p < 0.01$)
Russell et al. (1988)	Randomized to 3 groups	42 US women, mean age = 28, mean cig/day = 23	(a) Walk/jog: group/indiv., facility/home, 20–30 min, 70–80% HR max, [3, 9] + CP [4, 1]. (b) CP as (a) + HE [1, 9]. (c) CP as (a) Exercise	Abstinence criteria: not stated Validation: CO ET, 1, 4, 16 months	Contact time balanced between (a) and (b). Increase in tension-anxiety (POMS) for (a) only	(a + b + c) 83, 73, 49, 34 NS No difference between groups. Levels of abstinence for

Study	Sample/Recruitment	Intervention	Outcome measure	Comments	Results
Taylor *et al.* (1988)	Recruitment: inpatient volunteers, post-acute myocardial infarction. Randomization method: not stated. 58 US men (Excludes ×5 with abnormal fitness tests, ×28 experiencing cardiac events during program; ×10 dropouts and data unavailable for ×18. Exclusions included smokers and non-smokers: does not state which of those excluded were smokers)	began during the week after quit date (a) CV activity: various, group, facility, 30–40 min, 70–85% HR maximum, (i) [3, 23]; (ii) [3, 8] + CP × 1 session (b) (i, ii) as (a) home, 20 min, ×5/wk (c) Fitness test at end of treatment (d) Fitness test at baseline and ET + CP as (a)	Self report (definition of abstinence not stated) Validation: plasma thiocyanate <100 nmol/l Outcome data for end of treatment at 23 wk	For outcomes combined (a) with (b) and (c) with (d) Outcome data for end of treatment at 23 wk Contact time not balanced	separate groups not stated (a) + (b) 78 (b) + (d) 76 NS
Ussher *et al.* (2003)	Recruitment: public adverts. Randomized to 2 groups. 299 UK men and women. Mean age = 43 yrs mean cig/day = 22. <5 days of ex (30 mins) per wk	(a) NRT + ex. counseling [1, 7] (b) NRT + HE [1, 7]	CA using CO <10 ppm (ET)	(a) 23% versus (b) 7% active at ET, but no difference in weight gain. Walking most popular activity, had lower tension, anxiety and stress in wk 1, less irritability up to wk 2, less restlessness up to wk 3	Intent to treat: (a) 39.6% versus (b) 38.6% at ET, NS Among those (a) attending quit day: 14% greater abstinence at 2 wks for (a). No difference at ET

Notes: [*x; y*]: *x* = frequency (per wk); *y* = duration (wk); CP = cessation program; CV = cardiovascular; ET = end of treatment; HE = health education; NS = not significant; NRT = Nicotine Replacement Therapy; HRR = heart rate reserve; PPA = point prevalence abstinence; CA = continuous abstinence; ppm = parts per million; ex = exercise; yrs = years; wk = week.

with two major changes in health behavior (Emmons *et al.*, 1994; King *et al.*, 1996; Patten *et al.*, 2001). Furthermore, where the exercise program started after a period of smoking abstinence the potential for exercise to moderate withdrawal symptoms during this period was lost (Bock *et al.*, 1999; Grove *et al.*, 1993; Ussher *et al.*, 2001). The question remains, at what point should the smoker who is trying to quit begin an exercise program? Available evidence supports the recommendation for changes in exercise and smoking behavior being sequential rather than simultaneous (Emmons *et al.*, 1994; King *et al.*, 1996). However, it has been shown that abstaining smokers are more confident about adopting exercise than those preparing to quit (King *et al.*, 1996), which would support the notion of beginning an exercise program when already abstinent. Conversely, a recent quasi-experimental study has reported higher adherence rates for smokers who undergo an exercise regimen commencing eight weeks before the quit day compared with those starting exercise on the quit day (Patten *et al.*, 2001), although this difference may partly be due to the former regimen being of a longer duration. However, it may be unrealistic to expect someone to set a quit date several weeks away (except in conjunction with a specific date such as New Years Day or National No Smoking Day) and beginning an exercise program well in advance of a quit attempt.

With the provision of more extensive cessation programs the impact of the interventions may have been more pronounced. In one study, the treatment was limited to only a single counseling session (Taylor *et al.*, 1988). Furthermore, only one of the studies (Ussher *et al.*, 2003) described an intervention in which the smoking cessation and exercise components were integrated in such a way as to reinforce exercise as a coping strategy for smoking cessation (see Marlatt and Gordon, 1985). In other words, the potential for exercise to be used to reduce cigarette cravings and other withdrawal symptoms could have been made more explicit. While the study by Ussher *et al.* (2003) failed to show any effects on smoking abstinence (from the intention to treat analysis), there were significantly greater reductions in specific psychological symptoms in the exercise group versus the control group – up to three weeks of abstinence. If fewer withdrawal symptoms do predict better abstinence then such exercise-related changes should impact on quit rates. The lack of effects in the Ussher study may have been due to a relatively brief exercise counseling session. The study was designed to have good generalization to the normal care context in which brief counseling may be all that is possible. Nevertheless, it was encouraging to see significant increases in self-reported physical activity as a result of exercise counseling. Another explanation for no effect was that both the control and exercise groups were administered NRT. A comparison between exercise alone and a minimal control may well have shown exercise to be an effective intervention. Also, by only analyzing data from those who attended the quit date (rather than everyone who provided baseline data), the exercise did show positive effects on abstinence rates in the short term.

In most cases the exercise prescription was fitness oriented (ACSM, 1995), recommending at least 20 min of exercise on three days a week at a vigorous intensity of between 70% and 85% of maximal heart rate. A number of the trials reported an increase in fitness levels at the end of the treatment period within the active condition (Marcus *et al.*, 1991, 1995, 1999, 2003a; see also Albrecht *et al.*, 1998). Three studies showed an increase in fitness for the exercise conditions compared with the controls at the end of treatment (Marcus *et al.*, 1999, 2003a; Taylor *et al.*, 1988), while another showed no differences at the end of treatment or at a 4-month follow-up (Russell *et al.*, 1988).

Although some of the studies reported fitness measures for the control group during the treatment period (Hill, 1985; Marcus *et al.*, 1991, 1995, 1999; Russell *et al.*, 1988; Taylor *et al.*, 1988) only three of the investigations reported activity levels at this time (Hill, 1985; Marcus *et al.*, 2003b; Ussher *et al.*, 2003). Therefore, the relative increase in physical activity in the treatment group versus any spontaneous increase in activity in the control group could not be accurately monitored.

If an exercise program helps to prevent weight gain during cessation, with a knock on effect on cessation success, then it would make sense that the exercise program is maintained throughout the time when weight gain is most likely. Exercise programs can focus on providing regular structured exercise sessions or on lifestyle physical activity, or preferably a combination of the two (Pate *et al.*, 1995). As long as exercise is maintained after the intervention ends, the length of formal program should not matter. However, the fact that only two of the studies reported any post-intervention exercise programing (Hill *et al.*, 1993; Ussher *et al.*, 2003) may indicate that most interventions failed to support goals for long-term weight management.

During the treatment period a range of behavioral methods were employed to improve adherence to the exercise program. All but one of the studies (Ussher *et al.*, 2003) used group activities with full supervision of facility-based exercise and goal setting; six used self-monitoring (Hill, 1985; Marcus *et al.*, 2003b; Martin *et al.*, 1997; Russell *et al.*, 1988; Taylor *et al.*, 1988; Ussher *et al.*, 2003); one used reinforcement (Martin *et al.*, 1997); one telephone follow-up in the case of non attendance (Hill *et al.*, 1993), and one used remote monitoring of heart rate (Taylor *et al.*, 1988). All the studies reported activity levels for the treatment group during the treatment period with the exception of one study (Hill *et al.*, 1993). Compliance with the exercise program was high.

QUESTION 3: HOW MAY EXERCISE INTERVENTIONS WORK?

A number of explanations have been proposed for how exercise may aid smoking cessation. One suggestion is that exercise helps weight maintenance after quitting, which is a factor of common concern among quitters (Swan *et al.*, 1993). Of the 10 trials reviewed, only one reported a significantly smaller weight gain for those in the exercise condition compared with the controls at the end of treatment (Marcus *et al.*, 1999). However, those in the exercise condition by chance weighed more than the controls at baseline, which makes interpretation of the finding problematic. After a more recent 8-week trial (see Marcus *et al.*, 2003a), Lewis *et al.* (2004) reported significantly reduced weight concerns among those in the exercise intervention (compared with the control condition), who had successfully quit (compared with quitters in the control group). However, they observed no difference in weight gain between the exercise and control groups. Two important explanations were offered. First, the exercise dose (moderate intensity) was insufficient to aid weight maintenance, and second, the control group were using nicotine patches which attenuates weight gain during cessation (Jorenby *et al.*, 1996). The latter explanation was also offered by Ussher *et al.* (2003) when they reported no difference in weight gain between exercise and control groups in their trial. In a prospective study (Kawachi *et al.*, 1996), not included in the systematic review, the authors reported an association between weight gain and increase in exercise after quitting. Among women smoking less than 25 cigarettes per day, those who quit without changing their levels of exercise gained an average of 2.3 kg compared with non-quitters. This was reduced to 1.8 kg and 1.3 kg for those who increased exercise by between 8 and 16 MET-hours (the work metabolic rate divided by the resting metabolic rate) per week and those who increased exercise by more than 16 MET-hours per week, respectively. This gives some indication of how much exercise is needed to prevent weight gain following cessation.

If exercise is being used largely as a means of managing body weight of abstaining smokers, rather than as a means of increasing fitness, then an alternative recommendation for short and frequent bouts of moderate intensity activity may be the preferred option. This recommendation is consistent with the US Surgeon General's guidelines for health-benefiting exercise (USDHHS, 1996), although these were issued after the publication of most of the papers discussed. There appears to be no clear evidence that fitness change is linked to success in smoking cessation, but once again, the limitations of most of the studies prevents consensus.

Another explanation which has been investigated involves the role of exercise in the management of tobacco withdrawal symptoms (e.g., depression, irritability, restlessness, poor concentration) and nicotine cravings. Urges to smoke have been shown to reliably predict relapse to smoking (Piasecki et al., 2000; Shiffman et al., 1996), and withdrawal symptoms are a serious discomfort to smokers. Therefore, if exercise interventions were shown to ameliorate both cravings and discomforting withdrawal symptoms, such interventions would be attractive to smokers and may reduce rates of relapse.

Although the majority of the studies reviewed used psychological measures at baseline, only four of them investigated changes in affect (Marcus et al., 1999; Martin et al., 1997; Russell et al., 1988; Ussher et al., 2003). Russell et al. (1988) found a significant increase in tension-anxiety scores, as measured by the Profile of Mood States (POMs), for the active group compared with the control at four months post-intervention. Martin et al. (1997) found no significant treatment differences on mood (POMs) or depression (measured by the Beck Depression Inventory) when comparing measures taken at baseline and seven days post-treatment. Bock et al. (1999) found a significant acute effect of exercise on tobacco withdrawal but not a chronic effect. Ussher et al. (2003) observed that, relative to controls, those receiving an exercise counseling intervention reported less tension, anxiety, and stress (using the Mood and Physical Symptoms Scale (MPSS); West and Russell, 1985) during the first week of smoking abstinence, less irritability through two weeks of abstinence, and less restlessness through three weeks of abstinence.

QUESTION 4: DOES A SINGLE SESSION OF AEROBIC EXERCISE REDUCE URGES TO SMOKE AND TOBACCO WITHDRAWAL SYMPTOMS, DURING TEMPORARY ABSTINENCE?

We have identified five published, full peer-reviewed articles (Daniel et al., 2004; Pomerleau et al., 1987; Taylor et al., 2005; Thayer et al., 1993; Ussher et al., 2001), which have reported on the acute effects of aerobic exercise on urges to smoke and tobacco withdrawal symptoms, during temporary abstinence, as shown in Table 8.2. Temporary abstinence has been used to induce withdrawal symptoms to test the effects of other smoking cessation aids, such as glucose (West *et al.*, 1999). The severity of symptoms experienced may be associated with a number of factors, including degree of dependence, length of period of withdrawal, and presence of smoking cues, and this may influence the strength of observed effects of any intervention. Experimental procedures, relying solely on temporary abstinence, may not result in a replication of the withdrawal symptoms and nicotine cravings that are experienced in a more natural environment (Carter and Tiffany, 1999). Nevertheless, in the absence of many controlled studies with smokers who are trying to stop, such an approach may enable a better understanding of the acute effects of exercise during smoking cessation.

There was clear evidence that a single session of aerobic exercise reduced measures of desire for a cigarette (Tiffany and Drobes, 1991), strength of desire to smoke (West *et al.*, 1989), the urge to smoke, tobacco withdrawal symptoms on the MPSS (e.g., poor concentration, restlessness, irritability, depression), negative mood states, and increases positive affect. The lowest intensity of exercise to produce positive effects, relative to a passive control, was a 1-mile self-paced brisk walk (at 27% HRR) Taylor *et al.* (2005). The shortest duration of exercise to have a positive effect was 5 min (Daniel *et al.*, 2004; Thayer *et al.*, 1993). The longest lasting effect was 20 min (following a 17-min walk; Taylor *et al.*, 2005). The other studies also showed positive effects on withdrawal symptoms and cigarette cravings, with one study also reporting increased time until the next cigarette (Thayer *et al.*, 1993).

In addition to these studies which all involved aerobic exercise, Ussher *et al.* (submitted) reported that following 15 hours of abstinence a brief period of seated isometric exercise can reduce the urge to smoke and withdrawal symptoms, compared with a visualized isometric exercise condition and a passive control group. The exercise effects lasted 5 min. There were also reductions in self-reported poor concentration, stress, and tension for at least 10 min after the exercise. These findings therefore suggest that brief-seated isometric exercise may be useful for managing cigarette cravings in abstinent smokers. Given that abstainers may experience brief but strong cravings it appears that even seated exercise may be sufficient for immediate relief. The fact that the effects were greater than for an imagery condition (involving distraction) suggests that the mechanism for the observed effects was not through distraction. Exercise psychology research has focused on aerobic and resistance exercise, and to a lesser extent on Tai Chi and other slow moving forms of very light intensity exercise to observe effects on psychological well-being. If such a low exercise intensity can have even temporary effects, then further research is needed to understand the underlying mechanisms, as clearly more people may find this a convenient and acceptable form of activity.

In summary, there is accumulating evidence that a low–moderate dose of exercise has a moderating effect on smoking withdrawal symptoms and cravings that may help people cope with abstinence. Further work is needed to examine the psychological mechanisms associated with the acute effects of exercise in this context which consider methodological developments in exercise-related affect research involving non-smoking populations (Ekkekakis *et al.*, 2000), among different groups and conditions of abstinence.

Table 8.2 Acute effects of exercise on urges to smoke and withdrawal symptoms

AUTHOR	SUBJECTS CHARACTERISTICS	ABSTINENCE PERIOD	EXERCISE CHARACTERISTICS	MEASURES	DESIGN	OUTCOME
Pomerleau et al. (1987)	10 inactive healthy males. Mean age = 24 yrs. Mean cigs = 28 per day	30 min	(a) 80% VO$_2$max versus (b) 30% VO$_2$max Both 30 min cycling	POMS, Shiffman withdrawal scale	Within subject. Follow-up to 30 min post-exercise	(a) versus (b) NS for all measures
Thayer et al. (1993)	5 m and 11 f, Age = 18–44 years. Smoked 1–2 packs per day	45 min	(a) Brisk walk (b) Inactivity 5 min of either	Short AD-ACL (energy and tension), urge to smoke, time to next cig	Within subject. Follow-up immediately post-exercise	(a) Reduced urge to smoke, increased energy and time to next cig (17 versus 9 min delay)
Bock et al. (1999)	Group 1 = 24 f Group 2 = 44 f Both groups inactive. Mean cigs = 20 per day. Mean age = 38 yrs	During smoking cessation	(a) 30–40 min 60–85% HRR, aerobic activity (group 1 and 2) (b) Equal contact passive. All groups (a1, a2, and b) were involved in an 11 week cessation trial	PANAS, ESR, and cravings	Within (pre-/ post-exercise control) subject	(a) Group 1 and 2 reduced negative affect, nicotine withdrawal and cigarette cravings, in all wk (5–10) after quit date. No effect on positive affect

Study	Sample	Abstinence	Conditions	Measure	Design/follow-up	Results
Ussher *et al.* (2001)	78 inactive m and f. Mean cigs = 18 per day. Mean age = 36 yrs	15hrs	(a) 40–60% HRR, cycling + video; (b) video control; (c) passive control, all for 10 min	MPSS, plus Tiffany 'desire to smoke' item	Between groups. 10 min post-exercise follow-up	(a) Reduced desire to smoke, and withdrawal symptoms (irritability, restlessness, tension, depression, poor concentration, stress), cf. (b) and (c), up to 10 min post-ex
Daniel *et al.* (2004)	84 inactive m and f. Mean cigs = 17 per day. Mean age = 30 yrs	11–15 hrs	(a) 40–60% HRR cycling; (b) 10–20% HRR cycling; (c) passive control	MPSS, plus Tiffany 'desire to smoke' item	Between groups. Up to 10 mins post-exercise follow-up	(a) Reduced strength of desire to smoke (at 5 min post-ex.) and withdrawal (irritability, restlessness, tension, depression, poor concentration, stress) (at 10 min post-ex.) cf (b) and (c)
Taylor *et al.* (2005)	10 m and 5f, active. Mean cigs = 17 per day. Mean age = 26 yrs	15 hr	(a) Preferred intensity 1 mile treadmill brisk walk (means = 10.8 RPE; 30% HRR, 17 min), (b) passive rest	MPSS, plus 'strength of desire to smoke' item 32 item QSU	Within-subjects. 30 min post-exercise follow-up	(a) Reduced strength of desire to smoke, 2 QSU scales up to 20 min post-exercise

Notes: HRR = heart rate reserve; ESR = Evening Symptom Report; MPSS = Mood and Physical Symptom Scale; POMS = Profile of Mood States; PANAS = Positive and Negative Affect Scale; AD-ACL = Activation–Deactivation–Adjective Check List; QSU = Questionnaire on Smoking Urges; m = male; f = female.

QUESTION 5: DOES INVOLVEMENT IN SPORT AND EXERCISE REDUCE THE LIKELIHOOD OF PROGRESSION TO SMOKING?

Most people initiate smoking prior to 18 years of age, with critical periods of experimentation beginning in early adolescence between the ages of 13 and 16 years (Conrad *et al.*, 1992; Kessler *et al.*, 1997). While cross-sectional studies have consistently shown that adolescents who participate in greater levels of physical activity are less likely to smoke or smoke fewer cigarettes, only recently have studies investigated the protective effects of physical activity in prospective studies (Audrain-McGovern *et al.*, 2003, 2004; Rodriguez and Audrain-McGovern, 2004) reported that access to alternative or substitute reinforcers, such as physical activity and sports participation, reduced the risk of becoming a smoker (as a reinforcing behavior) by two-fold, and higher levels of physical activity reduced the odds of progressing to smoking or a higher level of smoking by nearly 1.5 (Audrain-McGovern *et al.*, 2003). This unique evidence is promising, but actually demonstrating a reduced risk of experimenting with or becoming a smoker, is complex (Peretti-Watel *et al.*, 2002).

The physical and psycho-social dimensions of different sports, exercise forms, and lifestyle physical activity make it difficult to identify the key components of importance for preventing progression to smoking. For example, Schneider and Greenberg (1992) reported that runners, joggers, and fast walkers were less likely to smoke and consume excessive alcohol than team sport participants. The additional pressure associated with competitive sport may result in a need for emotional and physical recovery, which may come from a cigarette for some smokers. In contrast, more moderate intensity physical activity may provide relaxation and invigorating effects, and create less of a need for a cigarette.

Nevertheless, evidence suggests that physical activity can have positive effects on a number of factors which have been identified as determinants of progression to smoking among adolescents including weight gain, negative affect, perceived stress, low self-perceptions, and low self-esteem. However, these mediators have yet to be investigated systematically.

Implications for the researcher

Most of the trials conducted have had significant methodological limitations. Adequately powered controlled trials are needed with specific groups (e.g., post-MI patients, those who have experienced weight gain or depression during previous quit attempts), that examine effects on continuous abstinence up to one year. Previous trials have focused on the adjunctive effects of exercise in combination with a behaviorally based smoking cessation program. However, most smokers attempt to stop smoking without enrolling in such a support program; therefore, a trial is needed to examine the effects of exercise alone on rates of smoking abstinence. This may be of particular importance to those who may be unable or unwilling to use pharmaceutical therapies, such as pre- and post-natal women (Ussher and West, 2003). Moreover, pregnant smokers express high levels of interest in using exercise as an aid to smoking cessation (Ussher *et al.*, 2004).

Further research is needed to identify the effects of adopting an exercise program prior to versus on the quit date. A growing literature has focused on the effectiveness of interventions designed to promote physical activity in different settings and among sub-groups of the population. Models for changing multiple behaviors are required and should be empirically tested. In the present context, in addition to smoking cessation, quitters may not only initiate an increase in physical activity but also attempt a dietary change for weight management.

A large proportion of cigarettes are smoked by people with a mental illness, such as depression, psychotic illness, and other addictions (Lasser *et al.*, 2000). Studies should consider intervention trials with such people, though these may involve non-experimental designs, without random assignment (Tkachuk and Martin, 1999).

There is a need to further investigate the factors influencing adoption and maintenance of exercise among quitters attempting to use exercise within a smoking cessation program, and this may involve qualitative research to draw consensus from individual experiences.

The mechanism(s) by which exercise may contribute to greater abstinence requires further investigation. For example, it is not known if those engaging in an exercise program and maintaining weight are more likely to be successful quitters than those who exercise but also gain weight. Also, considering the effects of weight gain may be too simplistic. Self-perceptions such as perceived body image or physical attractiveness may be more impor-tant, as a mediating factor. Improvements in physical self-perceptions are related to change in anthropometric measures and body weight, in the general population (Taylor and Fox, 2005), and appraisal of physical changes may link closely with cognitions responsible for smoking cessation relapse. Furthermore, if exercise is something that someone can initiate and maintain with confidence, then a quitter may feel more confident in his/her ability to avoid weight gain. These relationships require further investigation.

Further research is also needed to consider how single sessions of exercise can help quitters cope with withdrawal symptoms. The research paradigm in which smokers are asked to abstain from smoking for up to 24 hours has been used to induce withdrawal symptoms and then consider the acute effects of exercise of different intensities and duration. This design should be extended to understand the role of single sessions of exercise among people who are actually quitting and who are at different temporal stages in the attempt to quit. The relationship between exercise and nicotine cravings and urges to smoke also needs to be studied in naturalistic settings using real-time assessment (Shiffman *et al.*, 1996). Most previous studies have relied on single-item self-report measures of withdrawal. Future studies may need to consider whether meas-ures with multiple items have greater sensitivity than for single-item measures. Previous studies of exercise and smoking cessation have not blinded the investigator to the smokers' group assignment. If future studies could ensure this blinding experimental rigor would be enhanced. Further research should also consider the role of exercise in attenuating subsequent cue-elicited cravings (e.g., in response to natural and laboratory stressors), given the evidence that exercise can reduce acute responses to stressors (Hamer *et al.*, in press; Taylor, 2000).

Implications for the health professional and health service delivery

The inclusion of physical activity within smoking cessation programs appears to have fairly limited scientific support. This does not mean that there is no beneficial effect, only that there are insufficient studies of adequate quality to provide clear guidance.

The study with the greatest benefits initiated exercise prior to the quit date (Marcus *et al.*, 1997, 1999). An alternative view may be that the distraction of initiating exercise at the same time as quitting may be just as beneficial.

Smokers may have poor health status and contraindications to exercise due to lower levels of physical activity and fitness over a prolonged period of time. Care must be taken in prescribing exercise to people with medical conditions and low levels of fitness and physical activity. Unless a trained exercise professional is available, and screening has been undertaken by a health professional, general advice should be given to engage in low-moderate intensity exercise which raises overall energy expenditure and may aid coping with withdrawal symptoms.

There is inadequate evidence that exercise can help weight maintenance and management during quit attempts, but approaches to increase overall energy expenditure, rather than fitness (through vigorous exercise), should be the focus for practitioners. Exercise counseling should supplement dietary advice.

Exercise counseling should direct quitters to use exercise as a coping strategy for elevated cigarette cravings, and associated symptoms such as poor sleep, depression, poor concentration, and irritability, as often as necessary. Exercise prescriptions that focus on fitness change are probably not necessary, and may result in lower adherence to the exercise intervention.

WHAT WE KNOW SUMMARY

- The few rigorous trials reported have shown mixed effects of exercise on smoking cessation.
- There is evidence that interventions can increase exercise participation among smokers, pre-quitters and quitters, but the evidence that such change enables weight management among quitters is less clear.
- There is increasing evidence that single sessions of exercise, at low–moderate intensity (e.g., walking) can help temporary abstainers to cope with withdrawal symptoms and nicotine cravings, particularly in laboratory conditions.

WHAT WE NEED TO KNOW SUMMARY

- There is a need to better understand how exercise interacts with pharmaceutical interventions, with implications for managing weight and withdrawal symptoms.
- The effects of exercise on smoking cessation should be considered with other populations (e.g., adolescents, pregnant smokers) and in other settings, with rigorous trials.
- Lifestyle physical activity interventions (often through counseling) appear to cost less than structured exercise programs (Sevick *et al.*, 2000). We need to know if such counseling could be effectively integrated into standardized smoking cessation programs, as an adjunct to other therapies, at a relatively low cost.
- Further evidence is needed to understand how exercise may positively influence some of the established triggers to relapse during cessation, including psycho-social

stressors and cigarette cravings. Existing work should be extended with greater conceptual clarity when investigating the acute effects of exercise on mood and affect (Ekkekakis, 2003; Ekkekakis and Petruzzello, 2000, 2002). If smoking a cigarette provides both stimulation and relaxation, then the role of exercise within the context of a two-dimensional model of affect should be explored.

• Finally, it is also not known whether very high intensity exercise, as in competitive sport, elevates nicotine cravings for some people (perhaps as a result of competitive stress) and further research should examine the potential negative influence of exercise.

In summary, both smoking cessation and exercise counselors or practitioners should promote physical activity to aid cessation, particularly for weight management and mood regulation purposes. The additional health benefits from exercise make this an important behavioral change for smokers, but we need to know much more about how to engage potential smokers, smokers, and quitters in a more physically active lifestyle.

REFERENCES

Aarnio, M., Kujala, U. M., and Kaprio, J. (1997). Associations of health-related behaviors, school type and health status to physical activity patterns in 16 year old boys and girls. *Scandinavian Journal of Social Medicine, 25*, 156–167.

Aaron, D. J., Dearwater, S. R., Anderson, R., Olsen, T., Kriska, A. M., and Laporte, R. E. (1995). Physical activity and the initiation of high-risk health behaviors in adolescents. *Medicine and Science in Sports and Exercise, 27*, 1639–1645.

Abrams, K., Skolnik, N., and Diamond, J. J. (1999). Patterns and correlates of tobacco use among suburban Philadelphia 6th through 12th-grade students. *Family Medicine, 31*, 128–132.

ACSM (1995). *American College of Sports Medicine Guidelines for Exercise Testing and Prescription* (5th edn). London: Lea and Febiger.

Albrecht, A. E., Marcus, B. H., Roberts, M., Forman, D. E., and Parisi, A. F. (1998). Effect of smoking cessation on exercise performance in female smokers participating in exercise training. *American Journal of Cardiology, 82*, 950–955.

Ashelman, M. W. (2000). *Stop Smoking Naturally*. Lincolnwood, IL: Keats Publishing Inc.

Audrain-McGovern, J., Rodriguez, D., and Moss, H. B. (2003). Smoking progression and physical activity. *Cancer Epidemiology Biomarkers and Prevention, 12*, 1121–1129.

Audrain-McGovern, J., Rodriguez, D., Tercyak, K. P., Epstein, L. H., Goldman, P., and Wileyto, E. P. (2004). Applying a behavioral economic framework to understanding adolescent smoking. *Psychology of Addictive Behaviors, 18*, 64–73.

Baumert, P. W., Jr, Henderson, J. M., and Thompson, N. J. (1998). Health risk behaviors of adolescent participants in organized sports. *Journal of Adolescent Health, 22*, 460–465.

Bock, B. C., Marcus, B. H., King, T. K., Borrelli, B., and Roberts, M. R. (1999). Exercise effects on withdrawal and mood among women attempting smoking cessation. *Addictive Behavior, 24*, 399–410.

Boots Company PLC (1998). *Give up Smoking! Your Guide to a Brighter Future Without Smoking*. Nottingham, UK: The Boots Company PLC.

Boutelle, K. N., Murray, D. M., Jeffery, R. W., Hennrikus, D. J., and Lando, H. A. (2000). Associations between exercise and health behaviors in a community sample of working adults. *Preventive Medicine, 30*, 217–224.

Boyle, R. G., O'Connor, P., Pronck, N., and Tan, A. (2000). Health behaviors of smokers, ex-smokers, and never smokers in an HMO. *Preventive Medicine, 31*, 177–182.

Carter, B. L. and Tiffany, S. T. (1999). Meta-analysis of cue-reactivity in addiction research. *Addiction, 94*, 327–340.

Conrad, K. M., Flay, B. R., and Hill, D. (1992). Why children start smoking cigarettes: predictors of onset. *British Journal of Addiction, 87*, 1711–1724.

Coulson, N. S., Eiser, C., and Eiser, J. R. (1997). Diet, smoking and exercise: interrelationships between adolescent health behaviors. *Child: Care, Health and Development, 23*, 207–216.

Daniel, J., Cropley, M., Ussher, M., and West, R. (2004). Acute effects of a short bout of moderate versus light intensity exercise versus inactivity on tobacco withdrawal symptoms in sedentary smokers. *Psychopharmacology, 174*, 320–326.

Davis, T. C., Arnold, C., Nandy, I., Bocchini, J. A., Gottlieb, A., George, R. B. *et al.* (1997). Tobacco use among male high school athletes. *Journal of Adolescent Health, 21*, 97–101.

Derby, C. A., Lasater, T. M., Vass, K., Gonzalez, S., and Carleton, R. A. (1994). Characteristics of smokers who attempt to quit and of those who recently succeeded. *American Journal of Preventive Medicine, 10*, 327–334.

Doherty, S. C., Steptoe, A., Rink, E., Kendrink, T., and Hilton, S. (1998). Readiness to change health behaviours among patients at high risk of cardiovascular disease. *Journal of Cardiovascular Risk, 5*, 147–153.

Doll, R., Peto, R., Wheatley, K., Gray, R., and Sutherland, I. (1994). Mortality in relation to smoking: 40 years' observations on male British doctors. *British Medical Journal, 309*, 901–911.

Ekkekakis, P. (2003). Pleasure and displeasure from the body: perspectives from exercise. *Cognition and Emotion, 17*, 213–239.

Ekkekakis P. and Petruzzello, S. J. (2000). Analysis of the affect measurement conundrum in exercise psychology: fundamental issues. *Psychology of Sport and Exercise, 1*, 71–88.

Ekkekakis P. and Petruzzello, S. J. (2002). Analysis of the affect measurement conundrum in exercise psychology: a conceptual case for the affect circumplex. *Psychology of Sport and Exercise, 2*, 205–232.

Ekkekakis, P., Hall, E. E., Van Landuyt, L. M., and Petruzzello, S. J. (2000). Walking in (affective) circles: can short walks enhance affect? *Journal of Behavioural Medicine, 223*, 245–275.

Emmons, K. M., Marcus, B. H., Linnan, L., Rossi, J. S., and Abrams, D. B. (1994). Mechanisms in multiple risk factor interventions: smoking, exercise, and dietary fat intake among manufacturing workers. *Preventive Medicine, 23*, 481–489.

Fiore, M. C., Bailey, W. C., Cohen, S. J., Dorfman, S. F., Goldstein, M. G., Gritz, E. R. *et al.* (1996). *Smoking Cessation. Clinical Practice Guideline No 18*. AHCPR Publication No. 96-0692. Rockville, MD: Department of Health and Human Services, Public Health Service, Agency for Health Care Policy and Research.

Glasgow, R. E., Strycker, L. A., Eakin, E. G., Boles, S. M., and Whitlock, E. P. (1999). Concern about weight gain associated with quitting smoking: prevalence and association with outcome in a sample of young female smokers. *Journal of Consulting and Clinical Psychology, 67*, 1009–1011.

Grove, J. R., Wilkinson, A., and Dawson, B. T. (1993). Effects of exercise on stress related blood pressure responses: selected correlates of smoking withdrawal. *International Journal of Sports Psychology, 24*, 217–236.

Hamer, M., Taylor, A. H., and Steptoe, A. (in press). The effect of acute aerobic exercise on stress related blood pressure responses: a systematic review and meta-analysis. *Biological Psychology*.

Hedblad, B., Ogren, M., Isacsson, S. O., and Janzo, L. (1997). Reduced cardiovascular mortality risk in male smokers who are physically active. *Archives of Internal Medicine, 157*, 893–899.

Hill, J. S. (1981). Health behaviour: the role of exercise in smoking cessation. *Canadian Association of Health Physical Education and Recreation Journal, 28*, 15–18.

Hill, J. S. (1985). Effect of a program of aerobic exercise on the smoking behaviour of a group of adult volunteers. *Canadian Journal of Public Health*, *76*, 183–186.

Hill, R. D., Rigdon, M., and Johnson, S. (1993). Behavioural smoking cessation treatment for older chronic smokers. *Behavioral Therapy*, *24*, 321–329.

Hughes, J. R., Gulliver, S. B., Fenwick, J. W., Valliere, W. A., Cruser, K., Pepper, S. *et al.* (1992). Smoking cessation among self-quitters. *Health Psychology*, *11*, 331–334.

Hughes, J. R., Stead, L., and Lancaster, T. (2004). Antidepressants for smoking cessation. *The Cochrane Library*, Vol. 4. Oxford: Updated Software.

Hurt, R. D., Dale, L. C., Offord, K. P., Bruce, B. K., McClain, F. L., and Eberman, K. M. (1992). Inpatient treatment of severe nicotine dependence. *Mayo Clinic Proceedings*, *67*, 823–828.

Jonsdottir, D. and Jonsdottir, H. (2001). Does physical exercise in addition to a multicomponent smoking cessation program increase abstinence rate and suppress weight gain? An intervention study. *Scandinavian Journal of Caring Science*, *15*, 275–282.

Jorenby, D. E., Hatsukami, D. K., Smith, S. S., and Fiore, M. C. (1996). Characterisation of tobacco withdrawal symptoms: transdermal nicotine reduces hunger and weight gain. *Psychopharmacology*, *128*, 130–138.

Kawachi, I., Troisi, R. J., Rotnitzky, A. G., Coakley, E. H., Colditz, M. S., and Colditz, M. D. (1996). Can exercise minimise weight gain in women after smoking cessation. *American Journal of Public Health*, *86*, 999–1004.

Kessler, D. A., Natanblut, S. L., Wilkenfeld, J. P., Lorraine, C. C., Mayl, S. L., Gernstein, I. B. G. *et al.* (1997). Nicotine addiction: a pediatric disease. *The Journal of Pediatrics*, *130*, 518–524.

King, T. K., Marcus, B. H., Pinto, B. M., Emmon, K. M., and Abrams, D. B. (1996). Cognitive behavioural mediators of changing multiple behaviours: smoking and a sedentary lifestyle. *Preventive Medicine*, *25*, 684–691.

Lasser, K., Boyd, J. W., Wollhandler, S., Himmelstein, D. U., McCormick, D., and Bor, D. H. (2000). Smoking and mental illness: a population-based prevalence study. *Journal of the American Medical Association*, *284*, 2606–2610.

Levine, M. D., Perkins, K. A., and Marcus, M. D. (2001). The characteristics of women smokers concerned about post-cessation weight gain. *Addictive Behaviour*, *26*, 749–756.

Lewis, B., Bock, B., Albrecht, A., King, T., and Marcus, B. (2004). The effect of exercise and smoking cessation on weight concerns among women (Abstract). *Annals of Behavioral Medicine*, *27*(Suppl. 1), S101.

McMurdo, M. E. T. and Burnett, L. (1992) Randomised controlled trial of exercise in the elderly. *Gerontology*, *38*, 292–298.

Marcus, B. H., Albrecht, A. E., Niaura, R. S., Abrams, D. B., and Thompson, P. D. (1991). Usefulness of physical exercise for maintaining smoking cessation in women. *American Journal of Cardiology*, *68*, 406–407.

Marcus, B. H., Albrecht, A. E., Niaura, R. S., Taylor, E. R., Simkin, L. R., Feder, S. I. *et al.* (1995). Exercise enhances the maintenance of smoking cessation in women. *Addictive Behaviors*, *20*, 87–92.

Marcus, B. H., King, T. K., Albrecht, A. E., Parisi, A. F., and Abrams, D. B. (1997). Rationale, design and baseline data for Commit to Quit: an exercise efficacy trial for smoking cessation among women. *Preventive Medicine*, *26*, 586–597.

Marcus, B. H., Albrecht, A. E., King, T. K., Parisi, A. F., Pinto, B. M., Roberts, M. *et al.* (1999). The efficacy of exercise as an aid for smoking cessation in women: a randomised controlled trial. *Archives of Internal Medicine*, *159*, 1229–1234.

Marcus, B. H., Lewis, B., Hogan, J., King, T. K., Albrecht, A. E., Bock, B. *et al.* (2003a). The efficacy of moderate-intensity exercise as an aid for smoking cessation in women: a randomised controlled trial (Abstract). *Annals of Behavioral Medicine*, *25*(Suppl. 1), S047.

Marcus, B. H., Lewis, B., King, T. K., Albrecht, A. E., Hogan, J., Bock, B. *et al.* (2003b). Rationale, design and baseline data for Commit to Quit II: an evaluation of the efficacy of moderate-intensity physical activity as an aid to smoking cessation in women. *Preventive Medicine, 36*, 479–492.

Marcus, B. H., Hampl, J. S., and Fisher, E. B. (2004). *How to Quit Smoking Without Gaining Weight.* New York: Simon and Schuster.

Marlatt, G. A. and Gordon, J. R. (1985). *Relapse Prevention: Maintenance Strategies in the Treatment of Addictive Behaviors.* New York: Guildford.

Martin, J. E., Kalfas, K. J., and Patten, C. A. (1997). Prospective evaluation of three smoking interventions in, 205 recovering alcoholics: one-year results of project SCRAP-tobacco. *Journal of Consulting Clinical Psychology, 65*, 190–194.

Melnick, M. J., Miller, K. E., Sabo, D. F., Farrell, M. P., and Barnes, G. M. (2001). Tobacco use among high school athletes and non-athletes: results of the 1997 Youth Risk Behavior Survey. *Adolescence, 36*, 727–747.

Nishi, N., Jenicek, M., and Tatara, K. (1998). A meta-analytic review of the effect of exercise on smoking cessation. *Journal of Epidemiology, 8*, 79–84.

Paavola, M., Vartianen, E., and Puska, P. (2001). Smoking cessation between teenage years and adulthood. *Health Education Research, 16*, 49–57.

Pate, P. R., Pratt, M., Steven, S. N., Haskell, W. L., Macera, C. A., Bouchard, C. *et al.* (1995). Exercise and public health: a recommendation from the Centers for Disease Control and Prevention and the American College of Sports Medicine. *Journal of the American Medical Association, 273*, 402–407.

Pate, R. R., Heath, G. W., Dowda, M., and Trost, S. G. (1996). Association between physical activity and other health behaviors in a representative sample of US adolescents. *American Journal of Public Health, 86*, 1577–1581.

Pate, R. R., Trost, S. G., Levin, S., and Dowda, M. (2000). Sports participation and health related behaviors among US youth. *Archives of Pediatric Adolescent Medicine, 154*, 904–911.

Patten, C. A., Vickers, K. S., Martin, J. E., and Williams, C. D. (2001). Exercise interventions for smokers with a history of alcoholism: exercise adherence rates and effect of depression on adherence. *Addictive Behavior, 27*, 1–11.

Peretti-Watel, P., Beck, F., and Legleye, S. (2002). Beyond the U-curve: the relationship between sport and alcohol, cigarette and cannabis use in adolescents. *Addiction, 97*, 707–716.

Piasecki, T. M., Niaura, R., Shadel, W. G., Fiore, M. C., and Baker, T. B. (2000). Smoking withdrawal dynamics in unaided quitters. *Journal of Abnormal Psychology, 109*, 74–86.

Pomerleau, O. F., Scherzer, H. H., Grunberg, N. E., Pomerleau, C. S., Judge, J., Fetig, J. B. *et al.* (1987). The effects of acute exercise on subsequent cigarette smoking. *Journal of Behavioural Medicine, 10*, 117–127.

Rainey, C. J., McKeown, R. E., Sargent, R. G., and Valois, R. F. (1996). Patterns of tobacco and alcohol use among sedentary, exercising, nonathletic, and athletic youth. *Journal of School Health, 66*, 27–32.

Raw, M., McNeill, A., and West, R. (1998). *Smoking Cessation Guidelines for Health Professionals: A Guide to Effective Smoking Cessation Interventions for the Health Care System.* London: Health Education Authority.

Rodriguez, D. and Audrain-McGovern, J. (2004). Team sport participation and smoking: analysis with general growth mixture modeling. *Journal of Pediatric Psychology, 29*, 299–308.

Russell, P. O., Epstein, L. H., Johnson, J. J., Block, D. R., and Blair, E. (1988). The effects of exercise as maintenance for smoking cessation. *Addictive Behavior, 13*, 215–218.

Schneider, D. and Greenberg, M. R. (1992). Choice of exercise: a predictor of behavioral risks? *Research Quarterly for Exercise and Sport, 63*, 231–237.

Sedgwick, A. W., Davidson, A. H., Taplin, R. E., and Thomas, D. W. (1988). Effects of physical activity on risk factors for coronary heart disease in previously sedentary women: a five-year longitudinal study. *Australian and New Zealand Journal of Medicine, 18*, 600–605.

Sevick, M. A., Dunn, A. L., Morrow, M. S., Marcus, B. H., Chen, G. H., and Blair, S. (2000). Cost-effectiveness of lifestyle and structured exercise interventions in sedentary adults; results of Project Active. *American Journal of Preventive Medicine, 19*, 1–8.

Shiffman, S., Paty, J. A., Gnys, M., Kassel, J. D., and Hickcoc, M. (1996). First lapses to smoking: within-subjects analysis of real time reports. *Journal of Consulting and Clinical Psychology, 64*, 366–379.

Silagy, C., Lancaster, T., Stead, L., Mant, D., and Fowler, G. (2004). Nicotine replacement therapy for smoking cessation (Cochrane review). In *The Cochrane Library, 3*. Oxford: Updated Software.

Swan, G. E., Ward, M. M., Carmelli, D., and Jack, L. M. (1993). Differential rates of relapse in subgroups of male and female smokers. *Journal of Clinical Epidemiology, 46*, 1041–1053.

Taylor, A. H. (2000). Physical activity, stress and anxiety: a review. In S. J. H. Biddle, K. R. Fox, and S. H. Boutcher (Eds). *Physical Activity and Psychological Well-being* (pp. 10–45). London: Routledge.

Taylor, A. H. (2003). The role of primary care in promoting physical activity. In C. Riddoch and J. McKenna (Eds). *Perspectives in Health and Exercise* (pp. 153–180). London: MacMillan.

Taylor, A. H. and Fox, K. (2005). Changes in physical self-perceptions: findings from a randomised controlled study of a GP exercise referral scheme. *Health Psychology, 24*, 11–21.

Taylor, C. B., Houston-Miller, N., Haskell. W. L., and Debusk, R. F. (1988). Smoking cessation after acute myocardial infarction: the effects of exercise training. *Addictive Behaviors, 13*, 331–334.

Taylor, A. H., Doust, J., and Webborn, A. D. J. (1998). Randomised controlled trial to examine the effects of a GP exercise referral programme in Hailsham, East Sussex, on modifiable coronary heart disease risk factors. *Journal of Epidemiology and Community Health, 52*, 595–601.

Taylor, A. H., Katomeri, M., and Ussher, M. (2005). Acute effects of self-paced walking on urge to smoke during temporary smoking abstinence. *Psychopharmacology* (Epub ahead of print).

Thayer, R. E., Peters, D., Takahaski, P., and Birkhead-Flight, A. (1993). Mood and behaviour (smoking and sugar snacking) following moderate exercise: a partial test of self regulation theory. *Personality and Individual Differences, 14*, 97–104.

Thayer, R. E., Newman, J. R., and McClain, T. M. (1994). Self-regulation of mood: strategies for changing bad mood, raising energy and reducing tension. *Journal of Personality and Social Psychology, 67*, 910–925.

Tiffany, S. T. and Drobes, D. J. (1991). The development and initial validation of a questionnaire on smoking urges. *British Journal of Addiction, 86*, 1467–1476.

Tkachuk, G. A. and Martin, G. L. (1999). Exercise therapy for patients with psychiatric disorders: research and clinical implications. *Professional Psychology Research and Practice, 30*, 275–282.

United States Department of Health and Human Services (1990). *The Health Consequences of Smoking Cessation: A Report of the Surgeon General*. Rockville, MD: Public Health Service, Office on Smoking and Health.

United States Department of Health and Human Services, Centers for Disease Control and Prevention, National Center for Chronic Disease Prevention and Health Promotion (1996). *Physical Activity and Health: A Report of the Surgeon General*. Atlanta, GA: Centers for Disease Control and Prevention.

Ussher, M. (2005). Exercise interventions for smoking cessation (Cochrane review). In *The Cochrane Library, 4*. Oxford: Updated Software.

Ussher, M. and West, R. (2003) Interest in nicotine replacement therapy among pregnant smokers. *Tobacco Control, 12*, 108–109.

Ussher, M., Taylor, A. H., West, R., and McEwen, A. (2000). Does exercise aid smoking cessation? A systematic review. *Addiction*, *95*, 199–208.

Ussher, M., Nunziata, P., Cropley, M., and West, R. (2001). Effect of a short bout of exercise on tobacco withdrawal symptoms and desire to smoke. *Psychopharmacology*, *158*, 66–72.

Ussher, M. H., West, R., McEwen, A., Taylor, A. H., and Steptoe, A. (2003). Efficacy of exercise counselling as an aid for smoking cessation: a randomised controlled trial. *Addiction*, *98*, 523–532.

Ussher, M., West, R., and Hibbs, N. (2004). A survey of pregnant smokers' interest in different types of smoking cessation support. *Patient Education and Counseling*, *54*, 67–72.

Ussher, M., West, R., Doshi, R., and Sampuran, A. K. (submitted). Seated isometric exercise reduces desire to smoke. *Experimental Journal of Psychopharmacology*.

West, R. and Russell, M. (1985). Pre-abstinence smoke intake and smoking motivation as predictors of severity of cigarette withdrawal symptoms. *Psychopharmacology*, *87*, 407–415.

West, R., Hajek, P., and Belcher, M. (1989) Severity of withdrawal symptoms as a predictor of outcome of an attempt to quit smoking. *Psychology and Medicine*, *19*, 981–985.

West, R., Courts, S., Beharry, S., May, S., and Hajek, P. (1999). Acute effect of glucose tablets on desire to smoke. *Psychopharmacology*, *147*, 319–321.

Exercise and sleep

SHAWN D. YOUNGSTEDT AND
JULIE D. FREELOVE-CHARTON

Disturbed sleep is a common complaint. The global annual incidence of insomnia is estimated to be 20–40% (Mellinger *et al.*, 1985; Ohayon *et al.*, 1998). Sleep problems become increasingly prevalent with age, such that over 50% of the US population over the age of 60 experience some sleep-related complaint (Foley *et al.*, 1995). Moreover, poor or inadequate sleep has been linked to psychiatric disturbance (Mellinger *et al.*, 1985; Riemann and Voderholzer, 2003), decreased work productivity (National Commission on Sleep Disorders Research, 1993), and an increased risk of automobile accidents (Radun and Summala, 2004). For example, impairments in neurobehavioral performance and simulator driving performance following a night of sleep loss appear to be similar to those associated with blood alcohol levels of ~0.10 g/dl (Powell *et al.*, 2001). Epidemiological studies have shown a consistent association between short habitual sleep duration ($\leq$5 hr/night), as well as long sleep durations ($\geq$8 hr) and mortality (Youngstedt and Kripke, 2004). The result of insomnia, both directly and indirectly, is an annual economic burden in the US of approximately $13.9 billion (Walsh, 2004).

Despite the high prevalence and potentially tragic consequences, sleep problems remain largely untreated by clinicians. Self-help remedies for disrupted sleep (e.g., alcohol and melatonin) and its consequences (caffeine) are generally ineffective and can often exacerbate the existing condition. The regular use of sleeping pills, the most common treatment for insomnia, is associated with a substantial mortality risk (Kripke *et al.*, 1998). Usage is also associated with dependence and tolerance, along with a host of other side effects including nausea, prolonged daytime sedation, increased risk of falls, and cognitive impairment (Kripke, 2000). Although the use of sleeping pills beyond four weeks is discouraged by sleep experts, the majority of patients are chronic users (Kripke, 2000). Additionally, evidence suggests that this long-term usage cannot be explained by continued efficacy, since insomniacs who take sleeping pills chronically do not sleep better than non-medicated insomniacs. Rather, chronic usage could be attributed to the profound rebound insomnia that can occur with hypnotic discontinuation (Kripke, 2000).

Cognitive and behavioral treatments of insomnia such as sleep restriction therapy have been successful. Indeed, these treatments have been shown to be superior to hypnotics for the long-term management of insomnia (Morin *et al.*, 1999). Notwithstanding the success of cognitive-behavioral therapy, these treatments are expensive, labor-intensive, and require skilled clinical psychologists or psychiatrists with a broad knowledge of sleep medicine, and these individuals are in short supply. In contrast to both hypnotics and cognitive-behavioral treatments, exercise could be a relatively simple and inexpensive way of improving sleep quality and could be easily self-administered. There is also a general consensus among the general population (Vuori *et al.*, 1988), as well as sleep experts and physicians (American Academy of Sleep Medicine, 2004), that exercise promotes sleep. Indeed, exercise is often one of the first topics addressed in general recommendations about improving sleep.

The notion that exercise promotes sleep has also been consistent with both traditional and modern hypotheses regarding sleep function including energy conservation, body restitution, and temperature down-regulation hypotheses. Furthermore, there are both experimental and theoretical grounds for promoting exercise as an efficacious treatment or an adjuvant therapy for other sleep disorders including circadian rhythm disorders, mood-related sleep disorders, sleep apnea, and restless legs syndrome.

The primary aim of this review is to evaluate the evidence that exercise promotes sleep. We will focus sequentially on epidemiological evidence associating exercise with better sleep – experimental evidence that acute exercise promotes sleep, experimental evidence that chronic exercise promotes sleep, and the use of exercise for treating specific sleep disorders. We will attempt to critically consider each of these lines of evidence and identify possible moderating factors. However, the field of sleep research is complex. This is reflected in the many ways it is measured or reported. Rather than considering the nature of sleep and its measurement at this point, we have included more technical information in an appendix at the end of the chapter. For those less familiar with the literature, we feel that this provides a resource to critically assess the effects of exercise on sleep.

STRUCTURED REVIEW

The review was conducted by searching the PubMed, PsychLit, and Cochrane data bases since 1996, the date that a previous meta-analysis was performed (Youngstedt *et al.*, 1997).

In addition, citations within the located references were searched. We used the following key words: *exercise*, *physical activity*, *physical fitness*, *sleep*, and *sleep deprivation*. The literature included epidemiological studies and cross-sectional comparisons between physically active and inactive individuals, acute exercise studies, and exercise training or chronic studies.

EPIDEMIOLOGICAL STUDIES

In large population surveys, people report that exercise promotes their sleep (see Table 9.1). For example, a random sample ($n = 1,190$) of men and women living in Tampere, Finland were asked the following open-ended question: "Please state, in order of importance, three practices, habits, or actions which you have observed to best promote or improve your falling asleep immediately or your perceived quality of sleep." Both men and women listed exercise as the most important factor, more important than sauna exposure (even in Finland), quiet relaxation, or listening to music (Urponen et al., 1988). Epidemiological studies have consistently shown an association between self-reported exercise and better self-reported sleep (Arakawa et al., 2002; Kim et al., 2000; Morgan, 2003; Ohida et al., 2001; Sherrill et al., 1998; Uezu et al., 2000). For example, in a recent rigorous study, Morgan (2003) used interviews to study insomnia and physical activity in a representative sample of 1,042 adults over the age of 65, and included follow-up assessments at 4 years ($n = 673$) and 8 years ($n = 390$). Customary physical activity was assessed through an extensive interview. Insomnia was considered to be present if the respondent reported having "problems sleeping" "often" or "all the time" (other response choices ranged from "never" to "sometimes") and if that problem was experienced within the previous week. Logistic regression models, controlling for social engagement, physical health status, depressed mood, body mass index, gender, and age, consistently showed that low levels of physical activity were associated with a significantly higher prevalence of insomnia.

However, there are numerous limitations of the epidemiological studies associating exercise with sleep. First, they have often assessed both exercise and sleep using instruments with limited or unknown reliability and validity. For example, a typical question in these studies has been whether the respondent regularly engaged in habitual exercise, a question that is likely to have considerable variability in interpretation. Few of the studies have attempted to quantify exercise or physical activity using accepted metrics. Likewise, none of the epidemiological studies have included clinical diagnoses of sleep disorders, nor have they included questions that address accepted criteria for sleep disorders. Thus, the clinical relevance of these findings is unclear.

There are a number of plausible alternative explanations for the epidemiological association of exercise with better sleep and for survey respondents to have a false impression that exercise promotes their sleep. First, better sleep might be associated with a greater willingness and ability to exercise. When one is sleep-deprived, exercise might be one of the first things sacrificed. Research has suggested that a low level of physical activity is one of the most significant correlates of daytime sleepiness (Weaver et al., 1997; Whitney et al., 1998).

Second, people who exercise regularly tend to practice other healthy habits that could be conducive to sleep such as abstaining from tobacco, avoiding excessive caffeine

Table 9.1 Epidemiological studies examining exercise and sleep

AUTHOR	PARTICIPANTS n; AGES; LOCATION	DESIGN	TYPES OF QUESTIONS/ INSTRUMENTS	RESULTS AND COMMENT
Urponen et al. (1988)	n = 1,600	Random sample survey	Standardized questionnaires about sleep, exercise, sleep environment, lifestyle factors (e.g., sauna, stability in life)	Exercise rated most important behavior associated with better sleep Temporary lack of exercise associated with worse reported sleep
Vuori et al. (1988)	n = 1,190, ages 36–50 yrs, Finland	Random sample survey	Open-ended mail-in questionnaire about sleep, exercise, health, and other lifestyle factors	Exercise rated most important behavior associated with better sleep
Tynjala et al. (1993)	n = 40,202, ages 11–16 yrs, 11 mostly European countries	Representative survey	Standardized questionnaires on leisure time physical activity, fitness, sleep, lifestyle, health	Self-reported physical condition weakly correlated with reported difficulty falling asleep ($r \leq 0.10$)
Sherrill et al. (1998)	n = 722: n = 403 women, 59.9 ± 14.4 yrs; n = 319 men, 54.1 ± 2.3 yrs Arizona, US	Non-random survey	Self-administered questionnaire: questions regarding exercise, sleep	Multiple logistic regression: regular vigorous exercise and walking at least 6 blocks/day associated with significantly fewer complaints about sleep
Tynjala et al. (1999)	n = 4,187, 11–15 yrs, Finland	WHO Representative survey	Standardized questionnaires on leisure-time physical activity, sleep, health habits	Multiple logistic regression: significant association of physical activity with better sleep in girls, but not boys
Kim et al. (2000)	n = 3,030, ages 20+ yrs, Japan	Representative survey	Structured questionnaire including habitual exercise, insomnia, health, during previous month	Multiple logistic regression: lack of exercise associated with higher incidence of insomnia OR 1.7, controlling for other covariates

Liu et al. (2000)	n = 1,365, ages 12–18 yrs, China	Non-random survey	Self-administered questionnaire including habitual exercise (none, 1–2d, ≥3 d/wk), insomnia, health, life stress	Multiple logistic regression: progressively more insomnia reported with less habitual exercise OR for 0, 1–2 d/wk, ≥3 d/wk = 3.06, 2.77, 1.0, respectively, controlling for other covariates
Uezu et al. (2000)	n = 788, ages 60–93 yrs, Japan	Non-random survey Compared n = 150 with best versus 150 with worst reported sleep	Questionnaire regarding sleep, exercise, health	Good sleepers reported significantly more exercise than poor sleepers
Ohida et al. (2001)	n = 31,260, ages 20–90 yrs, Japan	Random survey	Questionnaire including lifestyle (exercise), insufficient sleep, health, occupation	Multiple logistic regression: lack of exercise associated with significantly more insufficient sleep
Arakawa et al. (2002)	n = 312, ages 71.9 ± 6.7 yrs	Non-random survey	Standardized questionnaire on sleep health and lifestyle	Daily habits such as short naps and taking appropriate exercise in the evenings contributed to good sleep, and that sleep health was related to the activities of daily living of the elderly
Morgan (2003)	n = 1,042, ages 65 + yrs, UK	Representative survey	Interviews at 4 yrs and 8 yrs: free-living physical activity and walking, social activity, insomnia, health status	Multiple logistic regression: lower physical activity associated with significant prevalence, incidence, and persistence of insomnia

Notes: yrs = years; d = day/s; wk = week/s.

and alcohol use, and maintaining a healthy diet (Dishman, 2001; Sun *et al.*, 2002). Third, it seems apparent that the notion that exercise promotes sleep is based partly on the assumption that sleepiness is synonymous with physical fatigue (Dawson and Fletcher, 2001; Lichstein *et al.*, 1997). However, there is no compelling support for this assumption. Although sleepiness and physical fatigue often occur simultaneously (e.g., at the end of the day), they are also commonly observed independent of each other. For example, long periods of bed rest are associated with more sleep (Campbell, 1984). Conversely, feelings of alertness are commonly self-reported following exercise.

Fourth, both cross-sectional and experimental evidence indicate that chronic exercise is associated with feelings of greater energy and less fatigue (Hong and Dimsdale, 2003; O'Connor and Youngstedt, 1995). Based upon these feelings, people could make the assumption that exercise must be promoting their sleep. However, feelings of greater energy could be attributed to physiological consequences of training, such as having a higher blood volume, and lower resting heart rate and respiratory rate.

Fifth, the epidemiological association between exercise and better sleep might be explained by a third factor, such as better physical health or better mental health. Both these constructs are associated with better sleep and higher levels of physical activity (Jones *et al.*, 2002). Another confounding factor could be bright light exposure. It has been shown that low levels of exposure to environmental illumination are associated with poor sleep and depression (Youngstedt *et al.*, 1999b). Additionally, experimental increases in bright light exposure can elicit dramatic sleep-promoting and antidepressant effects (Kripke, 1998). Research has demonstrated that the average adult spends >1 hour/day in outdoor light (Youngstedt *et al.*, 1999b), but people who exercise outdoors are obviously more likely to receive much more light. Considering that 30 min of bright light (equivalent to a bright outdoor light) is an effective antidepressant treatment, it can be speculated that regular outdoor exercise would promote better mood and sleep via light exposure (Partonen *et al.*, 1998).

ACUTE EXERCISE STUDIES

Laboratory studies

A meta-analysis of studies examining the influence of exercise versus sedentary control treatments on polysomnographic markers of sleep found that exercise produced a statistically significant increase in total sleep duration (mean effect size (95% CI) = 0.42 (0.17, 0.68)) (Youngstedt *et al.*, 1997). However, this effect represented a median increase in total sleep time of only 10 min. The practical relevance of a 10-min increase in sleep is not clear. There is no compelling evidence that such a change over a single night would have an impact on daytime sleepiness or functioning. Across the literature, exercise had virtually no mean effect on sleep latency (ES = −0.05 (−0.24, −0.15)) or wakefulness during the night (ES = 0.07 (−0.23, 0.37)), which are two of the better polysomnographic correlates of insomnia complaints.

The meta-analysis also found a significant increase in slow wave sleep (effect size = 0.19 (−0.03, 0.39)), though the median increase in slow wave sleep (SWS) was only 1.4 min (Youngstedt *et al.*, 1997). This finding was noteworthy because it is often assumed that exercise elicits large increases in SWS. Interestingly, the largest effects of acute exercise on stages of sleep were found for rapid eye movement (REM) sleep (ES = -0.49 (-0.72, -0.26)). Exercise elicited a median decrease in REM sleep of 6 min, and a median increase in the latency for REM sleep to first occur after sleep onset of 11.6 min (ES = 0.52 (0.27, 0.78)). As with SWS changes, the implications for these small (albeit significant) post-exercise decreases in REM sleep on a single night are not established. To our knowledge, there have been only a few laboratory studies of the effects of acute exercise on sleep since 1997.

Field studies

Three studies (of which we are aware) have examined the influence on sleep of acute exercise in one's usual environment (see Table 9.2). In a questionnaire-based study, Porter and Horne (1981) examined daily activity and sleep across seven consecutive days in 51 young, healthy normal sleepers. Daily variations in activity level did not have a significant effect on pre-sleep tiredness, nor on subjective sleep. Youngstedt *et al.* (2003) reported the results of two studies. The first study examined self-reported exercise durations and sleep diaries for 105 consecutive days in 31 college students who were normal sleepers. The main analysis revealed no significant within-subjects association between daily exercise and sleep. In the second study, 71 physically active, generally good sleepers were assessed ($n = 38$, ages 18–30 years; $n = 33$, ages 60–75 years). Over seven consecutive days, physical activity was assessed via actigraphy and a validated diary-derived estimate of energy expenditure, while sleep was assessed via actigraphy and diaries. No within-subject relationships were found, even when comparing sleep following the week's most active versus least active days.

In testing a group of young athletes ($n = 16$, mean age = 21.7 years), Hague *et al.* (2003) found that slow wave sleep was significantly greater, while sleep latency and REM sleep were significantly less, following an exercise day in the subjects' usual environment compared with a sedentary day, in which subjects were restricted to the laboratory. However, as discussed in the Appendix, there is little compelling evidence for interpreting the increase in slow wave sleep versus the decrease in REM sleep as a "positive" finding. Moreover, the results could have been confounded by extraneous factors (e.g., exposure to sunlight) between the treatments. In summary, as with the laboratory studies, the field studies do not provide compelling evidence that acute exercise promotes sleep to a substantial degree.

Potential explanations for small effects

The lack of more compelling evidence for acute exercise effects on sleep may be partially attributed to several experimental limitations. First, exercise and sleep recording in the laboratory cannot duplicate the exercise and sleep conditions that have been associated with better sleep in one's usual environment. Of course, separating the influence of exercise per se from environmental influences is important, but unique aspects of the laboratory environment (e.g., stress or boredom) could attenuate the usual effects of exercise.

Table 9.2 Acute exercise and sleep studies

AUTHOR	PARTICIPANTS n; AGES; FITNESS/ ACTIVITY; SLEEP HISTORY	DESIGN	MEASURES	RESULTS AND DISCUSSION
Porter and Horne (1981)	$n = 51$, 25–30 yrs, most were active, normal sleepers	Prospective study over 7 days General linear model comparing sleep following physical activity on days rated "less active," "normal," "greater than normal" activity	Daily diary measures including sleep latency, total sleep time, pre-sleep tiredness and post-sleep tiredness	No significant effects of activity on quality or quantity of sleep or post-sleep tiredness
O'Connor et al. (1998)	$n = 8$, 19–35 yrs, normal sleepers, physically active	Within-subjects, randomly completed: 1 hr cycling @60% VO_2max; 1 hr seated on cycle; 1 hr quiet reading; ending 30 min before bedtime	Verbal response to auditory stimulation: sleep latency, sleep efficiency, number of awakenings, total sleep time	No differences following exercise compared with control contrary to assumption that late-night exercise disturbs sleep
Kobayashi et al. (1999)	$n = 10$, 21 ± 0.7 yrs, sedentary normal sleepers	Within-subjects, cross over 1 hr @50–60% VO_2max at (1) 0740–0840 hr (2) 1630–1730 hr (3) 2030–2130 hr 15 hr, 6 hr, 2 hr before bedtime, respectively	Polygraphic sleep latency Subjective diary of ease of going to sleep, sleep satisfaction, sleep maintenance	Sleep latency significantly shorter after night exercise (mean 6.4 ± 3.1 SD min) versus morning (12.9 ± 6.9 min) or afternoon exercise (20.4 ± 13.2 min) Significantly better subjective sleep after evening versus other times No impairment in sleep following evening exercise even in sedentary subjects

Study	Sample	Design	Measures	Results
Youngstedt et al. (1999a)	n = 16, 27.3 ± 4.3 yrs, aerobically fit normal sleepers	Within-subjects, cross-over, (1) 3 hr cycling at 65–75% HRR ending 30 min before bedtime (2) sedentary control	Actigraphic assessment of SOL, TST, WASO; Sleep diary assessment of SOL, TST, WASO, insomnia	ANOVA compared with control: no significant changes in actigraphic or self-reported sleep. Evidence contradicting that late-night exercise impairs sleep
Hague et al. (2003)	n = 16, 21.7 ± 2.8 yrs, aerobically fit normal sleepers	Within-subjects, cross-over, (1) usual exercise day (2) sedentary day	Polygraphic: sleep latency, SWS, REM sleep, REM latency, stages 1 and 2	Significantly greater SWS and REM latency, but less REM sleep following exercise compared to sedentary day. Potential confound of staying indoors in the lab during sedentary day versus usual activities on exercise day
Youngstedt et al. (2003)	Study 1: n = 31, 22.9 ± 2.8 yrs, variable fitness normal sleepers; Study 2: n = 38, ages 18–30 yrs, n = 33, ages 60–75 yrs, aerobically fit normal sleepers	Study 1: within-subjects prospective study over 105 days; Study 2: within-subjects prospective study over 7 days	Study 1: self-reported daily diary of exercise duration and sleep (SOL, TST, WASO, sleep efficiency) for 105 days; Study 2: actigraphic and self-reported physical activity and sleep (SOL, TST, WASO)	Study 1: no within-subjects correlation of daily exercise and sleep; Study 2: no within-subjects association of daily physical activity with sleep

Notes: hr = hour/s; yr = year/s; min = minute/s; SOL = sleep latency; TST = total sleep time; WASO = wake after sleep onset; SWS = slow wave sleep.

Second, most acute exercise studies have examined exercise and sleep on only one or two days (Youngstedt *et al.*, 1997). Since sleep is sensitive to multiple factors, and has considerable inter-night variability, several experimental days may be necessary to delineate any beneficial effects of exercise. Undoubtedly, the greatest limitation of previous research has been the exclusive focus on good sleepers, for whom major improvements in sleep are not likely (i.e., ceiling/floor effects). In fact, the effects of exercise are similar to the effects of hypnotics when the comparisons are restricted to good sleepers (Youngstedt, 2003).

The obvious question that arises from this literature is "why have studies focused only on good sleepers?" There is no analogous extensive literature on other putative sleep treatments. The apparent answer is that much of the earlier research in this area, particularly prior to 1990, was driven by traditional hypotheses regarding sleep function. These theories predicted a unique role of exercise for enhancing sleep, but have since been largely discredited. One hypothesis, which is probably still accepted by the general public, is that sleep serves a function of energy conservation (Berger and Phillips, 1988). If this was in fact the case, then exercise would have a unique sleep-promoting effect because nothing, except perhaps starvation, elicits a greater depletion of energy stores. However, evidence contrary to an energy conservation function of sleep are that (1) energy savings are minimally greater (perhaps 5%) during sleep compared with relaxed wakefulness, and (2) continuous bedrest can produce profound increases in sleep (Rechtschaffen, 1998). Another hypothesis states that sleep serves a body restitution function, which would be particularly necessary following the tissue breakdown associated with exercise. However, there is no compelling evidence of a particular effect of sleep on protein synthesis or replenishment of ATP stores (Rechtschaffen, 1998). In actuality, recent research has shown that growth hormone is excreted in equal amounts in the absence of sleep (Brandenberger and Weibel, 2004).

A more recent hypothesis stating that sleep serves a body–brain cooling function (McGinty and Szymusiak, 1990) also predicts a uniquely potent effect of exercise because exercise elevates body temperature more readily than any other stimulus. This hypothesis is still being assessed.

It is noteworthy that there are some isolated studies showing extraordinary increases in total sleep time or slow wave sleep following marathon or ultramarathon events (Driver *et al.*, 1994; Shapiro *et al.*, 1975). However, there are potential caveats with these data. For example, sleep was not assessed on the nights prior to these events, and sleep may have been profoundly impaired on these nights due to nervous anticipation and having to wake up early for the competition. Conversely, in one study, sleep was permitted ad lib on the morning after the event, but restricted on other nights (Driver *et al.*, 1994). Also, there is evidence which suggests that sleep following these events is severely fragmented (Driver *et al.*, 1994). Nonetheless, the results could also reflect a unique effect of prolonged exercise on sleep. The practical implications of this research for the general population are dubious. However, prolonged or intermittent light-intensity physical activity conceivably could have similar effects in less physically active individuals.

FACTORS MODERATING ACUTE EFFECTS

There are many factors that could moderate the influence of exercise on sleep. Several selected factors will be reviewed.

Proximity to bedtime

It is often assumed that late-night exercise will impair sleep, presumably by increasing physiological arousal, particularly when the exercise is vigorous. Anecdotal reports on this matter run the gamut, and could reflect individuals' responses to exercise. These individual differences are unknown as most self-report data is conflicting. In a survey of 322 adults who exercised within 2 hours of bedtime, the majority reported no effect of the evening exercise on difficulty falling asleep (76%) or increased restlessness and nocturnal awakenings (95%) (Vuori *et al.*, 1988). On the other hand, a recent study found that among evening exercisers ($n = 36$, between 6:00 and 7:30 pm), those who exercised >180 min/week reported significantly more trouble falling asleep then those who exercised <180 min/week (Tworoger *et al.*, 2003). However, no data regarding bedtime were reported, and no comparisons with a control treatment were reported.

Experimental studies comparing exercise versus control treatments have generally failed to support the assumption that late-night exercise impairs sleep. Indeed, two studies found no impairments in sleep following 1–3 hours of vigorous exercise, ending 30 min before bedtime (O'Connor *et al.*, 1998; Youngstedt *et al.*, 1999a). Another recent study found that polysomnographically assessed sleep latency was 2–3 times faster following exercise (cycling 1 hr at 50–60% VO_2peak) completed 2 hours before bedtime, compared with morning or early evening exercise (Kobayashi *et al.*, 1999). This research is noteworthy because it utilized sedentary subjects, for whom particular sensitivity to sleep-impairing effects of evening exercise might be expected due to the unaccustomed stimulus (i.e., exercise). In contrast, there are theoretical rationales for expecting that late-evening exercise might be the best time for promoting sleep. Research has shown that both anxiolytic and thermogenic effects of exercise on sleep are likely to be greatest during the first 1–2 hours after exercise (Youngstedt, 2000).

Duration

Meta-analysis revealed that sleep duration was most influenced by exercise duration (Youngstedt *et al.*, 1997). However, the relative strength of this association may have resulted from a clearer description of duration, or information from which duration could be estimated (e.g., distance), compared with other moderator variables. Reliable effects of exercise were observed only for exercise of 1 hour. For example, the mean effect sizes for exercise bouts lasting <1, 1–2, and >2 hours were 0.07, 0.45, and 0.61, respectively. These findings raise questions about the practical usefulness of exercise for the general population as large numbers of the population are generally not physically active for periods >1 hour each day.

Intensity

Exercise intensity, which can be considered a proxy for temperature elevation in most studies, generally did not significantly moderate the influence of acute exercise on sleep

(Youngstedt et al., 1997). Indeed, in the meta-analysis, the only significant effect of intensity was a linear increase in wakefulness after sleep onset with increasing intensity. These data contradict the thermogenic hypothesis that exercise promotes sleep via temperature elevation.

Fitness

An individual's overall fitness level does not appear to moderate the influence of acute exercise on sleep (Youngstedt et al., 1997). This finding is consistent with survey reports from the general population (Kim et al., 2000; Vuori et al., 1988) and could potentially have positive implications for the use of exercise as a treatment for insomnia. For example, if the sleep-promoting effects of exercise were delayed until an adequate level of fitness was reached, people might be reluctant to adhere to an exercise treatment.

INFLUENCE OF ACUTE EXERCISE ON DAYTIME SLEEPINESS

Another important issue is whether acute exercise can reduce daytime sleepiness and functioning associated with sleep loss. Studies have shown that exercise can decrease sleepiness following sleep deprivation, but this effect disappears as early as 10–15 min post-exercise (Horne and Foster, 1995; LeDuc et al., 2000). In comparisons of exercise at 20%, 40%, and 70% VO_2max, only the most vigorous exercise was found to improve auditory vigilance (Horne and Foster, 1995).

CHRONIC STUDIES

Since the experimental literature on the influence of chronic exercise on sleep is less extensive than the acute exercise literature, this review will describe individual chronic exercise studies in greater detail (see Table 9.3).

Young, normal sleepers

As with the acute exercise studies, chronic exercise studies have generally failed to show compelling sleep-promoting effects of exercise in healthy, young normal sleepers (Driver et al., 1988; Meintjes et al., 1989). One study noted a dramatic improvement in sleep of soldiers from the beginning to the end of an 18-week boot camp which included extensive exercise (Shapiro et al., 1984). However, there was no control treatment so the results could be explained by profound chronic sleep deprivation or a host of other stressors associated with boot camp.

Table 9.3 Chronic exercise and sleep studies

AUTHOR	PARTICIPANTS n; AGES; NORMAL OR INSOMNIAC	DESIGN	MEASURES	RESULTS/DISCUSSION
Shapiro et al. (1984)	n = 8, 17–21 yrs, normal sleepers	Prospective, uncontrolled Baseline and after 9 and 18 wks of improved fitness with boot camp	Polygraphic: SOL, TST, sleep efficiency, WASO, SWS	SWS increased significantly at 9 wk and 18 wk versus baseline No significant changes in other sleep parameters Multiple uncontrolled confounds (e.g., prolonged sleep deprivation)
Driver et al. (1988)	n = 9, 24 ± 3 yrs, normal sleepers	Prospective, uncontrolled Baseline and after 4, 8, or 12 wks training programs	Polygraphic: SOL, sleep efficiency, SWS; subjective sleep quality, morning vigilance	Under baseline conditions, no changes in objective or subjective sleep at weeks 4, 8, or 12 versus wk 0
Meinjes et al. (1989)	n = 9, 20–28 yrs, normal sleepers	Prospective, uncontrolled 12 wks: cycling 3/wk; running 2/wk	Polygraphic: SOL, SWS Self-reported sleep	Under baseline conditions, no significant changes in polygraphic or self-reported sleep at wk 4, wk 8, or wk 12 compared with wk 0 Limitation: normal sleepers
Stevenson and Topp (1990)	n = 72, 63.9 ± 3.9 yrs, sleep status unknown	Random, prospective, uncontrolled 9 months (30 min, 3/wk): (1) moderate-intensity exercise (60–70% HRR) (2) low-intensity exercise (30–40% HRR)	Likert scales including sleep quality and quantity	Significant increase over time in sleep quantity No difference between treatments Instrument not validated No sedentary control treatment
Vitiello et al. (1994)	n = 30, 66.4 ± 0.8 yrs, normal sleepers	Prospective, random assignment 6 months (3 d/wk): (1) aerobic exercise (2) stretching	Polygraphic measures Subjective: Pittsburgh Sleep Quality Inventory (PSQI), Visual Analogue Retrospective Scale, Daily sleep diary	No significant improvement in polysomnographic sleep or any self-reported sleep following exercise versus stretching

(Table 9.3 continued)

Table 9.3 Continued

AUTHOR	PARTICIPANTS n; AGES; NORMAL OR INSOMNIAC	DESIGN	MEASURES	RESULTS/DISCUSSION
Alessi et al. (1995)	n = 65, 84.4 ± 7.2 yrs, poor sleepers in nursing home	Prospective, no sedentary control random assignment 9 wk (1) intensive exercise: sit-to-stand repetitions, walking, wheel-or chair propulsion, every 2 hr during day (5 d/wk) (2) moderate exercise: rowing + walking or wheelchair exercise once/day (3 d/wk)	Actigraphic: sleep duration, sleep efficiency, average duration of individual sleep episodes, daytime sleep	No significant improvement in night time sleep or reduction in daytime napping within or between groups
Guilleminault et al. (1995)	n = 30, 44 ± 8 yrs, primary insomnia	Prospect, random assignment 4 wk (1) sleep hygiene (SH) (2) SH + brisk walking (45 min/d) (3) SH + bright light (30 min/d)	Actigraphic and diary: SOL, TST, WASO	Only the light treatment group had a a significant improvement in actigraphic sleep Pattern suggested improvement with exercise
King et al. (1997)	n = 43, 50–76 yrs, moderate sleep complaints	Prospective random 16 wk: (1) aerobic exercise (4/wk, 30–40 min/d) (2) waiting list control	Pittsburgh Sleep Quality Index (PSQI) at baseline and 16 wk Daily sleep diary for 2 wks at baseline 8 wks or 16 wks	Exercise group improved significantly more on PSQI-assessed global sleep, sleep quality, sleep latency, and total sleep time Exercise group improved significantly more than control on diary-assessed: overall sleep quality, sleep latency, total sleep time, feeling rested upon awakening

Study	Sample	Design	Measures	Results
Singh et al. (1997)	$n = 32$, 71.3 ± 1.2 years, diagnosed depressives	Random assignment 10 wk: (1) weight training ($3\times$/wk) (2) health education control	Baseline and 10 wk: Pittsburgh Sleep Quality Inventory and Likert scales of sleep quality	Significantly greater improvement versus control in PSQI measures of: global sleep disturbance, sleep quality, daytime dysfunction; improvement in Likert-scales of sleep quality and quantity Exercise also significantly reduced depression
Naylor et al. (2000)	Experimental group $n = 14$, 75.2 ± 2.6 yrs, control group $n = 9$, 71.2 ± 2.6 yrs	Control group, but not random assignment: (1) 14, days mild social/physical activity (2) No change in social/physical activity	Assessment of circadian rhythmicity, nocturnal sleep, daytime functioning, mood, and vigor	The group exposed to structured activities had increased amounts of slow wave sleep and demonstrated improvement in memory-oriented tasks following intervention No significant changes were noted in the amplitude and phase of the body temperature rhythm or in subjective measures of vigor and mood
Tworoger et al. (2003)	$n = 173$, 50–75 yrs, mostly normal sleepers	Prospective, random assignment 1 yr: (1) Aerobic exercise (45 min, 5 d/wk (1030–1200 hr or 1800–1930 hr) (2) Stretching	Retrospective sleep quality estimation over previous month at baseline and 3, 6, 9, and 12 months	No significant difference between exercise and stretching condition (the prospectively chosen control) Post-hoc analysis among morning exercisers, those who exercised $\geq$225 min/wk had less trouble falling asleep than those who exercised <180 min/wk (OR 0.3, controlling for covariates) Among evening exercisers, those exercising 180–225 min/wk (OR3.5) or $\geq$225min/wk (OR3.3) had more trouble falling asleep
Young-McCaughan et al. (2003)	$n = 62$, 24–83 (mean 59 yrs), cancer patients	Uncontrolled 12 wks: 2/wk supervised walking; 3/wk home walking	Actigraphic sleep and questionnaire	No significant improvements in actigraphic sleep Significant improvement in reported "I have difficulty sleeping"

Notes; yr = year/s; d = day/s; wk = week; hr = hour/s; min = minute/s; SOL = sleep latency; TST = total sleep time; WASO = wake after sleep onset; SWS = slow wave sleep.

Older subjects

IMPLICATIONS FOR THE HEALTH PROFESSIONAL AND HEALTH SERVICE DELIVERY

Prospective uncontrolled chronic exercise studies of older individuals not specifically recruited for sleep complaints, have reported mixed results. Those studies utilizing self-report measures reveal more positive effects than those studies with more rigorous outcome measures. Stevenson and Topp (1990) found significant improvement in self-reported sleep quantity, but not self-reported sleep quality after 9 months of moderate or low intensity exercise training. However, a 12-week study of cancer patients (mean age = 59 years) found no significant changes in actigraphic sleep, though a significant decrease in self-reported sleeping difficulty was found (Young-McCaughan et al., 2003).

Controlled trials of older subjects, not necessarily selected for sleep problems, have generally yielded no positive effect from exercise. In a group of older healthy subjects (mean age = 66 years), researchers found no significant differences in subjective (Vitiello et al., 1994b) or polysomnographic sleep (Vitiello et al., 1994a) following a six-month aerobic exercise (n = 18) versus stretching control treatment (n = 21). Naylor et al. (2000) reported a significant increase in slow wave sleep following two weeks of exercise + social interaction in nursing home residents, but the statistical comparison with a control group was not reported. In a nine-week controlled trial (Alessi et al., 1995), physically restrained nursing home residents (n = 65, mean age = 85 years) were assigned to an extensive exercise regimen (i.e., several times per day × 5 days/week), involving sit-to-stand repetitions, walking, rowing, wheel-chair propulsion or a more moderate routine (i.e., aerobic activity, once per day, 3 times per week). The authors found no significant improvements in actigraphic sleep, even in those who showed dramatic improvements in exercise endurance.

A recent study compared the effects of a year-long exercise program (n = 87) versus a prospectively chosen control stretching program (n = 86) in overweight or obese post-menopausal women (ages 50–75 years) (Tworoger et al., 2003). The majority of the sample did not report sleep problems in baseline questionnaires. No significant improvements in self-reported sleep were found between the exercise and stretching treatments.

In summary, the available studies suggest that older adults without specifically diagnosed sleep problems do not show much improvement in sleep with chronic exercise.

OLDER SUBJECTS WITH SLEEP COMPLAINTS

A recent Cochrane review (Montgomery and Dennis, 2002) reviewed exercise studies meeting the following criteria: (1) randomized controlled trial; (2) subjects having insomnia; (3) over 80% of the sample was over age 60 years; (4) subjects had been screened for absence of dementia or depression. Only one study was identified (King et al., 1997). In that study, King and colleagues randomly assigned 43 older adults, complaining of moderate sleep disturbances, to a 16-week exercise training treatment or a waiting list control treatment. The treatment condition involved aerobic exercise (60–75% maximal capacity), 3–4 times per week (twice in a YMCA class, twice at home). The exercise group reported significantly greater improvements in self-reported sleep quality, sleep latency (net decrease versus control = 11.5 min), and total sleep time (net increase = 42 min) when compared with the control treatment.

Other controlled studies of older adults specifically recruited for sleep complaints have yielded promising results, although significant effects have been found only with self-report measures, and not objective sleep measures. In one investigation, depressed adults ($n = 32$, ages 60–84 years) were randomly assigned to a 10-week weight training treatment (3 times per week) or a health education control treatment (Singh *et al.*, 1997). Significant improvements in self-reported sleep and decreases in depression were found for the experimental group, and these effects were significantly correlated. Guilleminault *et al.* (1995) randomly assigned 30 middle-aged (mean age = 44 years) insomniacs to treatments involving sleep hygiene education (the control), sleep hygiene + exercise (brisk walking for 45 min/day), and bright light treatment (30 min/day) for a period of 4 weeks. Sleep was assessed via actigraphy and sleep logs. Whereas actigraphy revealed a mean increase in sleep latency (1 min) and decrease in total sleep time (3 min) in the control group, the exercise group had improvements in sleep latency and total sleep time of 7 min and 17 min, respectively. Interestingly, the bright light group had even greater decreases in sleep latency (8 min) and increases in total sleep time (44 min). Subjective sleep showed a similar pattern. However, due to the small number of subjects, the improvements in sleep were not significantly greater in the experimental versus control treatments.

In summary, chronic exercise studies have not provided much compelling evidence for improvements in sleep. As with the acute studies, much of this literature might be limited by ceiling–floor effects associated with testing normal sleepers. There is some evidence of larger effects of exercise among people with insomnia, but this is primarily limited to self-report data. Unfortunately, these measures can be confounded by the strong expectancies that people have regarding the sleep-promoting effects of exercise. The available evidence can also be challenged on other grounds. The Singh *et al.* (1997) study raises the question of whether exercise training can improve sleep independent of its antidepressant effects. Also, the waiting list control condition used by King *et al.* (1997) does not provide adequate control for a host of potential moderators including light exposure, social interaction, or Hawthorne effects. Finally, the Guilleminault *et al.* (1995) study reinforces the idea that light exposure could be an important confound in exercise studies. Overall, better controlled research is needed.

Other sleep problems

SLEEP APNEA

The majority of patients attending sleep disorder clinics have sleep apnea (Jordan and McEvoy, 2003). The most common type of this disorder is obstructive sleep apnea, which results from a collapse of the airway during sleep (Kuna and Remmers, 2000). The risks associated with sleep apnea are well-documented, including a high prevalence of hypertension, heart disease, and diabetes compared with the general population (Kuna and Remmers, 2000). Moreover, the constant arousal elicited by sleep apnea can cause profound daytime sleepiness and an increased risk of automobile accidents (George, 2001).

Loss of body weight is clearly a mechanism by which exercise could offer a preventive or adjunct treatment for sleep apnea. It has been hypothesized that engagement of the pharyngeal and glossal muscles during exercise could strengthen these muscles, making them less susceptible to collapse associated with upper airway obstruction (Giebelhaus et al., 2000). A recent epidemiological study ($n = 1,104$) found that hours of exercise per week was inversely associated with apnea-hypopnea severity, and this effect was independent of body mass index (BMI) (Peppard and Young, 2004). Moreover, a recent correlational study of apnea patients found that regular exercise was significantly associated with less fatigue, even after controlling for BMI and apnea severity (Hong and Dimsdale, 2003). In uncontrolled trials, exercise training alone, or in combination with caloric restriction, has been associated with significant decreases in disturbed breathing, which were not correlated with weight reduction.

RESTLESS LEGS SYNDROME

Restless legs syndrome (RLS) is associated with excruciating "creepy-crawly" sensations in the legs, which cause an irresistible urge to move the legs. The syndrome has been strongly linked to iron and dopamine deficiencies, and genetic factors (Montplaisir et al., 2000). People with RLS report anecdotally that moderate daytime exercise can prevent symptoms of RLS, and that leg movement is one of the most effective behavioral remedy for acute symptoms of RLS. These reports are supported by epidemiological evidence, which demonstrate that lack of exercise is a significant risk factor for RLS (Phillips et al., 2000).

In light of the side effects associated with pharmacologically treating RLS, which usually involves dopaminergic drugs, it is surprising that there has been such little research into the use of exercise as a treatment for RLS. Research by de Mello and colleagues has shown that vigorous acute exercise (de Mello et al., 1996), as well as chronic exercise training (de Mello et al., 2004), can significantly reduce RLS and periodic leg movements (PLMS), and that the effect of exercise on PLMS was no different than that of L-dopa (de Mello et al., 2004). These results are perhaps not surprising given the demonstrated dopaminergic effect of exercise. Further research into the effects of acute and chronic exercise on RLS patients is needed.

Mechanisms

ANXIOLYTIC AND ANTIDEPRESSANT EFFECTS

Perhaps the most plausible mechanism by which exercise could promote sleep is via anxiolytic or antidepressant effects. Anxiety disturbs sleep, almost by definition. Anxiolytic effects of exercise have been well established in dozens of studies over the past 40 years (see O'Connor et al., 2000 for a review). Acute bouts of exercise have been shown to reduce both subjective and physiological indices of anxiety (e.g., blood pressure), and these effects can persist for several hours. Likewise, chronic exercise has been shown to reduce symptoms of trait anxiety (O'Connor et al., 2000).

If anxiety reduction is the mechanism by which acute exercise promotes sleep, then the evening might be the preferred time to exercise, since anxiolytic effects of exercise are best-documented during the first few hours after exercise (O'Connor et al., 2000). The available evidence suggests no particular advantage (nor disadvantage) of evening exercise for sleep (Youngstedt et al., 1997), though studies have been limited to low-anxious people with little room for further anxiety reduction (i.e., floor effect). More recently, it was found that acute exercise significantly reduced state anxiety and blood pressure 20 min after exercise when compared with a control treatment; however, at bedtime, 4–6 hours later, there were no differences in anxiety between treatments, and there was no correlation between bedtime anxiety and sleep (Youngstedt et al., 2000). We are unaware of other tests of this hypothesis.

Depression is associated with sleep disturbance, which is alleviated by antidepressant treatments. Thus, the well-documented antidepressant effects of chronic exercise might be expected to result in better sleep (see Mutrie, 2000). As reviewed above, Singh et al. (1997) found evidence supporting this hypothesis. A number of antidepressant drugs also decrease REM sleep, and it has been posited that REM sleep suppression is the underlying mechanism (Vogel et al., 1990). Recent research has shown significant antidepressant effects of modest experimental restriction of REM sleep (approximately 25% decrease) (Cartwright et al., 2003). Thus, the decrease in REM sleep following acute exercise, repeated nightly, conceivably could moderate antidepressant effects of chronic exercise.

TEMPERATURE ELEVATION

Over the past two decades, the notion that exercise promotes sleep via a body heating effect has been the most widely accepted hypothesis regarding the influence of exercise on sleep (McGinty and Szymusiak, 1990). The anterior hypothalamus–preoptic (AHPO) area of the brain is closely involved in both sleep and temperature regulation. Indeed, some evidence suggests that some of the same neurons may be involved with both functions (McGinty and Szymusiak, 1990). For example, heating of warm-sensitive neurons in the AHPO can induce sleep. According to the hypothesis, manipulations that raise temperature may activate both temperature down-regulating and sleep mechanisms. Consistent with this hypothesis are studies showing that sleep can be promoted by warm water immersion a few hours before bedtime (Dorsey et al., 2000; Horne and Staff, 1983).

The most influential research supporting a thermogenic effect of exercise on sleep is that of Horne and colleagues at Loughborough University. An initial study (Horne and Staff, 1983) showed similar elevations in slow wave sleep following vigorous exercise and passive heating that elicited similar temperature elevations, and these slow wave sleep (SWS) increases were significantly greater than following moderate exercise which elicited lower temperature elevations. A subsequent study (Horne and Moore, 1985) showed that increases in SWS were significantly greater following an exercise condition in which temperature increase was augmented by having the subjects wear extra clothing compared with exercise in which temperature increase was blunted by having the subjects wear wet clothes in front of a fan.

However, there are a number of caveats to making definitive conclusions about the thermogenic hypothesis based on these data. First, while SWS increased, REM sleep decreased to a similar degree, and there is no compelling evidence that SWS is more indicative of "better" sleep than REM sleep. Moreover, there has not been a clear indication that SWS increases after exercise are associated with better subjective sleep. Indeed, a study by Driver and colleagues (1994) found a significant *negative* correlation between SWS and subjective sleep quality after exercise. Second, in the Horne and Moore (1985) study, exercise was performed approximately 6 hours before bedtime, which is enough time for body temperature to return to baseline levels. Third, as discussed above, meta-analytic data shows no consistent association between estimated temperature elevation and sleep changes following exercise (Youngstedt *et al.*, 1997). Nonetheless, this hypothesis is still tenable.

CIRCADIAN EFFECTS

Although bright light is believed to be the most important stimulus for shifting the circadian system, there is compelling evidence that exercise also has a significant phase-shifting effect. Current ongoing research is seeking to establish the ideal timing of exercise for shifting the circadian system (Buxton *et al.*, 2003; Youngstedt *et al.*, 2002b). Moreover, current research is exploring whether combining bright light and exercise can elicit synergistic phase-shifting effects (Youngstedt *et al.*, 2002a). Another potential effect of regularly timed exercise is that it could promote stabilization of the circadian system, promoting sleep via consistent sleep timing. Research suggests that circadian stabilization might be the primary means by which bright light treatment enhances sleep. Notably, bright light can elicit dramatic improvements in sleep, but these improvements do not correlate with phase-shifting effects (Campbell, 1998).

ADENOSINE

Adenosine has been strongly implicated in sleep regulation. For example, injections of adenosine have been shown to enhance sleep, while adenosine levels increase in proportion to the length of wakefulness in rodents (Porkka-Heiskanen *et al.*, 1997). Of course, exercise elicits dramatic increases in circulating adenosine. In support of an adenosine mechanism mediating exercise effects on sleep, our study found that SWS increases following exercise were nearly three times greater when subjects had previously consumed placebo treatment (ES = 0.85) compared with caffeine (ES = 0.36), which blocks adenosine receptors (Youngstedt *et al.*, 2000).

Implications for researchers

There are a number of weaknesses in the epidemiological studies associating exercise with sleep. Often, they have used relatively small samples and nonvalidated exercise and sleep measures, and have lacked adequate control for many potential confounds, such as the health and health habits of the subjects. However, there are existing data bases such as the Womens' Health Initiative Study (a 15-year NIH-sponsored study of the most common causes of death, morbidity, and poor quality of life in post-menopausal women) with hundreds of thousands of respondents, adequate measurement of both exercise and sleep, and careful documentation of dozens of potential confounds, which could yield more compelling epidemiological tests of the association of exercise and sleep.

The predominant shortcoming of experimental studies of the influence of exercise on sleep has been the paucity of research on individuals with disturbed sleep. Future experimental research should focus on people with insomnia who have more room for observable improvement. In addition, both acute and chronic effects of exercise should be examined. In order to gain a full understanding of the effects of exercise on sleep, there is also a need for randomized controlled trials comparing exercise with hypnotics and other behavioral treatments. We all experience insomnia occasionally. Further research, including the experimental induction of insomnia, will be needed to assess the potential role of exercise in preventing this condition.

Although experimental studies have generally focused on acute bouts of exercise, it is plausible that total amount of physical activity is the more important predictor of enhanced sleep. Meta-analytic data suggest that total duration might be the most important predictor (Youngstedt et al., 1997). Which condition would one expect to promote better sleep (assuming equivalent light exposure): 1 hour of vigorous exercise but otherwise sedentary behavior or 6 hours of slow, intermittent walking at the zoo? Based upon interviews with our research volunteers, it seems apparent that surveys associating exercise with better sleep can be partly attributed to total daily physical activity, not necessarily planned exercise. This issue might best be addressed by measuring associations of sleep with total energy expenditure using rigorous measures such as doubly labeled water.

An underlying implication in much of the lay literature is that people need more sleep after exercise. However, were this to be the case, then post-exercise improvements in sleep might have little relevance regarding daytime functioning and fatigue. This issue could be examined experimentally by manipulating time-in-bed as well as exercise.

Implications for practitioners

Individuals can be advised that exercise seems to modestly improve sleep, and that we have reason to believe that this effect could be substantial in people with disturbed sleep. Time-of-day is an important issue when considering exercise because it could have implications for exercise adherence. Conventional wisdom is that evening exercise, particularly vigorous exercise, will disturb sleep. However, individuals should be told that there is no compelling experimental evidence to support this assumption. Individuals should be encouraged to exercise whenever they find it to be most convenient. Furthermore, individuals should be advised that even if evening exercise disturbs their sleep initially, with experience they might become accustomed to evening exercise without negative sleep effects.

It seems prudent to recommend that exercise be performed outdoors, when possible. There are well-established antidepressant and sleep-promoting effects associated with bright light. Indeed, antidepressant effects of exercise are greater when exercise is performed in bright versus dim light (Partonen et al., 1998), and it seems reasonable to suppose a similar interaction of light with sleep and exercise. Finally, individuals can be advised that exercise need not be very intense to promote sleep; rather longer, moderate duration exercise should be advised.

WHAT WE KNOW SUMMARY

- People believe that exercise is an important sleep-promoting behavior.
- Individuals who exercise regularly have a lower risk of disturbed sleep but causal effects are less well established.
- Chronic exercise training may elicit significant improvements in sleep in individuals with disturbed sleep although there is no clear consensus.
- Acute exercise elicits a modest improvement in sleep among good sleepers. This effect is greater for longer exercise durations. The influence of acute exercise on sleep is similar for fit and unfit individuals. Exercise intensity or time-of-day of exercise do not have much moderating influence.

WHAT WE NEED TO KNOW SUMMARY

- We need to establish whether acute and/or chronic exercise promotes sleep in individuals with impaired sleep. Moreover, it is important to establish how exercise compares with other sleep treatments, including hypnotics and cognitive–behavioral therapy. Also, it will be important to establish whether exercise could be an effective adjuvant sleep treatment.
- There is currently a complete absence of data indicating whether acute exercise can promote sleep in insomniacs. This is an important issue because these individuals might not be willing to continue exercising if they do not realize sleep benefits quickly.
- There is a need for research exploring dose-response effects of various exercise parameters such as intensity and duration. Also, interactions of these parameters should be assessed.

APPENDIX

The nature of sleep and its measurement

Sleep has been defined as "a reversible behavioral state of perceptual disengagement from and unresponsiveness to the environment" (Carskadon and Dement, 2000, p. 15). Sleep is typically also defined by species-dependent stereotypic posture and behavior (e.g., recumbency, closed eyes, and quiescence in humans). The reversible nature of sleep distinguishes it from other states of unconsciousness (e.g., coma) (Carskadon and Dement, 2000). Sleep is also increasingly defined by its regulation by homeostatic and circadian mechanisms (Borbely, 1982; Dijk and Edgar, 1999). The homeostatic drive for sleep is evidenced by proportional increases in sleepiness and rebound increases in sleep with increasing durations of sleep loss. Circadian regulation of sleep in humans is indicated by rhythm in sleep propensity, which peaks at approximately the time of the circadian temperature minimum. In order to best understand the influence of exercise on sleep it is helpful to understand how sleep is measured. Different methods have different strengths and weaknesses that influence the interpretation of the scientific evidence associating exercise with better sleep. In humans, polysomnography is considered the "gold standard" marker of sleep.

Polysomnography

Standard polysomnographic measurement includes recording of electroencephalography (EEG) from occipital and temporal sites, electromyography (EMG) from the chin, oculomotor and leg muscles, respiration from abdominal and thoracic stain gauge sensors, and electrocardiography (ECG). During active engagement in physical or mental activity of wakefulness, the fast frequency (14–40 Hz), low amplitude beta waves are noted in the EEG. Quiet, relaxed wakefulness is characterized by a greater proportion of alpha brain waves of lower frequency (8–13 Hz) and higher amplitude.

The transition from wake to sleep is typically characterized by slow rolling eye movements, theta brain wave activity (4–8 Hz), deeper breathing, and reduction in EMG activity, as the individual enters stage 1 sleep. Stage 1 is the lightest sleep stage, and people who are aroused during stage 1 are often not aware that they had fallen asleep. Stage 1 sleep typically lasts between 1–7 min, followed by entrance into deeper, stage 2 sleep.

Stage 2 sleep is characterized by two easily recognized sleep patterns: 12–14 Hz, low amplitude sleep spindles that last 1–3 sec, and large amplitude (150 μv) sharp bipolar K-complexes, which typically appear in single bursts. The first episode of stage 2 sleep typically lasts about 30–40 min, and is followed by entrance into stage 3 and stage 4 sleep, which last approximately 50–60 min.

Stages 3 and 4 are commonly combined and called slow wave sleep (SWS), characterized by low frequency (2–4 Hz) brain waves of ≥75 μv. Stages 3 and 4 are distinguished by the prevalence of these slow waves. If >25% but <50% of a 30-sec epoch contains slow waves, the epoch is scored as stage 3; if the epoch contains >50%, it is scored as stage 4 sleep. Together, stages 1–4 sleep are called non-REM (NREM) sleep.

Following the first episode of slow wave sleep, sleep gradually becomes lighter, entering stage 2 and stage 1, followed by entrance into the first episode of rapid eye movement (REM) sleep (Carskadon and Dement, 2000). REM sleep is distinguished by obvious eye movements, as well as by an inhibition of EMG activity (typically measured at the chin), and by the appearance of low voltage fast-frequency EEG activity. Because this EEG activity resembles that observed during wakefulness, REM sleep is often called "paradoxical sleep." The average latency for the first appearance of REM sleep is approximately 90 min. The majority of dreams occur during REM sleep, particularly the most vivid dreams. An abnormally short REM latency, and early morning awakening, are common features of major depression (Benca et al., 1992).

The NREM-REM cycle is repeated throughout the night at approximately 90 min intervals (Carskadon and Dement, 2000) stages 1, 2, SWS, and REM sleep comprise approximately 5%, 50%, 20%, and 25% of the total sleep period, respectively. However, the duration of the various sleep stages varies across the night. For example, most SWS appears in the first third and most REM sleep appears in the last third of the sleep period.

Scoring of polysomnographic sleep typically follows standardized procedures developed by Rechtschaffen and Kales (1968). An updated scoring consensus is currently being developed. Scoring involves deciding the stage of sleep for every 30-second epoch throughout the sleep period. The process can take several hours and requires a great deal of skill. Automated computer software has simplified the storage and scoring of the records, but experienced scorers are still needed for editing the results.

The criteria for "good sleep" are based upon associations with feeling well rested, and having high levels of energy and behavioral functioning during the daytime. The best-documented EEG features of good sleep are short sleep latency, few awakenings, and minimal time spent awake after sleep onset (WASO), and minimal amounts of stage 1 sleep (Bliwise, 1992). Sleep quality is also associated with total sleep time, but this association is less robust compared with that associated with WASO (Carskadon et al., 1982; Stepanski et al., 1984).

Although it is often assumed that SWS is most indicative of sleep quality, this assumption is based upon questionable lines of evidence. For example, one argument for a particular value of SWS, is that 24-hour sleep deprivation results in a preferential "rebound" in SWS when sleep is resumed (Rechtschaffen et al., 1999). However, interestingly, more prolonged sleep deprivation results in a preferential rebound in REM sleep (Rechtschaffen et al., 1999). Further research contradicting SWS as the most restful sleep are findings that pharmacologic increases in SWS are correlated neither with subjective reports of better sleep, nor with improvements in neurobehavioral performance (Landolt et al., 1999). Conversely, hypnotically induced improvements in self-reported sleep and in sleep by other criteria often produce no changes or decreases in SWS.

Quantitative EEG

The standard procedures for scoring sleep stages are based upon arbitrary criteria, which could conceivably obscure important information. For example, spectral analysis could reveal substantial amounts of delta waves that could be scored as absent, if the amount of delta waves over 30-second epochs does not meet the 25% criterion. Attempts to quantify sleep with more quantitative methods have not proved more valid with respect to daytime functioning and sleepiness, although efforts in this direction are ongoing.

Actigraphy

Wrist actigraphic estimation of sleep has become increasingly more common in both clinical and experimental settings. Indeed, actigraphy has become an accepted means of diagnosing sleep problems and detecting clinical improvement (Littner et al., 2003; Sadeh et al., 1995). All-night and 24-hour min-by-min comparisons between actigraphic and EEG recordings in dozens of subjects have led to sophisticated algorithms that can estimate whether one is asleep or awake with better than 90% accuracy (Jean-Louis *et al.*, 2001a,b). Although not as accurate as EEG, actigraphy has several important advantages over polysomnography. First, actigraphic recording is far less expensive than polysomnographic recording, which can cost up to $2,000 per night in many hospitals. Second, actigraphs, which are approximately the size and weight of a wrist watch, allow sleep to be estimated non-invasively. Third, since daytime polysomnographic recording is not feasible in most settings – certainly not in one's usual home–work environment – actigraphy provides the best objective method for assessing napping. Although actigraphic recording cannot reveal differences between stages of sleep, it is noteworthy that there is little compelling evidence for differences between stages 2, 3, 4, or REM sleep in terms of reported sleep quality, daytime sleepiness, or neurobehavioral functioning.

Questionnaires

Sleep has also been measured with self-report questionnaires. These measures are viewed skeptically by many sleep researchers because they often correlate poorly with objective measures (Baker *et al.*, 1999; Carskadon *et al.*, 1976). As well, they are dependent upon the willingness and ability of subjects to report how they slept and are more susceptible to experimental behavioral artifacts, such as expectancy effects. Within the realm of self-reports, general retrospective recalls of sleep are probably less accurate than prospective sleep assessments. Despite the limitations of self-reports, it is important to bear in mind that both the clinical definition of insomnia and the established efficacy of various treatments are generally determined completely by self-report measures.

REFERENCES

Alessi, C. A., Schnelle, J. F., MacRae, P. G., Ouslander, J. G., Al-Samarrai, N., Simmons, S. F. *et al.* (1995). Does physical activity improve sleep in impaired nursing home residents. *Journal of the American Geriatrics Society*, *43*, 1098–1102.

American Academy of Sleep Medicine (2004). *Sleep Hygiene*. Chicago, IL: American Academy of Sleep Medicine.

Arakawa, M., Tanaka, H., Toguchi, H., Shirakawa, S., and Taira, K. (2002). Comparative study on sleep health and lifestyle of the elderly in the urban areas and suburbs of Okinawa. *Psychiatry and Clinical Neurosciences*, *56*, 245–246.

Baker, F. C., Maloney, S., and Driver, H. S. (1999). A comparison of subjective estimates of sleep with objective polysomnographic data in healthy men and women. *Journal of Psychosomatic Research*, *47*, 335–341.

Benca, R. M., Obermeyer, W. H., Thisted, R. A., and Gillin, J. C. (1992). Sleep and psychiatric disorders: a meta-analysis. *Archives of General Psychiatry*, *49*, 651–668.

Berger, R. J. and Phillips, N. H. (1988). Comparative aspects of energy metabolism, body temperature and sleep. *Acta Physiologica Scandinavica*, *133*(S574), 21–27.

Bliwise, N. G. (1992). Factors related to sleep quality in healthy elderly women. *Psychology and Aging*, *7*, 83–88.

Borbely, A. A. (1982). A two process model of sleep regulation. *Human Neurobiology*, *1*, 195–204.

Brandenberger, G. and Weibel, L. (2004). The 24-h growth hormone rhythm in men: sleep and circadian influences questioned. *Journal of Sleep Research*, *13*, 251–255.

Buxton, O. M., Lee, C. W., L'Hermite-Baleriaux, M., Turek, F. W., and Van Cauter, E. (2003). Exercise elicits phase shifts and acute alterations of melatonin that vary with circadian phase. *American Journal of Physiology*, *284*, R714–R724.

Campbell, S. S. (1984). Duration and placement of sleep in a "disentrained" environment. *Psychophysiology*, *21*, 106–113.

Campbell, S. S. (1998). Bright light treatment of sleep maintenance insomnia and behavioral disturbance. In R. W. Lam (Ed.). *Seasonal Affective Disorder and Beyond: Light Treatment for SAD and Non-SAD Conditions* (pp. 289–304). Washington, DC: American Psychiatric Press, Inc.

Carskadon, M. A. and Dement, W. C. (2000). Normal human sleep: an overview. In M. H. Kryger, T. Roth, and W. C. Dement (Eds). *Principles and Practice of Sleep Medicine* (3rd edn, pp. 15–25). New York: W. B. Saunders Company.

Carskadon, M. A., Dement, W. C., Mitler, M. M., Guilleminault, C., Zarcone, V. P., and Spiegel, R. (1976). Self-reports versus sleep laboratory findings in 122 drug-free subjects with complaints of chronic insomnia. *American Journal of Psychiatry*, *133*, 1382–1388.

Carskadon, M. A., Brown, E. D., and Dement, W. C. (1982). Sleep fragmentation in the elderly: relationship to daytime sleep tendency. *Neurobiology of Aging*, *3*, 321–327.

Cartwright, R., Baehr, E., Kirby, J., Pandi-Perumal, S. R., and Kabat, J. (2003). REM sleep reduction, mood regulation and remission in untreated depression. *Psychiatry Research*, *121*, 159–167.

Dawson, D. and Fletcher, A. (2001). A quantitative model of work-related fatigue: background and definition. *Ergonomics*, *44*, 144–163.

de Mello, M. T., Lauro, F. A., Silva, A. C., and Tufik, S. (1996). Incidence of periodic leg movements and of the restless legs syndrome during sleep following acute physical activity in spinal cord injury subjects. *Spinal Cord*, *34*, 294–296.

de Mello, M. T., Esteves, A. M., and Tufik, S. (2004). Comparison between dopaminergic agents and physical exercise as treatment for periodic limb movements in patients with spinal cord injury. *Spinal Cord*, *42*, 218–221.

Dijk, D. J. and Edgar, D. M. (1999). Circadian and homeostatic control of wakefulness and sleep. In F. W. Turek and P. C. Zee (Eds). *Regulation of Sleep and Circadian Rhythms* (pp. 111–147). New York: Marcel Dekker.

Dishman, R. K. (2001). The problem of exercise adherence: fighting sloth in nations with market economies. *Quest*, *53*, 279–294.

Dorsey, C. M., Teicher, M. H., CohenZion, M., Stefanovic, L., Satlin, A., Tartarini, W. *et al.* (2000). Core body temperature and sleep of older female insomniacs before and after passive body heating. *Sleep*, *22*, 891–898.

Driver, H. S., Meintjes, A. F., Rogers, G. G., and Shapiro, C. M. (1988). Submaximal exercise effects on sleep patterns in young women before and after an aerobic training programme. *Acta Physiologica Scandinavica*, *133*, 8–13.

Driver, H. S., Rogers, G. G., Mitchell, D., Borrow, S. J., Allen, M., Luus, H. G. *et al.* (1994). Prolonged endurance exercise and sleep disruption. *Medicine and Science in Sports and Exercise*, *26*, 903–907.

Foley, D. J., Monjan, A. A., Brown, S. L., Simonsick, E. M., Wallace, R. B., and Blazer, D. G. (1995). Sleep complaints among elderly persons: an epidemiologic study of three communities. *Sleep*, *18*, 425–432.

George, C. F. P. (2001). Reduction in motor vehicle collisions following treatment of sleep apnea with nasal CPAP. *Thorax*, *56*, 508–512.

Giebelhaus, V., Strohl, K. P., Lormes, W., Lehmann, M., and Netzer, N. (2000). Physical exercise as an adjunct therapy in sleep apnea – an open trial. *Sleep and Breathing*, *4*, 173–176.

Guilleminault, C., Clerk, A., Black, J., Labanowski, M., Pelayo, R., and Claman, D. (1995). Nondrug treatment trials in psychophysiologic insomnia. *Annals of Internal Medicine*, *155*, 838–844.

Hague, J. F. E., Gilbert, S. S., Burgess, H. J., Ferguson, S. A., and Dawson, D. (2003). A sedentary day: effects on subsequent sleep and body temperatures in trained athletes. *Physiology and Behavior*, *78*, 261–267.

Hong, S. and Dimsdale, J. E. (2003). Physical activity and perception of energy and fatigue in obstructive sleep apnea. *Medicine and Science in Sports and Exercise*, *35*, 1088–1092.

Horne, J. A. and Foster, S. C. (1995). Can exercise overcome sleepiness? *Sleep Research*, *24A*, 437.

Horne, J. A. and Moore, V. J. (1985). Sleep EEG effects of exercise with and without additional body cooling. *Electroencephalography and Clinical Neurophysiology*, *60*, 33–38.

Horne, J. A. and Staff, L. H. E. (1983). Exercise and sleep: body-heating effects. *Sleep*, *6*, 36–46.

Jean-Louis, G., Kripke, D. F., Cole, R. J., Assmus, J. D., and Langer, R. D. (2001a). Sleep detection with an accelerometer actigraph: comparisons with polysomnography. *Physiology and Behavior*, *72*, 21–28.

Jean-Louis, G., Kripke, D. F., Mason, W. J., Elliott, J. A., and Youngstedt, S. D. (2001b). Sleep estimation from wrist movement quantified by different actigraphic modalities. *Journal of Neuroscience Methods*, *105*, 185–191.

Jones, A. Y., Dean, E., and Lo, S. K. (2002). Interrelationships between anxiety, lifestyle self reports and fitness in a sample of Hong Kong University students. *Stress*, *5*, 65–71.

Jordan, A. S. and McEvoy, R. D. (2003). Gender differences in sleep apnea: epidemiology, clinical presentation and pathogenic mechanisms. *Sleep Medicine Reviews*, *7*, 377–389.

Kim, K., Uchiyama, M., Okawa, M., Liu, X., and Ogihara, R. (2000). An epidemiological study of insomnia among the Japanese general population. *Sleep*, *23*, 41–47.

King, A. C., Oman, R. F., Brassington, G. S., Bliwise, D. L., and Haskell, W. L. (1997). Moderate intensity exercise and self-rated quality of sleep in older adults. A randomized controlled trial. *Journal of the American Medical Association*, *277*, 32–37.

Kobayashi, T., Yoshida, H., Ishikawa, T., and Arakawa, K. (1999). Effects of the late evening exercise on sleep onset process. *Sleep Research Online*, *2* (Suppl. 1), 233.

Kripke, D. F. (1998). Light treatment for nonseasonal depression: speed, efficacy, and combined treatment. *Journal of Affective Disorders*, *49*, 109–117.

Kripke, D. F. (2000). Chronic hypnotic use: deadly risks, doubtful benefit. *Sleep Medicine Reviews*, *4*, 5–20.

Kripke, D. F., Klauber, M. R., Wingard, D. L., Fell, R. L., Assmus, J. D., and Garfinkel, L. (1998). Mortality hazard associated with prescription hypnotics. *Biological Psychiatry*, *43*, 687–693.

Kuna, S. and Remmers, J. E. (2000). Anatomy and physiology of upper airway obstruction. In M. H. Kryger, T. Roth, and W. C. Dement (Eds). *Principles and Practice of Sleep Medicine* (3rd edn, pp. 840–858). New York: W. B. Saunders Company.

Landolt, H. P., Meier, V., Burgess, H. J., Finelli, L. A., Cattelin, F., Achermann, P. *et al.* (1999). Serotonin – 2 receptors and human sleep: effect of a selective antagonist on EEG power spectra. *Neuropsychopharmacology*, *21*, 455–466.

LeDuc, P. A. Jr, Caldwell, J. A. Jr, and Ruyak, P. S. (2000). The effects of exercise as a countermeasure for fatigue in sleep-deprived aviators. *Military Medicine, 12,* 249–266.

Lichstein, K. L., Means, M. K., Noe, S. L., and Aguillard, R. N. (1997). Fatigue and sleep disorders. *Behavior Research and Therapy, 35,* 733–740.

Littner, M., Kushida, C. A., Anderson, W. M., Bailey, D., Berry, R. B., Davilla, D. G. *et al.* (2003). Practice parameters for the role of actigraphy in the study of sleep and circadian rhythms: an update for 2002. *Sleep, 26,* 337–341.

Liu, X., Uchiyama, M., Okawa, M., and Kurita, H. (2000). Prevalence and correlates of self-reported sleep problems among Chinese adolescents. *Sleep, 23,* 27–34.

McGinty, D. and Szymusiak, R. (1990). Keeping cool: a hypothesis about the mechanisms and functions of slow wave sleep. *Trends in Neurosciences, 13,* 480–487.

Meintjes, A. F., Driver, H. S., and Shapiro, C. M. (1989). Improved physical fitness failed to alter the EEG sleep patterns of sleep in young women. *European Journal of Applied Physiology, 59,* 123–127.

Mellinger, G. D., Balter, M. B., and Uhlenhuth, E. H. (1985). Insomnia and its treatment. Prevalence and correlates. *Archives of General Psychiatry, 42,* 225–232.

Montgomery, P. and Dennis, J. (2002). Physical exercise for sleep problems in adults aged 60+. *Cochrane Database Systematic Reviews, 4, CD003404.*

Montplaisir, J., Nicolas, A., Godbout, R., and Walters, A. (2000). Restless legs syndrome and periodic limb movement disorders. In M. H. Kryger, T. Roth, and W. C. Dement (Eds). *Principles and Practice of Sleep Medicine* (3rd edn, pp. 742–752). New York: W. B. Saunders Company.

Morgan, K. (2003). Daytime activity and risk factors for late-life insomnia. *Journal of Sleep Research, 12,* 231–238.

Morin, C. M., Colecchi, C., Stone, J., Sood, R., and Brink, D. (1999). Behavioral and pharmacological therapies for late-life insomnia. A randomized controlled trial. *Journal of the American Medical Association, 281,* 991–999.

Mutrie, N. (2000). The relationship between physical activity and clinically defined depression. In S. J. H. Biddle, K. R. Fox, and S. H. Boutcher (Eds). *Physical Activity and Psychological Well-being* (pp. 46–62). London: Routledge.

National Commission on Sleep Disorders Research (1993). *Wake Up America: A National Sleep Alert. Executive Summary and Executive Report.* Washington, DC: US Government Printing Office.

Naylor, E., Penev, P. D., Orbeta, L., Janssen, I., Ortiz, R., Colecchia, E. F. *et al.* (2000). Daily social and physical activity increases slow-wave sleep and daytime neuropsychological performance in the elderly. *Sleep, 23,* 87–95.

O'Connor, P. J. and Youngstedt, S. D. (1995). Influence of exercise on human sleep. In J. O. Holloszy (Ed.). *Exercise and Sport Sciences Review* (23rd edn, pp. 105–134). Baltimore, MD: Williams and Wilkins.

O'Connor, P. J., Breus, M. J., and Youngstedt, S. D. (1998). Exercise-induced increase in core temperature does not disrupt a behavioral measure of sleep. *Physiology and Behavior, 64,* 213–217.

O'Connor, P. J., Raglin, J. S., and Martinsen, E. W. (2000). Physical activity, anxiety and anxiety disorders. *International Journal of Sport Psychology, 31,* 136–155.

Ohayon, M. M., Caulet, M., and Guilleminault, C. (1998). How a general population perceives its sleep and how this relates to the complaint of insomnia. *Sleep, 20,* 715–723.

Ohida, T., Kamal, A. M. M., Uchiyama, M., Kim, K., Takemura, S., Sone, T. *et al.* (2001). The influence of lifestyle and health status factors on sleep loss among the Japanese general population. *Sleep, 24,* 333–338.

Partonen, T., Leppamaki, S., Hurme, J., and Lonnqvist, J. (1998). Randomized trial of physical exercise alone or combined with bright light on mood and health-related quality of life. *Psychological Medicine*, *28*, 1359–1364.

Peppard, P. E. and Young, T. (2004). Exercise and sleep-disordered breathing: an association independent of body habitus. *Sleep*, *27*, 480–484.

Phillips, B., Young, T., Finn, L., Asher, K., Hening, W. A., and Purvis, C. (2000). Epidemiology of restless legs syndrome in adults. *Archives of Internal Medicine*, *24*, 2137–2141.

Porkka-Heiskanen, T., Strecker, R. E., Thakkar, M., Bjorkum, A. A., Greene, R. W., and McCarley, R. W. (1997). Adenosine: a mediator of the sleep-inducing effects of prolonged wakefulness. *Science*, *276*, 1265–1268.

Porter, J. M. and Horne, J. A. (1981). Exercise and sleep behaviour. A questionnaire approach. *Ergonomics*, *24*, 511–521.

Powell, N. B., Schechtman, K. B., Riley, R. W., Li, K., Troell, R., and Guilleminault, C. (2001). The road to danger: the comparative risks of driving while sleepy. *The Laryngoscope*, *111*, 887–893.

Radun, H. and Summala, H. (2004). Sleep-related fatal vehicle accidents: characteristics of decisions made by multidisciplinary investigation teams. *Sleep*, *27*, 224–227.

Rechtschaffen, A. (1998). Current perspectives on the function of sleep. *Perspectives in Biology and Medicine*, *41*, 359–390.

Rechtschaffen, A. and Kales, A. (1968). *A Manual of Standardized Terminology, Techniques and Scoring System for Sleep Stages of Human Subjects*. Los Angeles, CA: Brain Information Service, Brain Research Institute, UCLA.

Rechtschaffen, A., Bergmann, B. M., Gilliland, M. A., and Bauer, K. (1999). Effects of method, duration and sleep stage on rebounds from sleep deprivation in the rat. *Sleep*, *22*, 11–31.

Riemann, D. and Voderholzer, U. (2003). Primary insomnia: a risk factor to develop depression? *Journal of Affective Disorders*, *76*, 255–259.

Sadeh, A., Hauri, P. J., Kripke, D. F., and Lavie, P. (1995). An American Sleep Disorders Association Review: the role of actigraphy in the evaluation of sleep disorders. *Sleep*, *18*, 288–302.

Shapiro, C. M., Griesel, R. D., Bartel, P. R., and Jooste, P. L. (1975). Sleep patterns after graded exercise. *Journal of Applied Physiology*, *39*, 187–190.

Shapiro, C. M., Trinder, P. M. W., Paxton, S. J., Oswald, I., Flenley, D. C., and Catterall, J. R. (1984). Fitness facilitates sleep. *European Journal of Applied Physiology*, *53*, 1–4.

Sherrill, D. L., Kotchou, K., and Quan, S. F. (1998). Association of physical activity and human sleep disorders. *Archives of Internal Medicine*, *158*, 1894–1898.

Singh, N. A., Clements, K. M., and Fiatarone, M. A. (1997). A randomized controlled trial of the effect of exercise on sleep. *Sleep*, *20*, 95–101.

Stepanski, E., Lamphere, J., Badia, P., Zorick, F., and Roth, T. (1984). Sleep fragmentation and daytime sleepiness. *Sleep*, *7*, 18–26.

Stevenson, J. S., and Topp, R. (1990). Effects of moderate and low intensity long-term exercise by older adults. *Research in Nursing and Health*, *13*, 209–218.

Sun, Y. H., Yu, T. S., Tong, S. L., Zhang, Y., Shi, X. M., and Li, W. (2002). A cross-sectional study of health-related behaviors in rural eastern China. *Biomedical and Environmental Science*, *15*, 347–354.

Tworoger, S. S., Yasui, Y., Vitiello, M. V., Schwartz, R. S., Ulrich, C. M., Aiello, E. J. *et al.* (2003). Effects of a yearlong moderate-intensity exercise and a stretching intervention on sleep quality in postmenopausal women. *Sleep*, *26*, 830–836.

Tynjälä, J., Kannas, L., and Välimaa, R. (1993). How young Europeans sleep. *Health Education Research. Theory and Practice*, *8*, 69–80.

Tynjälä, J., Kannas, L., Levälahti, E., and Välimaa, R. (1999). Perceived sleep quality and its precursors in adolescents. *Health Promotion International*, *14*, 155–166.

Uezu, E., Taira, K., Tanaka, H., Arakawa, M., Urasakii, C., Toguchi, H. *et al.* (2000). Survey of sleep-health and lifestyle of the elderly in Okinawa. *Psychiatry and Clinical Neurosciences*, *54*, 311–313.

Urponen, H., Vuori, I., Hasan, J., and Partinen, M. (1988). Self-evaluation of factors promoting and disturbing sleep: an epidemiological survey in Finland. *Social Science Medicine*, *26*, 443–450.

Vitiello, M. V., Prinz, P. N., and Schwartz, R. S. (1994a). Slow wave sleep but not overall sleep quality of healthy older men and women is improved by increased aerobic fitness. *Sleep Research*, *23*, 149.

Vitiello, M. V., Prinz, P. N., and Schwartz, R. S. (1994b). The subjective sleep quality of healthy older men and women is enhanced by participation in two fitness training programs: a nonspecific effect. *Sleep Research*, *23*, 148.

Vogel, G. W., Buffenstein, A., Minter, K., and Hennessey, A. (1990). Drug effects on REM sleep and on endogenous depression. *Neuroscience and Biobehavioral Reviews*, *14*, 49–63.

Vuori, I., Urponen, H., Hasan, J., and Partinen, M. (1988). Epidemiology of exercise effects on sleep. *Acta Physiologica Scandinavica*, *133*(S574), 3–7.

Walsh, J. K. (2004). Clinical and socioeconomic correlates of insomnia. *Journal of Clinical Psychiatry*, *65*, 13–19.

Weaver, T. E., Laizner, A. M., Evans, L. K., Maislin, G., Chugh, D. K., Lyon, K. *et al.* (1997). An instrument to measure functional status outcomes for disorders of excessive sleepiness. *Sleep*, *20*, 835–843.

Whitney, C. W., Enright, P. L., Newman, A. B., Bonekat, W., Foley, D., and Quan, S. F. (1998). Correlates of daytime sleepiness in 4578 elderly persons: the cardiovascular health study. *Sleep*, *21*, 27–36.

Young-McCaughan, S., Mays, M. Z., Arzola, S. M., Yoder, L. H., Dramiga, S. A., Leclerc, K. M. *et al.* (2003). Changes in exercise tolerance, activity and sleep patterns, and quality of life in patients with cancer participating in a structured exercise program. *Oncology Nursing Forum*, *30*, 441–452.

Youngstedt, S. D. (2000). Late-night exercise and sleep. *The American Journal of Medicine and Sports*, *2*, 220–221.

Youngstedt, S. D. (2003). Ceiling and floor effects in sleep research. *Sleep Medicine Reviews*, *7*, 351–365.

Youngstedt, S. D. and Kripke, D. F. (2004). Long sleep and mortality: rationale for sleep restriction. *Sleep Medicine Reviews*, *8*, 159–174.

Youngstedt, S. D., O'Connor, P. J., and Dishman, R. K. (1997). The effects of acute exercise on sleep: a quantitative synthesis. *Sleep*, *20*, 203–214.

Youngstedt, S. D., Kripke, D. F., and Elliott, J. A. (1999a). Is sleep disturbed by vigorous late-night exercise? *Medicine and Science in Sports and Exercise*, *31*, 864–869.

Youngstedt, S. D., Kripke, D. F., Elliott, J. A., Baehr, E. K., and Sepulveda, R. S. (1999b). Light exposure, sleep quality, and depression in older adults. In M. F. Holick and E. G. Jung (Eds). *Biologic Effects of Light 1998* (5th edn, pp. 427–435). Boston, MD: Kluwer Academic Publishers.

Youngstedt, S. D., O'Connor, P. J., Crabbe, J. B., and Dishman, R. K. (2000). The influence of acute exercise on sleep following high caffeine intake. *Physiology and Behavior*, *68*, 563–570.

Youngstedt, S. D., Kripke, D. F., and Elliott, J. A. (2002a). Circadian phase-delaying effects of bright light alone and combined with exercise in humans. *American Journal of Physiology*, *282*, R259–R266.

Youngstedt, S. D., Kripke, D. F., Elliott, J. A., Huegel, G. O., and Rex, K. M. (2002b). Exercise phase-response curves in young and older adults. *Society for Research on Biological Rhythms*, *8*, 110.

Youngstedt, S. D., Perlis, M. L., O'Brien, P. M., Palmer, C. R., Smith, M. T., Orff, H. J. *et al.* (2003). No association of sleep with total daily physical activity in normal sleepers. *Physiology and Behavior*, *78*, 395–401.

Sport, social inclusion, and crime reduction

FRED COALTER

CHAPTER 10

SPORT AND SOCIAL INCLUSION: NEW LABOUR AND THE THIRD WAY

Since the 1997 election of the "new" Labour government in the United Kingdom, sport has become more central to the broader social policy agenda, largely because of the presumed externalities, or benefits, associated with participation. For example, Policy Action Group 10 (Department of Culture, Media and Sport, 1999) stated that "sport can contribute to neighborhood renewal by improving communities' perform-ance on four key indicators – health, crime, employment, and education." A more detailed set of aspirations was provided by the Scottish Office (1999, p. 22), which claimed that:

Arts, sport and leisure activities . . . have a role to play in countering social exclusion. They can help to increase the self-esteem of individuals; build community spirit; increase social interaction; improve health and fitness; create employment and give young people a purposeful activity, reducing the temptation to anti-social behavior.

Vague and unexamined claims about sport's externalities have always underpinned public investment in sport (Coalter, 1998). However, the increased importance of sport can be explained by certain aspects of "new" Labour's agenda, especially their desire to create a "Third Way" between the perceived failures of "old" Labour policies of state control, state provision and anti-individualism and the Thatcherite neo-Liberal, free-market policies, with their extreme individualism. The Third Way is a relatively amor-phous term associated with the writings of Giddens (1998, 2001) and represents an attempt to modernize and reform all aspects of government and civil society. Drawing loosely on the communitarian ideas of Etzioni (1997), Putnam's (1993, 2000) concepts of social capital, and Hutton's (1995) notions of a "stakeholder" society, the Third Way seeks to strengthen civil society and empower communities. This is to be achieved by promoting "active citizenship" and reducing social exclusion. Social exclusion is a much wider concept than poverty. For example, Room (1995) proposes that, whereas poverty was distributional, social exclusion is relational – it refers to inadequate social participa-tion, lack of social integration, and lack of power. Forrest and Kearns (1999) suggest that "social exclusion arises from a combination of unemployment, low income, marital breakdown, and a generally resource-poor social network . . . trapped within or chan-nelled into specific neighbourhoods" (p. 1). The Social Exclusion Unit (1998) defined it as a shorthand label for a combination of linked problems-unemployment, poor skills, low income, poor housing, high crime environment, bad health, and family breakdown.

Central to this agenda is the rather diffuse concept of social capital, which is taken to refer to various social and moral relations that bind communities together. It is viewed as having three main components – strong social networks and civic infrastruc-ture; strong social norms (i.e., informal and formal rules about personal and social behavior and associated sanctions); and mutual trust and reciprocity among members of a community. Although the concept is not new, the recent work of Putnam (2000) on the decline of community in the United States has lead to increased policy interest. Evidence suggests that communities high in social capital tend to have a number of desired conditions – lower crime rates, better health and lower rates of child abuse (Office of National Statistics, 2001; Performance and Innovation Unit, 2002). For example, the Acheson report on inequalities and health (quoted in Health Education Authority, 1999, pp. 2–3) states that:

Opportunities afforded by exercise might also lead to wider networks and social cohesion . . . it has been suggested that people with good social networks live longer, are at reduced risk of coronary heart disease, are less likely to report being depressed or to suffer a recurrence of cancer, and are less susceptible to infectious illness than those with poor networks.

Within this context, the "new" Labour government has emphasized the potential role of sport, both via participation and volunteering. The presumption that participation in sport can contribute to the development of "active citizenship" is clear in the statement that "people who participate in sports and arts activities are more likely to play an active role in the community in other ways" (Scottish Office, 1999, p. 22). This new emphasis has been described as marking a shift from the traditional approach of developing sport *in* the community, to developing communities *through* sport (Coalter *et al.*, 2000; Houlihan and White, 2003).

SPORTS AND THEIR PRESUMED PROPERTIES

The presumption that sport can contribute to community development, urban regeneration, and social inclusion implies that participation in sport can produce outcomes which serve to strengthen and improve certain weak, or negative, aspects of processes, structures, and relationships thought to characterize deprived urban areas. A number of writers have listed the supposed structural and processual aspects of sport that can produce sociopsychological benefits (Coalter *et al.*, 2000; Collins *et al.*, 1999; Keller *et al.*, 1998; Svoboda, 1994; Wankel and Sefton, 1994).

In summary, the potential benefits of sports participation are:

- Physical fitness and health.
- Improved mental health and psychological well-being, leading to the reduction of anxiety and stress (see Biddle *et al.*, 2000).
- Personality development via improved self-concept, physical and global self-esteem/ confidence, self-confidence, and increased locus of control.
- Sociopsychological benefits such as empathy with others, tolerance, co-operation, and the development of social skills.
- Sociological impacts such as increased community identity, social coherence, and integration.

The logic of this process is outlined in Figure 10.1 (see also Coalter, 2002). Traditional sports development has largely been concerned with providing sufficient opportunities to achieve certain *sporting outcomes* – increased and more equitable participation. In this approach participation – sport for all – was the only measure of effectiveness.

However, in the new social inclusion agenda, the tests of effectiveness have shifted from "sport for all" to what Richard Caborn, Minister of Sport, has referred to as "sport for good" – the government now invests in sport for its contributions to the wider social agenda. Consequently the assumption (as outlined in Figure 10.1) is that increased participation in sport will lead to *intermediate* (individual) *impacts* – such as fitness, sense of well-being, self-esteem, social skills, and social involvement. Such impacts are then likely to lead to *intermediate outcomes* (changes in behavior) – decreased drug use, decreased anti-social behavior, increased healthy lifestyle, and improved educational

Figure 10.1 The social impacts of sport: a logic model.

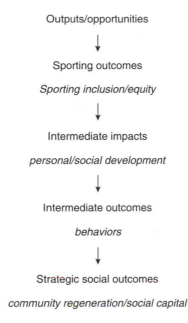

performance. The accumulation of such behaviors, plus the more general impact of an improved sporting infrastructure (i.e., clubs, teams, volunteers etc.), will produce strategic social outcomes such as increased social capital, community cohesion, and social regeneration. However, such rather functionalist analyses ignore a number of significant issues.

THE DIVERSITY OF SPORT

Sport is a collective noun that hides more than it reveals. For example, there are individual, partner, and team sports; contact and non-contact sports; motor-driven or perceptually dominated sports and those that place different emphases on strategy, chance and physical skills. This diversity is illustrated by the acceptance by all sports councils in the United Kingdom of the all-encompassing definition of "sport" contained in the Council of Europe's European Sports Charter (quoted in Sport England, 2004):

Sport means all forms of physical activity which, through casual or organized partici-pation, aim at expressing or improving physical fitness and mental well-being, forming relationships or obtaining results in competitions at all levels.

(p. 3)

Consequently, in terms of producing intermediate impacts and outcomes, it is best to regard sports as a series of different *social relationships* and *social processes* in which it is assumed that certain types of learning, or "socialization," occur. From this perspective the main issues are what *sports processes* produce what *outcomes* for which *sections of the population* and in what *circumstances*.

NECESSARY AND SUFFICIENT CONDITIONS

Clearly, participation in sport is a necessary condition to obtain any of the potential benefits. However, as these outcomes are "only a possibility" (Svoboda, 1994) there is a need to consider sufficient conditions (the conditions under which the potential outcomes are achieved). It cannot be assumed that any, or all, participants will automatically obtain the presumed benefits in all circumstances. Such outcomes remain only a possibility because:

1   Participation in sport is just one of many things that people do. Therefore, its impact will depend on the relative salience of the experience compared to other factors (e.g., criminal sub-cultures).
2   The nature and extent of any effects will depend on the nature of the experience. Sport is not a homogenous, standardized product, or experience.
3   Effects will be determined by the frequency and intensity of participation and the degree of participants' adherence over time. Although these factors are especially important for fitness and health benefits, they also have clear implications for the development of technical and social skills and attitudes and values.
4   Even if sports participation does assist in the development of certain types of personal competence, confidence, and attitudes (intermediate impacts), this cannot simply be taken to imply that these will be transferred to wider social or community benefits (intermediate and social outcomes).
5   It is often difficult to disentangle the effects of participation in sport from parallel social influences and developmental processes.

Therefore, the measurement of cause and effect, of the relationship between inputs and desired outcomes, presents a number of difficulties. Until recently, such problems have largely been ignored, with the emphasis being placed on the *theoretical* possibilities associated with sports participation. The apparent theoretical strength and coherence of the description of sports' potentially positive contributions partly explains widespread failures to undertake systematic monitoring and evaluation of the outcomes of sport or physical activity-based projects – theory permitted the assumption of such outcomes.

However, such a lack of robust evidence has become an increasing problem for sport in an era of "welfare effectiveness" and so-called "evidence-based policy making." From this perspective, public investment in sport is undertaken to achieve wider social policy aims and evidence of outcomes and impacts is required. Further, the increased pressure for evidence of effectiveness and examples of "best practice" also relate to a need to understand processes that lead to successful outcomes to enable providers to "manage for outcomes" – that is, provide the optimal sporting experiences to achieve desired outcomes, rather than simply assume that such outcomes will be an inevitable consequence of participation.

The problem for sport is that its claims range from the physiological via the socio-psychological to the social (each with different methodological traditions and criteria of proof), include a number of indirect effects (crime reduction, increased educational achievement; social cohesion), and has a non-cumulative evidence base in which a wide range of key terms have been operationalized in variety of ways. As a consequence, the evidence base for both practice and outcomes is generally weak, providing little guidance for policy and provision. However, although such a situation is often used to question sports' contributions, it is one not confined to sport. For example,

much primary care clinical activity, including the way care is organized, is unsupported by any substantial body of evidence. The primary care "evidence gap" is not a single entity – it encompasses evidence gaps about implementation, effectiveness and applicability, as well as gaps in basic scientific knowledge.

(Department of Health, 1999, p. 3)

Such issues and dilemmas will be illustrated via an analysis of the literature on the potential role of sport in the reduction of anti-social behavior and crime. Sport and crime reduction is a useful example for a number of reasons – it has always been a central rationale for public investment in sport, it has an increasingly high policy priority (with widespread concerns about youth crime), crime is taken to symbolize community fragmentation and the absence of "social capital," and is often viewed as a major consequence of social exclusion. For example, the definitions of social exclusion offered by the Cabinet Office and in Social Exclusion: Opening the Door to a Better Scotland (Scottish Office, 1999) both include "living in a high crime environment."

SPORT AND CRIME

Many policy-related reviews of the potential social value of sport (Collins *et al.*, 1999; Department of Culture, Media and Sport, 1999; Sport England, 1999) list the prevention of youth crime as an issue to which sports can make a contribution. This reflects a widespread belief in the "therapeutic" potential of sport (Coalter, 1988; Collins *et al.*, 1999; Nichols and Taylor, 1996; Taylor *et al.*, 1999).

For example, Schafer (1969) outlines five elements underpinning the presumed therapeutic potential of sport and its ability to reduce criminal behavior:

- By "differential association" young people at risk are removed from the criminal culture of their peer groups and mix with more positive role models.
- Sport provides an alternative to educational underachievement, blocked aspirations and low self-esteem.
- Sport encourages the development of self-discipline.
- Sport provides catharsis and an antidote to adolescent boredom.
- Sport addresses certain adolescent development needs for adventure, excitement, autonomy and identity formation.

To critically review the claims regarding the therapeutic potential of sport in reducing crime, an extensive search of several reference databases (Ingenta, SportDiscus, Cabi Online Abstract Journal Service, and Swetswise) was performed from 1996–2003 and included the search terms: sport; crime; anti-social behavior; delinquency; rehabilitation; young offenders; deterrence; prevention; drug abuse. In addition, two major reviews undertaken by the author (Coalter, 1988, 1996) were drawn on. Substantive reviews are identified in Table 10.1 and relevant empirical studies are identified in Table 10.2.

Table 10.1 Research reviews examining sport/physical activity and anti-social behavior

AUTHOR	REVIEW DESIGN AND SCOPE	CONCLUSIONS
Coalter (1989)	Literature review via searches of on-line databases and one in-depth case study	The efficacy of sport as an antidote to delinquency is not proven. Issues of self-selection, the nature of the learning process and lack of longitudinal evidence remain unresolved
Coalter (1996)	Literature review via searches of on-line databases	Necessary to acknowledge both the complexity/diversity of causes of crime and sporting-processes. Sports-therapy approaches tend to ignore issues of gender. Context and process seems more important than sporting activity. Voluntary attendance is essential. Sport must be accompanied with broader development programs
West and Crompton (2001)	A review of 26 published evaluations of outdoor adventure programs. Some of the studies measured recidivism rates and some assessed the psychological benefits of participation on self-concept	The consistency of the findings supports notion that outdoor adventure programs contribute to alleviating negative behaviors But, only tentative support because of suspect internal validity, different operationalization of concepts, post-facto development of hypotheses, and over-concentration on self-concept
Taylor et al. (1999)	A review of 54 Probation Services demanding physical activity programs in England and Wales, plus 10 case studies	Evaluating outcomes is a complex and difficult task. Identified key ingredients, including: a clear rationale; suitable activities and locations; longer term perspective required; high quality staff; explicit acknowledgement of participants' achievements; post-program support
Robins (1990)	Literature review and interview-based evaluations of 8 crime prevention and 7 rehabilitation schemes	Little systematic evaluation of outcomes and limited theoretical understanding of causes of crime. Need for educational development, a focus on job training and community development
Utting (1996)	Review of a range of approaches and programs seeking to reduce crime among young people, including sport	Lack of empirical research means that important practice issues remain unresolved. Effective programs will include: careful assessment of needs; clear and simply defined outcomes; a logic model; target specific at-risk groups; skilled staff; involve participants in planning, implementation, and evaluation

The identified studies are mainly related to specific programes which seek to use sport to address issues of crime and divide broadly into prevention (or diversion) and rehabilitation of offenders. However, before looking at these in detail it is worth referring to one study which sought to measure relationships between general participation in sport and delinquency (Begg *et al.*, 1996) A longitudinal, cohort study measured the relationship between self-reported sports participation and self-reported "serious delinquency" (i.e., shop-lifting, car theft, burglary, assault etc). The authors concluded that, after controlling for delinquent behavior and psychosocial factors at age 15, females with moderate or high levels of sporting activity were significantly more likely to be delinquent at age 18 than those with low levels of sporting activity. Males with high levels of sporting activity were significantly more likely to be delinquent at age 18 than those with low levels of sporting activity. The authors concluded that the best predictor of delinquent behavior at age 18 was delinquent behavior at age 15, irrespective of sporting involvement. They argue that deterence requires a range of strategies which take into account the special needs and norms of delinquents, illustrating the problematic nature of simple assumptions about the relationship between sports participation and reduced anti-social behavior.

DIVERSIONARY PROGRAMS AND THE PREVENTION OF CRIME

These studies tend to be relatively large-scale community-based sports programs targeted at specific areas and/or during specific time periods (e.g., summer sports programs) and aim "at the casual integration of youth at risk, in order to reduce delinquency rates by encouraging the positive use of their leisure time" (Robins, 1990, p. 19). An example of this is the Splash programs that run during school holidays, and concentrate on a core of at-risk 13–17-year olds. These programs are provided in high-crime housing estates in England and Wales and seek to engage young people in constructive activities. A wide range of activities are offered, although sport is the largest single category (i.e., football, basketball, rounders, climbing, sailing, roller hockey, and skateboarding). Other activities include music/dance/drama, residential (i.e., camping, forest orienteering), arts/crafts, and day trips (i.e., zoos, museums etc).

Evaluations in 2002 and 2003 claim that the schemes had led to an aggregate reduction in "youth crime" (Cap Gemini Ernst and Young, 2003; Loxley *et al.*, 2002). For example, in 2003 it was reported that in ten areas, total recorded crime was reduced by 7.4% and juvenile nuisance increased by only 0.1% (compared to 13.2% in an equivalent period prior to the scheme). It is interesting to note that, as these schemes have developed, it has been deemed necessary to go beyond simply providing activities and include developmental activities such as advice on anger management, alcohol and drug abuse, personal health and hygiene, and vocational training, greatly reducing the ability to identify the precise contribution of sport.

However, it was admitted that the analysis of local crime figures was difficult because of changes in recording and different sizes of areas covered, and that the conclusions were based on relatively small samples. In addition, large-scale diversionary programs often have a number of common weaknesses (Coalter *et al.*, 2000; Robins, 1990; Utting, 1996), such as vague rationales or over-ambitious objectives, vague definitions

Table 10.2 Empirical studies examining sport/physical activity and crime reduction

AUTHOR	COUNTRY	PARTICIPANTS	DESIGN	INTERVENTION	FINDINGS
Crompton and Witt (1996b)	USA	6–19 at-risk year olds	Interviews with managers and leaders	Outreach leaders providing activities	Leadership is critical
Begg et al. (1996)	New Zealand	800 15–18 year old	Longitudinal cohort study based on self-reported delinquency. Logistic regression analysis		Females with moderate/high levels of sporting activity and males with high levels of activity at 15 were significantly more likely to be delinquent at 18 than those with low levels of activity. Deterrence hypothesis not supported
Nichols and Taylor (1996)	UK	49 16–25-year old voluntary attenders referred by Probation Service	Interviews, survey of participants, case studies, documentary analysis. Participants and control group reconviction scores compared over 2 years	12 week one to one sports counselling and support to encourage independent participation	(1) Effect related to length of involvement in program (2) Elements contributing to success included: voluntary participation, sports leaders, improved self-esteem and fitness, new peer group, access to vocational training
Cap Gemini Ernst and Young (2003)	UK	13–17 year olds in high crime estates in England and Wales	Analysis of crime and incidents statistics. Interviews with participants, parents, and staff	Multi-activity holiday programs	Limited, but statistically significant decreases in crime in some areas; variations in practice and impacts across schemes

Study	Country	Sample	Method	Activities	Findings
Andrews and Andrews (2003)	UK	20 young people (10–17 year of age) in a secure unit	8 month participant observation study	Organised PE classes and formal and informal sporting activities	Supports use of sporting activities which de-emphasize regulations and winning and permits choice and provides positive feed-back
Farrell et al. (1995)	USA	96 18–25-year old African American males	Questionnaire survey	Basketball league, educational programs, mentoring	(1) Reduced crime rates by 30% in target area (2) Created safe haven for positive social activities (3) Directed energies in positive direction (4) Improved educational and career aspirations
Loxley et al. (2002)	UK	13–17 year olds living in deprived-housing estates	Case studies	Six summer activity programs	(1) Not wholly successful in attracting at-risk youth (2) Only one scheme showed a decline in incidents reported to the police (3) Modest additional interventions can have a diminishing impact in areas with a reasonable level of existing provision

of "anti-social behaviors" and rather simplistic theories of the causes of crime (see Asquith *et al.* (1998) for a comprehensive list of socio-psychological "high-risk factors"). A Home Office review of such programs (Utting, 1996) concluded that "it is difficult to argue that such activities have in themselves a generalizable influence on criminality. The lack of empirical research means important practice issues remain unresolved" (p. 84).

The notion that this was a widespread problem was indicated by Robins (1990) in a review of 11 UK schemes designed to use sport to divert young people from criminal behavior. Robins concluded that "information about outcomes was hard to come by" (p. 1). In a review of 120 programs for at-risk youth in the United States, Witt and Crompton (1996a) found that 30% undertook no evaluation and only 4% undertook pre/post evaluation of participation-related changes. They also pointed to the lack of clear objectives in most programs, stating that "the lack of specific objectives written in an operational format leads to the inference that many agencies have not identified specific standards by which to evaluate the success of their programmes" (Witt and Crompton, 1996a, p. 12).

Further, many academic studies are methodologically very weak and the generic issue of the problems of measuring inter-dependent and secondary effects of sports participation is present. Taylor (1999) suggests that the major problem in identifying and measuring the effects of sport on crime is that the influence on crime is indirect, working through a number of intermediate outcomes or processes, such as improved fitness, self-esteem, self-efficacy and locus of control, and the development of social and personal skills. It is clearly not sufficient simply to measure outcomes and assume that these are "sports effects." These acknowledged difficulties in evaluating outcomes in more general, larger scale "diversionary" programs are also present in small-scale, targeted rehabilition schemes.

SPORT AND THE REHABILITATION OF OFFENDERS

These approaches tend to be less "product-led" and based on intensive counselling, in which the needs of offenders are identified and programs adapted to suit their needs. This is usually via outdoor adventure activities, or demanding physical activity programs, aimed at such intermediate impacts as the development of personal and social skills, improving self-confidence, self-efficacy and locus of control – which it is hoped will result in the intermediate outcome of reduced offending behavior (Coalter, 1988; Taylor *et al.*, 1999).

An evaluation of the West Yorkshire Sports Counselling Project (Nichols and Taylor, 1996) compared reconviction rates over two years of participants and a control group. The project was a 12×3 hours per week voluntary sports program based on a one-to-one participant-centered approach in which trained sports leaders counseled participants in particular activities, introduced them to appropriate clubs and encouraged independent participation. Participants, who had completed eight or more weeks, were significantly less likely to be reconvicted. Various aspects of the program were identified as contributing to its success – the voluntary nature of participation, the skills of sports leaders, improved self-esteem and perceptions of fitness, the length of the course, new peer group, and access to employment-orientated training courses.

In a recent North American review of the role and effectiveness of 21 outdoor recreation programs in reducing recidivism rates, West and Crompton (2001) found that of 14 programs reporting recidivism rates, 8 reported reduced rates; of the 16 reporting changes in self-concept, 14 showed significant positive changes. However, despite these results, the authors give only tentative support to such approaches because of several methodological concerns – lack of internal validity, lack of consistency in defining recidivism and self-concept, lack of control groups, and too narrow a focus on self-concept rather than measuring the impact on multiple-protective factors. Protective factors include such elements as participants knowing that there is at least one adult supporting their positive development; the existence of places to spend free time in a positive, productive environment in their home area; opportunities to work together in a group and learn how to resolve conflicts constructively; the opportunity to be around peers consistently who are demonstrating positive conventional behavior; and placing a value on achievement (Witt and Crompton, 1997).

More generally, concern has been expressed about low completion rates and the possibility of "self-selection," with those most positively affected being those least likely to re-offend. Further, returning participants to their original peer environment after short periods of time inevitably means that for some there will be a return to criminal or anti-social behavior. For example, Taylor *et al.* (1999) point to evidence that the relative success of such programs was in part related to the length of the program, with the longer programs being most successful.

A major study of British programs concluded that evaluation was variable and that performance indicators ranged from the simple monitoring of attendance via the use of anecdotal evidence, to a few who estimated reconviction rates (Taylor *et al.*, 1999). This led the researchers to conclude that:

Programme managers . . . feel that quantitative indicators are insufficient to capture the essence of the outputs [and] that this reflects the difficulty of not only determining the significant variables but also measuring the precise effect they have . . . there is a problem finding qualitative evaluation techniques which are feasible with limited resources but which adequately monitor the complex outcomes which most of the programmes aspire to. All programmes agree that physical activities do not by themselves reduce offending. All agree that there are personal and social development objectives that form part of a matrix of outcomes. These developments may, sooner or later, improve offending behaviour, but their impact is unpredictable in scale and timing. To expect anything more tangible is unrealistic.

(Taylor *et al.*, 1999, p. 50)

In a Home Office review of such programs Utting (1996, p. 56) concluded that:

there is a shortage of reliable information regarding which aspects of sport, adventure and leisure pursuit programmes are most effective and for how long. It is not clear which interventions are most appropriate for different groups of young people.

Further, there is strong evidence to suggest that not all sports will be relevant for many vulnerable young people. For example, there is some evidence of the need for small-group or individual activities that are non-competitive, emphasize personally constructed goals and have a minimum of formal rules and regulations. Sugden and Yiannakis (1982) suggest that certain adolescents reject organized, competitive mainstream sport because it contains components similar to those which they have already failed to resolve – adherence to formal rules and regulations, achievement of externally defined goals and competitive and testing situations. This analysis is supported by an 8-month participant observation study of 20 residents (aged 12–17, including 5 girls) in a secure unit in the United Kingdom (Andrews and Andrews, 2003). The authors illustrate the potentially threatening nature of "traditional" sports for such volatile young people. The ethos of sport and exercise provision involved small group and individual lessons. Where games were played, they had minimal rules and a strong emphasis on fun as an escape from the strict regulations governing the unit. Autonomy and ownership were encouraged by letting the young people construct their own gym program, based on individual aims and goals and their appraisal of their abilities. To foster self-esteem, peer comparison of physical abilities was not encouraged, emphasis was placed on task mastery, support was not contingent upon performance and feedback was fair and appropriate. Further, the authors argue that care needs to be taken when providing aggressive sports which re-affirm adolescent masculine aggression. The authors suggest that traditional sport may not be as effective in cultivating principled moral judgment as theories suggest. Their general conclusion was that sporting activities should de-emphasize regulations and winning, place an emphasis on choices, with programs tailored to suit individual needs and the regular use of positive feedback (see also Witt and Crompton, 1997).

SPORT, INTEGRATED DEVELOPMENT, AND REDUCING CRIME

Evaluations of both diversionary and rehabilitative approaches suggest that the therapeutic potential of sport is maximized by working in partnership with other agencies as part of integrated development programs that seek, systematically, to achieve improvements in cognitive and social skills, to reduce impulsiveness and risk-taking behavior, raise self-esteem and self-confidence, and improve education and employment prospects (Asquith *et al.*, 1998; Utting, 1996).

We have already noted the increasing use of this approach in the UK Splash program and Wilkins (1997) offers an example from the United States. It is claimed that the Kansas City Night Hoops program has led to "an overall 25% decrease in crime" and that "other cities who run hoops programs report similar results" (Wilkins, 1997, p. 60). This is part of the so-called Midnight Basketball movement aimed at young men in high-crime neighborhoods, with games scheduled at various times around midnight when many gang and drug-related crimes are most likely to occur. However, such positive results are not simply a function of participation in sport, but of a much more complex program. Although, the strong salience of basketball for urban youth is the key to making contact with those at-risk, "the most urgent objective" is education and life learning (Wilkins, 1997, p. 60). The highly structured program includes non-traditional education components which seek to develop employment skills, personal development, self-esteem, conflict resolution, health awareness, and substance abuse prevention (see also Farrell *et al.*, 1996). Consequently, while sport plays a central role in this program, the clear conclusion is that *diversion* must be complemented by *development* and that sport cannot achieve the desired outcomes on its own, especially among those most at-risk (for a British example see Deane, 1998). As a recent Cabinet Office (2002, p. 60) report on sport concluded, ". . . playing sport will not lead to a permanent reduction in crime by itself. Successful programmes require a variety of other support mechanisms to be in place."

In addition to using the salience of sport to attract at-risk youth to integrated development programs, research indicates that the quality of leadership and social relationships are vitally important factors. For example, Witt and Crompton (1996b, p. 16) demonstrated that "leadership is perhaps the most important element in determining the positive impact of a program, since it shapes what participants derive from their experience." In his review of UK initiatives, Utting (1996) also stresses the important role of youth workers in the delivery of sporting programs. Reporting on a program in the United States, Feldman *et al.* (1983) suggest that the type of treatment, leadership experience, and group composition all had an influence on behavioral measures.

More generally, programs seem to be most successful when they are "bottom-up" (Deane, 1998; Witt and Crompton, 1996b). Also, evidence suggests that the potential for success is increased if young people are involved both in influencing the nature of the provision and in its management (Coalter and Allison, 1996; Fitzpatrick *et al.*, 1998; West and Crompton, 2001). In an analysis of diversionary sports programs in the United States, Witt and Crompton (1996a, p. 22) stated that "empowerment is an important theme that runs through these case studies. Empowerment enables youth to take ownership and responsibility for their recreational and social activities."

Consequently, for those most at-risk, the evidence suggests that traditional approaches and forms of provision may not be effective. In a report to the Sports Council for Wales, The Leisure and Environmental Protection Department of the Newport County Borough Council (1999, p. 4) concluded that:

While sport can have a positive role to play in addressing social cohesion, this is unlikely to happen if it is organized, or promoted along conventional lines. Engaging the most disaffected . . . can best be achieved through the deployment of a combination of community development and sports development resource.

IMPLICATIONS FOR RESEARCHERS

There are strong theoretical arguments for the potentially positive contribution which sport can make to reduce the propensity to commit crime if used in a targeted and systematic manner. However, there is an absence of robust research data on the extent and nature of *intermediate impacts* and their influence on subsequent behavior (*intermediate outcomes*), especially for large scale sports diversionary projects. There are widespread issues of validity (with a variety of definitions of key terms being used) and reliability (because of poor design) that significantly limit an accumulation of comparable evidence. For example, West and Crompton (2001) comment that, in many of the studies that they reviewed, the authors failed to offer details of the variables or procedures involved.

There is a need for a much more systematic approach to research (before and after studies; the use of treatment and control groups, although this is often difficult) to measure the nature of the intermediate impacts produced by different types of programs (e.g., improved fitness, self-esteem, self-efficacy and locus of control, and the development of cognitive, personal, and social skills). West and Crompton (2001) suggest that there is a need to measure the differential effects of various aspects of the process – the location and duration of activities, the optimal size of groups, participant/staff ratios, the skills of leaders, the importance of voluntary participation, the role of peer acceptance, and the importance of various "protective factors" (e.g., adult support and affirmation).

The measurement of intermediate outcomes presents two types of difficulties. First, measuring the effectiveness of such programs in reducing crime requires longitudinal and follow-up studies which raise a variety of resource and ethical issues. Second, and much more problematic, is the fact that the effects of sport on crime are indirect, working through a number of intermediate outcomes or processes. Further, such processes are also subject to a range of intervening variables (e.g., normal, adolescent development processes) and confounding variables (other environmental factors) – issues often ignored in current research.

In the absence of more robust longitudinal studies, one possible approach would be a more widespread use of logic models or "theories of change" (Centres for Disease Control and Prevention, 1999; Granger, 1998). The notion of a "theory of change" relates to such, often unexamined, questions as why do we assume that sport can have certain impacts on participants and communities; what are the properties and processes of sports participation which may lead to such outcomes; can we define clearly the theory of the relationship between participation in sport and a range of outcomes (i.e., improved fitness, health, changed attitudes to crime, and increased self-esteem)? In other words, a "logic model" requires us to demonstrate the nature of hypothetical links between the design and content of a program, its intermediate impacts (mostly measurable) and the presumed intermediate outcomes (much more difficult to measure).

A logic model reveals assumptions concerning conditions for program effectiveness and provides a frame of reference for one or more evaluations of the program. A detailed logic model can also strengthen claims for causality and be the basis for estimating the program's effect on endpoints that are not directly measured, but are in a causal chain supported by prior research (Centres for Disease Control and Prevention, 1999). In such an approach there is an urgent need for a much more precise definition and measurement of the key terms that are central to the process (e.g., anti-social behavior, self-esteem).

This approach is related to that proposed by Nichols and Crow (2004) who argue that the definitions of outcomes and appropriate methods of evaluation will vary between three broad ideal types of programs – primary programs aimed at simple diversion through large-scale open access sports programs; more targeted secondary programs aimed at deterring criminal behavior among at-risk youth; and finally, highly selective tertiary programs which systematically seek to emphasize social development. They suggest that there are substantial methodological problems relating to the evaluation of effectiveness of both primary open access programs and secondary, at-risk, programs because of difficulties in collecting details of participants, the limitations of recorded crime statistics, and the general problem of seeking to impute causal relations between programs and crime statistics. In such circumstances they suggest in-depth interviews, case studies of individuals and surveys of residents – while admitting the limitations and limited generalisability of such data. Tertiary, social development, programs have targeted and easily identifiable participants and offer the possibility of before and after testing (e.g., self-esteem, locus of control, and cognitive skills), although the identification of a comparable control group often poses difficulties. Further, the measurement of such intermediate impacts would need to be accompanied by a longitudinal tracking of recidivism rates.

IMPLICATIONS FOR POLICY AND PRACTICE

Both rehabilitative and diversionary programs need to adopt a participant-centered and proactive, "managing for outcomes", approach. They should be based on an in-depth understanding of the causes of criminality (see e.g., Asquith *et al.*, 1998) and acknowledge that different types of sports, with differing emphases on rules and performance, will be relevant for different types of individuals. A needs-based youth work approach may be more appropriate than a product-led sports development approach. Evidence suggests that traditional facility-based programs will have little impact. Outreach approaches, locally recruited credible leadership, "bottom-up" approaches and non-traditional, local, provision appear to have the best chance of success with the most marginal at-risk groups.

Although the salience of sport appears to be effective in attracting at-risk youth to programs, in general, sport cannot do it on its own. Sport needs to be part of a broader integrated, structured, and developmental approach. The programs need to be structured to provide access to a range of protective factors (Witt and Crompton, 1997) and opportunities for personal, cognitive, and social development (Utting, 1996) – diversion must be complemented by development.

WHAT WE KNOW SUMMARY

Because of a widespread lack of robust, cumulative, and comparative research data it is very difficult to be precise about the relationship between sports participation and reduced anti-social behaviour and crime. For example, one in-depth study of a number of sports-centred rehabilitation schemes concluded that their impact is unpredictable in scale and timing and to expect any more definite conclusion is unrealistic (Taylor *et al.*, 1999). Additionally, a review of US rehabilitation schemes could provide only tentative support to such approaches because of several methodological concerns (West and Crompton, 2001). However, taking the balance of probabilities the following conclusions can be drawn:

- The most effective use of sport to address systematically anti-social and criminal behavior is in combination with programs that seek to address wider personal and social development.
- Sports' salience can be used to attract young people to integrated programs that offer formal programs in personal development, health awareness, and employment training.

- Leadership is perhaps the most important element in determining the positive impact of a program.
- Locally recruited leaders and a bottom-up approach maximize the chances of success.

WHAT WE NEED TO KNOW SUMMARY

In a paper for the Council of Europe, Parkinson (1998) argued that:

Sport, like most activities, is not a priori good or bad, but has the potential of producing both positive and negative outcomes. Questions like "what conditions are necessary for sport to have beneficial outcomes?" must be asked more often.

Utting (1996) concluded that we lack clarity about which interventions are most appropriate for different groups of young people. Consequently, the most pressing requirements are:

- We need to understand the elements of the process required to maximize desired intermediate impacts – the various combinations of such factors as voluntary participation, leadership, the mixture of rules and regulations, task versus ego orientation, protective factors (Witt and Crompton, 1997), personal and vocational development, length of program and post-program support.
- Such information should inform the design of programs, the training of personnel and permit the optimal allocation of resources.
- More longitudinal studies which track participants in a variety of programs to assess the long-term behavioral outcomes of (possibly) short-term attitude change.
- More generally (especially in relation to the broader social-inclusion agenda), we need to understand how sports can broaden their appeal. Consequently, the general policy desire to use sport to build social capital, reduce social exclusion and contribute to neighborhood renewal (Department of Culture, Media and Sport, 1999) and more targeted polices to reduce crime and anti-social behavior both need to address similar issues. There is a need for better understanding of a range of issues in order to enable a more proactive approach to "managing for outcomes." Such issues include the implications of the current nature and organization of sport, the varying degrees of attractiveness of particular types of sport to particular target groups, the extent to which sport can achieve any of the presumed externalities "on its own" or needs to be embedded in wider programs of personal and social development and the extent to which such programs can be product-led or needs-based.

REFERENCES

Andrews, J. P. and Andrews, G. J. (2003). Life in a secure unit: the rehabilitations of young people through the use of sport. *Social Science and Medicine*, 56, 531–550.

Asquith, S., Buist, M., Loughran, N., MacAuley, C., and Montgomery, M. (1998). *Children, Young People and Offending in Scotland: a Research Review*. Edinburgh: The Scottish Office.

Backman, S. J. and Crompton, J. L. (1984). Do outdoor education experiences contribute to cognitive development? *Journal of Environmental Education, 16*, 4–13.

Begg, D., Langley, J., Moffitt, T., and Marshall, S. (1996). Sport and delinquency: an examination of the deterrence hypothesis in a longitudinal study. *British Journal of Sports Medicine, 30*, 335–341.

Best, J. (1999). *Making the Case for the Benefits of Sport: Research Programme Proposal.* Hong Kong: Hong Kong Sports Development Board.

Biddle, S., Fox, K., and Boutcher, S. (Eds) (2000). *Physical Activity and Psychological Well-being.* London: Routledge.

Cabinet Office (2002). *Game Plan: a Strategy for Delivering Government's Sport and Physical Activity Objectives.* London: Cabinet Office.

Cap Gemini Ernst and Young (2003). *Splash 202. Final Report.* London: Youth Justice Board.

Centres for Disease Control and Prevention (1999). *Framework for Program Evaluation in Public Health* (No. RR–11). Retrieved October 18, 2004 from www.cdc.gov/eval/framework.htm

Coalter, F. (1988). *Sport and Anti-social Behaviour: a Literature Review.* Edinburgh: Scottish Sports Council.

Coalter, F. (1996). *Sport and Anti-social Behaviour: a Policy Analysis* (Research Digest, 41). Edinburgh: Scottish Sports Council.

Coalter, F. (1998). Leisure Studies, leisure policy and social citizenship: the failure of welfare or the limits of welfare? *Leisure Studies, 17*, 21–36.

Coalter, F. (2002). *Sport and Community Development: a Manual* (Research Report, 86). Edinburgh: Sport Scotland.

Coalter, F. and Allison, M. (1996). *Sport and Community Development* (Research Digest, 42). Edinburgh: Scottish Sports Council.

Coalter, F., Allison, M., and Taylor, J. (2000). *The Role of Sport in Regenerating Deprived Urban Areas.* Edinburgh: Scottish Office Central Research Unit.

Collins, M., Henry, I., and Houlihan, B. (1999). *Sport and Social Inclusion: a Report to the Policy Action Team 10.* London: Department of Culture, Media and Sport.

Crompton, J. L. and Witt, P. A. (1997). Programs that work: the Roving Leader Program in San Antonio. *Journal of Park and Recreation Administration, 15*, 84–92.

Deane, J. (1998). Community Sports Initiatives – An evaluation of UK policy attempts to involve the young unemployed – The 1980's Action Sport Scheme. *Sport in the City: Conference Proceedings, Loughborough, 1*, 140–159.

Department of Culture, Media and Sport (DCMS) (1999). *Policy Action Team 10: Report to the Social Exclusion Unit – Arts and Sport.* London: HMSO.

Department of Health (1999). *NHS R and D Strategic Review Primary Care: a Report of Topic Working Group.* London: The Stationary Office.

Etzioni, A. (1997). *The New Golden Rule: Community and Morality in a Democratic Society.* New York: Basic Books.

Farrell, W., Johnson, R., Sapp, M., Pumphrey, R., and Freeman, S. (1996). Redirecting the lives of urban black males: an assessment of Milwaukees's Midnight Basketball League. *Journal of Community Practice, 2*, 91–107.

Feldman, R. A., Caplinger, T. E., and Wodarsk, J. S. (1983). *The St. Louis Conundrum: the Effective Treatment of Antisocial Youths.* Englewood Cliffs, NJ: Prentice Hall.

Field, J. (2003). *Social Capital.* London: Routledge.

Fitzpatrick, S., Hastings, A., and Kinkree, K. (1998). *Including Young People in Urban Regeneration: a Lot to Learn?* Bristol, England: The Policy Press.

Forrest, R. and Kearns, A. (1999). Joined-up places? *Social Cohesion and Neighbourhood Regeneration.* York, England: Joseph Rowntree Foundation.

Giddens, A. (1998). *The Third Way: the Renewal of Social Democracy.* London: Polity Press.

Giddens, A. (Ed.) (2001). *The Global Third Way Debate.* London: Polity Press.

Granger, R. C. (1998). Establishing causality in evaluations of comprehensive community initiatives. In K. Fulbright-Anderson, A. C. Kubisch, and J. P. Connell (Eds). *New Approaches to Evaluating Community Initiatives, 2: Theory, Measurement, and Analysis.* Washington, DC: Aspen Institute.

Hastad, D. N., Segrave, J. O., Pangrazi, R., and Petersen, G. (1984). Youth sport participation and deviant behavior. *Sociology of Sport Journal, 1,* 366–373.

Heal, K. and Laycock, G. (1987). *Preventing Juvenile Delinquency: the Staffordshire Experience, Crime Prevention Unit Paper 8.* London: Home Office.

Health Education Authority (1999). *Physical Activity and Inequalities: a Briefing Paper.* London: Health Education Authority.

Houlihan, B. and White, A. (2002). *The Politics of Sport Development.* London: Routledge.

Hutton, W. (1995). *The State We're In.* London: Jonathan Cape.

Keller, H. (1982). A historical review. *Journal of Physical Education Recreation and Dance,* Nov–Dec, 26–27.

Keller, H., Lamprocht, M., and Stamm, H. (1998). *Social Cohesion through Sport.* Strasbourg: Committee for the Development of Sport, Council of Europe.

Leeds United Community (1999). *Playing for Success: the Leeds United Study Support Centre 1998–1999.* Leeds: United Football Club.

Leisure and Environment Protection Department (1999). *The Role of Sport in Tackling Social Exclusion.* Wales: Newport County Borough Council.

Long, J. and Sanderson, I. (1998). Social benefits of sport: Where's the proof? *Sport in the City: Conference Proceedings, Loughborough, 2,* 295–324.

Loxley, C., Curtin, L., and Brown, R. (2002). *Summer Splash Schemes 2000: Findings from Six Case Studies, Crime Reduction Research Series Paper 12.* London: Home Office.

McDonald, D. and Tungatt, M. (1992). *Community Development and Sport.* London: Sports Council.

Nichols, G. and Crow, I. (2004). Measuring the impact of crime reduction interventions involving sports activities for young people. *The Howard Journal, 43,* 267–283.

Nichols, G. and Taylor, P. (1996). *West Yorkshire Sports Counselling: Final Evaluation Report.* Sheffield: University of Sheffield Management Unit.

O'Brien, K. A. (1992). Effective programming for youth at-risk. *The Voice,* Summer, 16–17, 47–48.

Office for National Statistics (2001). *Social Capital: a Review of the Literature.* London: Office for National Statistics.

Parkinson, M. (1998). *Combating Social Exclusion: Lessons from Area-based Programmes in Europe.* Bristol: The Policy Press.

Perfomance and Innovation Unit (2002). *Social Capital: a Discussion Paper.* London: Cabinet Office.

Putnam, R. (1993). The prosperous community: social capital and public life. *The American Prospect, 4,* 11–18.

Putnam, R. (2000). *Bowling Alone: the Collapse and Revival of American Community.* New York: Simon and Schuster.

Robins, D. (1990). *Sport as Prevention: the Role of Sport in Crime Prevention Programmes Aimed at Young People* (University of Oxford, Centre for Criminological Research occasional paper no. 12). Oxford: The Centre.

Room, G. (Ed.) (1995). *Beyond the Threshold: the Measurement and Analysis of Social Exclusion.* Bristol: Policy Press.

Schafer, W. (1969). Some social sources and consequences of inter-scholastic athletics: the case of participation and delinquency. *International Review of Sport Sociology, 4,* 63–81.

Scottish Office (1999). *Social Inclusion: Opening the Door to a Better Scotland*. Edinburgh: Scottish Office.

Segrave, J. and Hastad, D. N. (1984). Interscholastic athletic participation and delinquency behaviour: an empirical assessment of relevant variables. *Sociology of Sport Journal, 1*, 96–111.

Sharp, C., Mawson, C., Pocklington, K., Kendal, L., and Morrison, J. (1999). *Playing for Success National Evaluation*. Slough: National Foundation for Educational Research.

Social Exclusion Unit (1998). *Truancy and Social Exclusion: a Report by the Social Exclusion Unit, Cm3957*. London: The Stationery Office.

Sport England (1999). *Best Value through Sport: the Value of Sport to Local Authorities*. London: Sport England.

Sport England (2004). *The Framework for Sport in England*. London: Sport England.

Sugden, J. and Yiannakis, A. (1982). Sport and juvenile delinquency: a theoretical base. *Journal of Sport and Social Issues, 6*, 22–30.

Svoboda, B. (1994). *Sport and Physical Activity as a Socialisation Environment: Scientific Review Part 1*. Europe: Committee for the Development of Sport (CDDS).

Taylor, P. (1999). *External Benefits of Leisure: Measurement and Policy Implications*, Paper presented to Tolern Seminar DCMS, November, London, England.

Taylor, P., Crow, I., Irvine, D., and Nichols, G. (1999). *Demanding Physical Activity Programmes for Young Offenders under Probation Supervision*. London: Home Office.

Utting, D. (1996). *Reducing Criminality among Young People: a Sample of Relevant Programmes in the United Kingdom*. London: Home Office Research and Statistics Directorate.

Wankel, L. and Sefton, J. M. (1994). Physical activity and other lifestyle behaviours. In C. Bouchard, R. J. Shephard, and T. Stephens (Eds). *Physical Activity, Fitness and Health* (pp. 531–50). Champaign, IL: Human Kinetics.

West, S. T. and Crompton, J. L. (2001). A review of the impact of adventure programs on at-risk youth. *Journal of Park and Recreation Administration, 19*, 113–140.

Wilkins, N. O. (1997). Overtime is better than sudden death. *Parks and Recreation*, March, 54–61.

Witt, P. A. and Crompton, J. L. (Eds) (1996a). *Recreation Programs that Work for at Risk Youth*. Pennsylvania, PA: Venture Publishing Inc.

Witt, P. A. and Crompton, J. L. (1996b). The at-risk youth recreation project. *Journal of Parks and Recreation Administration, 14*, 1–9.

Witt, P. A. and Crompton, J. L. (1997). The protective factors framework: a key to programming for benefits and evaluating results. *Journal of Parks and Recreation Administration, 15*, 1–18.

CHAPTER 11

From emerging relationships to the future role of exercise in mental health promotion

ADRIAN H. TAYLOR AND
GUY E. J. FAULKNER

The purpose of this edited collection was to develop evidence-based conclusions for researchers and health professionals and to further the consideration of physical activity as a strategy for improving mental health. In this final chapter, we summarize the key findings from each research area examined in the book. Much of this is based on the statements in each chapter that represent "what we know" about the field based on available evidence. We then provide a brief editorial commentary to place the summary in the broader context. Finally, we consider some of the limitations of the existing evidence base, summarize what we need to know, and lastly conclude by identifying key issues facing researchers and health professionals.

SUMMARY OF RESEARCH FINDINGS

In this section, the key findings from the respective chapters are summarized. We then briefly provide an editorial commentary on the "what we know" summaries.

DEMENTIA: WHAT WE KNOW SUMMARY

- Physical activity has been shown to be inversely associated with cognitive decline.
- Case-control studies tend to show a slight beneficial influence of physical activity against Alzheimer's disease (AD).
- Prospective analyses tend to show a more convincing protective effect of physical activity against AD and all combined forms of dementia.
- No association is evident between physical activity and Vascular dementia (VaD).
- Physical activity has been shown to improve functional status in frail nursing home residents with dementia including AD.
- No evidence of harmful effects of physical activity or exercise is evident (including vigorous exercise).

Editorial commentary

The early focus of research on the effects of sport, exercise, and physical activity on information processing speed and reaction time largely concerned younger people (see Boutcher, 2000). Chapter 2 by Danielle Laurin, René Verreault, and Joan Lindsay on physical activity and dementia highlights the rapidly growing field of exercise science and gerontology. It also reflects future challenges in public health as a larger proportion of the population advances toward old age, the prevalence of these medical conditions will continue to increase as they are primarily associated with this cohort. Advances in medical technology are allowing better insights into the neuro-cognitive ageing process, and, as a result, exercise scientists now have the opportunity to examine just how physical activity influences these processes. Research involving animal models is also revealing important advances in how exercise may enhance brain health and plasticity (Cotman and Berchtold, 2002).

Current evidence for the beneficial effects of exercise is limited. While cross-sectional relationships have been reported, and a few prospective studies show encouraging results, there are a number of alternative explanations for physical inactivity having a causal effect on the development of dementia, and conversely, a more active lifestyle preventing or slowing down progression. If being physically active does have a protective role, then there is insufficient evidence to take us much beyond speculation about the type and dose of exercise necessary. Progression in dementia may be slow and intermittent and this compounds the opportunity to demonstrate causal effects. Given the range of other health benefits from physical activity, even among the very old, regular daily aerobic physical activity that involves neuropsychological processes and enhanced cerebral blood flow in the prefrontal and frontal brain regions is likely to be justified in an attempt to prevent cognitive decline.

SCHIZOPHRENIA: WHAT WE KNOW SUMMARY

- There is a high incidence of obesity and other morbid conditions strongly related to physical inactivity in this population.
- Exercise interventions are possible.
- The existing research examining the psychological benefits of exercise participation does have many methodological flaws and tends to be of pre-experimental design.
- There is some tentative support that participating in exercise is associated with an alleviation of negative symptoms associated with schizophrenia, such as depression, low self-esteem, and social withdrawal.
- There is less evidence that exercise may be a useful coping-strategy for dealing with positive symptoms, such as auditory hallucinations.

Editorial commentary

Surprisingly, little attention has been given to the physical health needs of people with a diagnosis of schizophrenia. Indeed, early treatment involved physical restraint and confinement to small physical spaces. The identification of a shorter life expectancy and prevalence of cardiovascular disease, largely resulting from a poor lifestyle, has driven recent interest in promoting physical activity for this population. Evidence for any psychological benefit is therefore embryonic, although it is clear from the review by Guy Faulkner that enhancing physical health can impact psychological well-being in this population. Research designs that involve adequately powered sample sizes, carefully controlled exercise interventions, and follow-ups are likely to remain rare with this population for ethical and pragmatic reasons. This should not detract from the need to provide evidence-based interventions drawn from non-experimental work. Such studies have provided important information about activity levels and the influence of medical, environmental, and social factors on motivation and behavior. This information can drive the development of tailored approaches to promote physical activity.

DRUG AND ALCOHOL REHABILITATION: WHAT WE KNOW SUMMARY

- There is unequivocal support that physical exercise regimens have a positive effect on aerobic fitness and strength if administered as an adjunct in alcohol rehabilitation.
- There is unsubstantial evidence for the benefits of exercise on fitness during drug rehabilitation.

- The link between improvements in self-esteem and exercise with alcohol and drug rehabilitation at this time is equivocal.
- There is limited support that exercise regimens have a positive effect on reducing anxiety and depression if administered as an adjunct in alcohol and drug rehabilitation.
- There is experimental evidence from one study to suggest that alcohol cravings may be alleviated during exercise.
- The evidence for exercise improving abstinence levels or controlling drinking levels is at this time equivocal.

Editorial commentary

Dependence on alcohol and drugs is a common problem. For example, one out of every 10 Canadians aged 15 and over, about 2.6 million people, reported symptoms consistent with alcohol or illicit drug dependence (Statistics Canada, 2003). As Marie Donaghie and Michael Ussher write, the current treatment for such dependence is far from perfect which necessitates the examination of innovative strategies, such as exercise, for rehabilitation. As with most of the issues covered in this text, the rationale for considering exercise is convincing because of the well-accepted physical health benefits associated with physical activity. In this case, the role of physical activity in improving cardiorespiratory fitness and muscle strength, which may be compromised for many individuals receiving treatment, makes intuitive sense. More evidence is required concerning the psychological outcomes of participating in exercise programs; although, anecdotal reports are promising (see Hays, 1999). This lack of evidence highlights the underdeveloped nature of this research area and the rich potential for developing research programs that systematically addresses the use of exercise as a coping strategy for alcohol and drug rehabilitation.

There are clearly special challenges associated with the use of physical activity with these populations in terms of initiating and maintaining exercise participation. More critically, these authors also highlight a recurring theme (also raised in relation to smoking-cessation): are multiple health behavior changes possible? Are we expecting too much in asking individuals to make two or even three major changes in health behavior, particularly if those changes are attempted simultaneously? Non-pharmacological interventions that assist abstinence efforts, also contributing other significant health outcomes, at the same time deserve urgent research and practice attention.

CONGESTIVE HEART FAILURE: WHAT WE KNOW SUMMARY

- Patients with Congestive Heart Failure (CHF) show evidence of anxiety and depression and often experience a dramatic reduction in their quality of life (QOL).
- Significant improvements in exercise capacity have been demonstrated in CHF patients included in clinical trials.
- The evidence suggests that exercise can play an important role in improving the function and QOL of patients with CHF.

Editorial commentary

The treatment of physical medical conditions has often disregarded psychological factors in terms of the etiology, rehabilitation, and the enhancement of mental health. This is clearly true for people experiencing CHF. Progressive physical deconditioning associated with CHF may leave people tired, anxious, depressed, and feeling functionally inadequate. Partially reversing this deconditioning is clearly possible with appropriate exercise programs, and may bring with it improvements in function and QOL as Ffion Lloyd-Williams and Frances Mair highlight. Less is known about how exercise may reduce fear and depression, specifically among this population. As our understanding of how patients experience and respond to CHF treatment improves, then interventions, including exercise-based programs, can be designed to maximise the psychosocial benefits. For example, rumination about the condition and the implications for dependents and occupational demands may elicit anxiety and depression. In this case, exercise as a distraction may be more important than the physical dose in rehabilitation. Alternatively, an exercise bout may simply highlight an individual's low functional capability and subsequently exacerbate any negative perceptions they may have regarding their QOL. When we know more about how exercise may improve the QOL and psychological well-being of individuals with CHF, then interventions may be designed to optimise the likelihood of demonstrating positive effects.

HUMAN IMMUNODEFICIENCY VIRUS (HIV) AND ACQUIRED IMMUNODEFICIENCY SYNDROME (AIDS): WHAT WE KNOW SUMMARY

- HIV and AIDS markedly increase the incidence and prevalence of depressive symptoms.
- Aerobic exercise training has been associated with quantifiable improvements in aerobic fitness; however, the effects on psychological well-being are less certain.
- There is a decrease in the rate of depressive symptoms and improved QOL/ psychological well-being in HIV$^+$ subjects (regardless of the disease stage) using a very wide variety of QOL instruments.
- The exercise program (e.g., dose) to improve fitness should consist of 45 minutes, three times per week of aerobic exercise combined with a smaller component of resistance training. It is important to note that for deconditioned individuals there should be a progressive increase in dose.
- The optimal "dose" (length × duration × intensity) for changes in psychological well-being have not been determined from existing studies.
- "Dropouts" are a significant problem with exercise programs in HIV/AIDS patients and should engender adequate preplanning to prospectively identify barriers to continued participation.
- Aerobic exercise appears to provide greater improvements in psychological well-being when compared to resistance exercises in some studies.

Editorial commentary

A diagnosis of HIV can be viewed as a chronic stressor. As a result, exercise may be a strategy for coping with the diagnosis, impairments, and treatment of this condition. An intriguing element in the rationale for promoting exercise for individuals with HIV, is the development of the psychoneuroimmunologic model (see Figure 6.1). As others have noted, this model is potentially applicable to chronic diseases where psychological stress and immune functioning have been implicated in disease progression (Perna and Bryner, 2002). In terms of HIV, William Stringer concludes that aerobic exercise interventions may result in improved psychological well-being for individuals with this disease, although there is no evidence to suggest that exercise training may lead to a decrease in morbidity or mortality. However, there is clear support for aerobic exercise improving aerobic fitness, which may be particularly important for maintaining activities of daily living and enhancing QOL. Underpinning both these conclusions is the problem of dropout from exercise programs and how little we know about enhancing compliance within this population.

CANCER: WHAT WE KNOW SUMMARY

- The number of cancer survivors will continue to increase in the coming decades.
- Cancer and its treatments often have negative effects on QOL.
- Exercise has been shown to improve QOL, especially in breast cancer survivors and especially after treatments have been completed.
- Exercise may improve QOL in cancer survivors beyond the benefits of group psychotherapy.
- Reduced fatigue may be one of the key factors explaining why exercise enhances QOL in cancer survivors.
- Exercise interventions that increase physical fitness may result in even greater improvements in QOL.

Editorial commentary

The diagnosis of cancer often brings fear and uncertainty for victims and caregivers. There may be stages (with different periods of time) of emotional response, from denial to anger and depression, before one eventually accepts the diagnosis. Individual responses are highly variable, from passive and accepting to active coping and determination to overcome the disease. Making simple statements about the benefits of exercise for enhancing QOL for cancer patients is not easy, given the range of responses and coping strategies used across the duration of the diagnosis. As a result, it may be easier to say that being physically inactive is unlikely to be beneficial for a number of reasons. The chapter by Kerry Courneya provides some promising evidence that exercise may improve QOL for breast cancer patients, after conventional treatments have been completed, beyond that provided by psychotherapy. Reversing the deconditioning associated with cancer treatment appears to be the most plausible mechanism by which exercise impacts an individual's QOL (e.g., daily energy levels). Much less attention has been given to the role of exercise in reducing anxiety and enhancing physical self-perceptions, with possible psychoimmunological implications.

SMOKING CESSATION: WHAT WE KNOW SUMMARY

- The few rigorous trials reported have shown mixed effects of exercise on smoking cessation.
- There is evidence that interventions can increase exercise participation among smokers, pre-quitters and quitters, but the evidence that such change enables weight management (a common cause of relapse) among quitters is less clear.
- There is increasing evidence that single sessions of exercise, at a low to moderate intensity (e.g., walking) can help temporary abstainers to cope with withdrawal symptoms and nicotine cravings, particularly in laboratory conditions.

Editorial commentary

Adrian Taylor and Michael Ussher conclude that both smoking cessation and exercise practitioners should promote physical activity to aid cessation while acknowledging the limited number of studies and many methodological limitations. An important conclusion is that such interventions can increase the physical activity levels of smokers. This in itself should be seen as a positive outcome in smoking-cessation trials and could be considered in the light of an alternative approach to help smokers reduce or discontinue their smoking behavior (see Hatsukami *et al.*, 2004). Referred to as harm reduction, it can refer to a policy, strategy, or a particular intervention that assumes continued use of an undesired behavior and aspires to lower the risk of adverse consequences associated with the continuation of the addictive behavior of smoking. Specific risks to the health and well-being of individuals are not expected to be eliminated; however, steps are taken to diminish the adverse effects (Hirschhorn, 2002).

With the exception of medicinal nicotine, harm reduction methods have yet to demonstrate a reduction in morbidity and mortality rates (McNeill, 2004). Therefore, it is essential that new and innovative harm reduction strategies be developed. Potentially, physical activity could be considered in such a role. Most critically, regular physical activity appears to delay the occurrence of disease and death initiated by tobacco consumption. Epidemiological evidence consistently demonstrates an association between physical fitness, physical activity, and all-cause mortality risk even after statistical adjustment for smoking habits (e.g., Blair *et al.*, 1989; Myers *et al.*, 2002; Paffenbarger *et al.*, 1986). Simplistically, this evidence indicates that physically active smokers live longer than inactive smokers. Further epidemiological research is undoubtedly required to prove such a proposition. This chapter undoubtedly adds to the case for physical activity as a harm-reduction strategy. The reviewed research appears to demonstrate that smokers can increase their physical activity, and that such an increase may be an effective coping strategy for those smokers desiring to achieve cessation, while also assisting others with cessation attempts.

SLEEP: WHAT WE KNOW SUMMARY

- People believe that exercise is an important sleep-promoting behavior.
- Individuals who exercise regularly have a lower risk of disturbed sleep but causal effects are less well established.
- Chronic exercise training may elicit significant improvements in sleep among individuals with disturbed sleep although there is no clear consensus.
- Acute exercise elicits a modest improvement in sleep among good sleepers. This effect is greater for longer exercise durations. The influence of acute exercise on sleep is similar for fit and unfit individuals. Exercise intensity or time-of-day of exercise do not have much of a moderating influence.

Editorial commentary

There is clear evidence that sleep is a comorbid factor associated with a variety of physical and mental health problems, and it therefore makes sense that there is an optimum need; the purpose of which is not so clear. Of all self-help behaviors, exercise has been identified as important for promoting attainment of that need for sleep. Many critical questions emerge from this notion that exercise is beneficial for sleep. These are largely addressed in the chapter and result in a far from clear relationship as determined by a systematic review of research evidence by Shawn Youngstedt and Julie Freelove-Charton. The methodological complexities of examining the effects of exercise on psychological well-being are no more evident than it is in this chapter. Operational definitions of physical activity and exercise have been inconsistent and sometimes vague, while the measurement of sleep appears to be a science in and of itself. As well, the relationship between acute and chronic effects of exercise have not yet been adequately considered. For example, do chronic improvements in sleep reflect an increasing volume in single doses of exercise (with improved aerobic capacity over time)? Intuitively, laboratory studies may allow better control over measurement and interventions, but do they remove the daily events that also play an important role in our sleep patterns? A major shortcoming inherent in the research conducted in this area is the overwhelming focus on good sleepers: Far less is known about the acute and chronic effects of exercise on poor sleepers and those with sleep disorders. Importantly, this chapter considers this limited evidence.

Sleep research engages a wide range of academic interests, from sociologists and psychologists to immunologists and endocrinologists. If exercise is viewed as a stressor, with exercise training eliciting an adaptation to this stressor, then it would make sense to understand the effects of exercise on sleep in the context of stress and sleep. The literature unfortunately has not considered the relative dose of exercise, but rather has focused on absolute doses and the timing of such doses, in an attempt to identify moderating factors which strengthen the observed relationship between acute exercise and sleep. Familiarity with a dose of exercise may be more important than the actual dose itself. For example, when exercising just before bedtime, one person may be able to quickly recover and therefore experience a rapid onset of sleep, whereas another person may experience sleep disturbance from the same dose. The lack of a consensus in some of the findings presented in this chapter may reflect a need for more sophisticated research that considers interactions between hypothesized moderating variables, and focuses primarily on poor sleepers.

SPORT AND SOCIAL INCLUSION: WHAT WE KNOW SUMMARY

- The most effective use of sport, to systematically address anti-social and criminal behavior, is to combine with programs that seek to address wider personal and social development.
- The salience of sport can be used to attract young people to integrated programs that offer formal programs in personal development, health awareness, and employment training.
- Appropriate leadership is perhaps the most important element in determining the positive impact of a program.
- Locally recruited leaders and a bottom-up approach maximize the chances of success.

Editorial commentary

The effects of physical activity on social outcomes, such as those related to social exclusion, remain a challenge for evaluation. Social outcomes by their very nature are difficult to define and delimit. Randomized controlled trials (RCTs) (see Chapter 1), such an important element of evidence-based medicine, will rarely be appropriate as the effects need to be observed in real settings where control of the intervention will be very difficult, if not impossible. This requires innovation in research design, but also, an acceptance of other forms of evidence in supporting the role of physical activity in reducing social exclusion. Overall, the impact of physical activity on such outcomes may be greater than the limited evidence-base suggests (Department of Health, 2004). Many community-based programs involving physical activity have been, and are being, delivered with the goal of enhancing a myriad of social outcomes. Yet these programs are rarely evaluated rigorously, nor do they reach scientific outlets of dissemination such as academic journals. The evidence that does exist is certainly not convincing. However, there are sound reasons to believe that physical activity remains a viable process for reducing social exclusion and improving social well-being with one important caveat. To paraphrase Fred Coalter from an earlier review, it is most likely that sport and physical activity are in themselves not *the* solution. As part of wider ranging development initiatives, they could be *part* of the solution when addressing issues of crime, education and employment, and community development and social exclusion (Coalter, 2001).

LIMITATIONS OF THE RESEARCH

The evidence for physical activity having a positive effect on outcomes related to psychological well-being does appear weak or at best in their infancy in some of the areas presented. RCTs are in the minority and much of what we know is based on less robust research designs. Biddle *et al.* (2000) identified a range of research questions that need addressing with respect to physical activity and mental health. Many of these still remain unanswered (see Table 11.1). We now draw attention to generic issues that were raised in this collection regarding measurement, populations, research design, exercise, and physical activity programing, and mechanisms.

Table 11.1 What we need to know summary points

Measurement
- Are current psychometric measures adequate for capturing the range of affective responses in physical activity and for assessing change over time?
- How much change in scores is necessary for a meaningful impact on functioning, behaviors and well-being? To date, insufficient evidence is available in many areas to develop clinical criteria and targets of change.

Populations
- How do special groups (e.g., the obese with social physique anxiety, asthmatics and chronic obstructive pulmonary disease (COPD) patients who experience fears about breathing; older people with a fear of failing) differ in the benefits of a program of exercise?
- Is the mental health effects the same across all ages and both genders?
- More information is needed on those who do not volunteer for studies or who drop out and do not feature in the results.

Exercise and physical activity programing
- What are the long-term effects of accumulated doses of activity (in line with current recommendations for physical activity for cardiovascular disease prevention)?
- What are the longer-term effects (i.e., over 4 months) of physical activity? We need to know, for example, whether a 10-week exercise program will have lasting effects, and if not what is necessary to maintain the effects?
- What are the effects of short bouts (<15 min) of free-living, unsupervised aerobic physical activity, which can be most easily integrated into an active lifestyle, as a low-cost intervention?
- What are the social effects of exercise on mental well-being?
- We need to know whether exercise practitioner manipulations of self-efficacy, outcome expectancy, perceived competence, goal setting, feedback, attentional focus and perceived exertion and enjoyment can have effects, particularly among inactive and inexperienced exercisers.
- Adherence to exercise training appears to be greater when it is of moderate intensity (e.g., walking), and integrated into an active lifestyle. What are the determinants of adherence to free-living and facility-based exercise programs?
- What are the competencies and skills required by exercise professionals to most effectively promote physical activity for psychological well-being? What is the role of other mental health professionals?
- Are the psychological effects of physical activity the same for different modes of activity (e.g., aerobic, strength-based, flexibility-based)?
- Do different intensities and durations of physical activity make a difference and do fitness levels modulate that effect?
- When might high intensity exercise produce positive affective responses?

(Table 11.1 continued)

Table 11.1 Continued

Economic issues

- The cost-effectiveness of physical activity as a treatment for mental health has not been considered. More studies need to compare physical activity with other interventions, not only in terms of mental health but also cost. Related to this would be careful consideration of adherence to the respective interventions.

Mechanisms

- How do the potential mechanisms underlying the effects interact?
- How do effects of exercise compare to those of drug treatments and what adjunctive value does exercise have along with drug treatment?
- If drugs are also administered is the interaction of drug and exercise safe?
- Under what conditions are the associations between physical activity and psychological well-being causal?
- What mechanisms explain the link between activity and psychological well-being?
- We need information on the dynamics of change. Little is known about how long it takes to produce changes and how long they last.
- Is it necessary to develop physiological adaptations to an exercise regimen before psychological well-being increases occur?

Source: Adapted from Biddle *et al.* (2000).

MEASUREMENT

There needs to be a clearer rationale for both physical activity and psychological outcome measures which reflect conceptual and theoretical understanding. For example, if psychosocial processes (e.g., perceptions of mastery, greater positive social interaction or distraction) appear most influential in the relationship between physical activity and mental health, then these dimensions of physical activity participation should be measured and manipulated into, or controlled within, the intervention.

Future research efforts should make attempts to link participation in physical activity to broader health outcomes such as the use of health services or days of hospitalization. If the evidence in this book is to become practice, then the outcomes must be salient to those operating the specific health service. Increasingly, QOL measures have become routinely used in health care; however, there may still be some way to go to break out of the biomedical model. This is particularly true for those conditions with predominantly physical symptoms (e.g., CHF, HIV, Cancer). For conditions involving a mental illness, the biomedical model may still drive the treatment, but there appears to be more willingness to understand the psycho-social dimensions experienced by patients. Nevertheless, clinical psychologists and psychiatrists may minimize the role and value of physical activity in providing psychological benefits (see Faulkner and Biddle, 2001).

No study presented in this collection has examined the cost-effectiveness of exercise interventions and the language of economic analysis is still notably absent in the exercise science literature (Biddle *et al.*, 2000). The issue of cost-effectiveness may ultimately decide if exercise will formally be adopted by health services as a strategy for enhancing mental health. However, most studies presented here involve relatively small sample sizes. One implication of studies involving small samples is that conducting economic evaluations alongside clinical trials can be problematic. The sample size required to detect a meaningful difference in costs may be much larger than that required to detect a clinically meaningful difference (Gray *et al.*, 1997). Another increasingly used indicator of effectiveness in clinical decision-making is the notion of numbers needed to treat (NNT) in order to see a single positive clinical outcome. The greater the likelihood of a positive outcome, then a smaller number of patients is needed to receive a treatment or intervention (including promotion of physical activity). For example, if NNT was 30, it would mean that we may expect 30 people to be treated to prevent one additional bad outcome or to achieve one desirable outcome. As such, clinicians may be guided by the likely effectiveness of an intervention in their decision making. It is unlikely that for most conditions described in this collection this figure would be small enough to merit physical activity as a stand-alone treatment option. In fact, it is questionable whether a figure could even be calculated, due to a lack of information on absolute and relative risk or likelihood of a positive outcome (Weeks and Noteboom, 2004). Awareness of how treatment plans are decided upon may be important for exercise scientists if evidence is to be accumulated to influence policy makers and clinicians. Importantly, NNT is used when the outcome variable is dichotomous. Although some outcome variables (resulting from exercise interventions) in this collection are not clinically defined as present or absent (e.g., successful or failed quitter in smoking cessation), many outcome variables are not.

POPULATIONS

Most of the populations of interest in this book do less physical activity than the general population. This may be a result of a medical condition, and the advice and treatment provided. For some medical conditions, physical inactivity may well have been one of the influential factors. Most of the exercise psychology literature has focused on determinants of behavior among moderately active people: We know relatively little about the utility of traditional social psychology theories for predicting behavior and exploring the determinants of exercise in these particular populations is necessary. We also need to know the effects of exercise for different subpopulations within the general populations covered. For example, effects of exercise may vary depending on the stage of HIV progression, or the stage of recovery from drug and alcohol addiction.

Attrition and drop-out also appear to be high in some populations (e.g., individuals with HIV) and we need to examine and report the differences between adherers and nonadherers on important variables of interest. The side effects of some medications may be a barrier to regular participation in physical activity. One specific issue emerging across the collection is how little we know about the interaction between exercise and pharmacological treatment. Consequently, this area requires urgent academic attention.

RESEARCH DESIGN

Clearly we have focused this book on areas of work that are emerging rather than the traditional foci in the exercise and mental health literature. As anticipated, the evidence presented may not always provide clear consensus, often as a result of too few studies, or rather broad attempts to address research questions with small samples or inadequate designs. It is perhaps easy to recommend larger studies with carefully controlled interventions and longer follow-up periods to determine effectiveness. However, we may well see smaller effects from exercise interventions, in the future. For ethical reasons, participants in an exercise intervention trial must be allowed to receive 'standard health care'. As standard care improves with new pharmacological and other therapies, it becomes increasingly more difficult to demonstrate any additional benefits from exercise.

Pragmatic RCTs have in the past randomized all patients suitable and willing to enter a trial, rather than identifying only those willing to try exercise, then randomizing participants into exercise or no-exercise (and no treatment) (Tai and Iliffe, 2000). Giving patients (and clinicians) a choice of interventions, as occurs in equipoise trials (Lavori *et al.*, 2001), and then randomizing on the basis of that choice, may reveal larger beneficial effects from exercise. This is a recent development and such trials are expensive due to the large sample sizes needed to adequately consider the range of patient preferences. Funding may also not be available for many of the outcomes considered in this book, but at best, the measures are assessed as additional to the main outcomes in a trial. In this case, a physical outcome (with less measurement error) may require a smaller sample size, leaving the study underpowered to detect statistically significant effects for the psychological outcome measures.

It is evident that RCTs will remain at the top of the hierarchy of research designs (see Tai and Iliffe (2000) for a discussion of RCTs in the context of exercise promotion). However, it is also important to acknowledge growing awareness of the limitations of this approach (see Harris *et al.*, 2001) and that the adoption of public health programs and policies can be based on a range of evidential criteria (see Briss *et al.*, 2004).

Returning to issues discussed in Chapter 1, we support the acceptance of a diversity of research designs and methodological approaches in examining physical activity, and mental health. A narrow theoretical or methodological approach risks *excluding* important factors in mental health change and may hinder investigation of the unexpected or novel benefits experienced by the range of individuals who participate in physical activity.

Many of the benefits from increasing physical activity could be enhanced with changes in other health behaviors. Conversely, promotion of physical activity could be added to existing health promotion messages about diet and other health behaviors. Changing multiple habits at the same time may be too challenging for some people and it is important to understand how best to time advice and behavior change strategies, particularly among the least active. In relation to smoking cessation at least, becoming more physically active may serve as a "gatekeeping" function, increasing the likelihood of health behavior changes such as subsequent smoking cessation attempts (Bock *et al.*, 1998; Boudreaux *et al.*, 2003; Doherty *et al.*, 1998).

Exercise and physical activity programing

One of the criteria for demonstrating the causal effects of a treatment is to observe a dose-response effect (see Hill, 1965). Practitioners driven by a biomedical model will want to know what dose of exercise will have the optimum effect (and what doses may be insufficient to have an effect or even, at the other extreme, a detrimental effect). Given that most populations considered in this book will be less physically active than the general population it is better to focus on the lower end of the dose–response relationship (if there is one). The assumption that there is a dose–response relationship between physical activity and any dimension of mental health is a biomedical one. It assumes that physiological processes and adaptation (e.g., neuro-endocrine changes) are involved in causing the effects, and that these processes will be dependent on the frequency, intensity, and duration of exercise. Studies described in Chapters 4 and 9 on the acute effects of exercise on drug cravings and on sleep are examples of a biomedical approach. These chapters refer to recent studies aimed at identifying optimal effects, from just the physical exercise, without consideration of the social-psychological processes.

Current public health messages for the promotion of lifestyle physical activity refer to increasing energy expenditure in small but achievable doses such as three 10-min periods (or a session of 30 min) of low to moderate intensity exercise on at least 5 days per week. Practitioners may want to know if such a message is equally applicable to mental health promotion as it is to reducing coronary heart disease risk factors such as obesity, or whether 3 sessions per week of structured exercise of moderate to vigorous intensity is necessary. Given the likelihood that the populations described in the preceding chapters will be less active than average, the critical response is that it doesn't matter, as long as it is sustainable. If structured exercise requires organization (i.e., a setting, a booking, a group, a leader, travel) it may provide more barriers to participation, but it may also provide the necessary incentive, reinforcement, and social support to be sustained. Having said that, we know little about the use of exercise as a coping strategy. For example, if something is worrying or a craving is strong, then an interactional approach is needed to cope with stress or the urge to smoke during a quit attempt. Exercise should be promoted as a coping strategy, and the individual given the skills to develop it as such in a convenient and confident manner.

The importance of becoming more physically active may appear obscure for many of the populations considered in this book. Evidence that exercise may influence dimensions of psychological well-being, as described in this book, has not yet been synthesized for and assimilated by practitioners, caregivers, and most importantly individuals living with these conditions. Motivating practitioners to promote, and individuals to engage in, physical activity is therefore likely to be an ongoing challenge. We therefore need to know much more about how to effectively promote exercise to those with existing, or an increased risk of, mental health problems. When considering a health problem, it may be tempting to link recovery and well-being to the need to exercise more. Threat messages that imply a failure to become more active will result in no improvement in health status and may not work if the individual does not have the necessary confidence to make the appropriate changes in behavior (Berry, 2004).

Mechanisms

A consistent conclusion from all the chapters is that no single mechanism has yet been found to adequately explain the diverse range of mental health effects possible through physical activity participation. A key reason for this is that the occurrence of, and recovery from, mental health problems is influenced by a large number of diverse factors. Nevertheless, if we are to reliably prescribe and manage exercise provision across a range of mental health contexts, it may ultimately be necessary to understand how, why, and under what conditions does psychological change occur. In acknowledging the huge variety of potential triggers (e.g., exercise type, environment, social context) and individual circumstances (e.g., state of mental health, needs, preferences, and personal background), Fox (1999) suggests that several mechanisms most likely operate in concert with the precise combination being highly individual-specific. That is, different processes operate for different people at different times.

One approach to understanding the causes or mechanisms of mental health change through physical activity is to take an *inclusive process* approach (see Carless and Faulkner, 2003). This kind of approach, which includes consideration of the broad range of biological and psychosocial factors that impact mental health, is more likely to lead to an understanding of the causes of mental health change than can be achieved through consideration of any individual mechanism in isolation. Recent theories characteristic of a process approach may be particularly useful in this regard, such as Cloninger and colleague's (1994) psychobiological theory of personality, self-determination theory (see Ryan and Deci, 2000), and La Forge's (1995) integrative model.

It is also worth noting the growing body of research that has investigated the effects of exercise on issues related to mental health with animals. Whereas it may be easy to dismiss this work with suggestions that we can not tap the subjective experiences of animals, implicit in our definition of mental health, exciting discoveries are emerging. For example, exercise impacts on the neural anatomy of the brain and is associated with biochemical changes in the mesolimbic system where emotions are controlled. This book only briefly identifies such research (e.g., see Chapters 2, 4, 8, and 9) but work with animals may help to identify some important psychophysiological mechanisms involved in this area of inquiry. Further work will undoubtedly extend the very few human studies that have pharmacologically blocked specific neural and biochemical pathways in the brain to determine if exercise has the same psychological outcomes. In a similar vein, further research will subsequently extend our understanding of psychopharmacokinetics and the interactions between exercise and prescribed medication.

TAKING THE FIELD FORWARD

What impact would we like to achieve from this book? With today's web-based access to information, many health and exercise practitioners, and students can locate reviews and trials on just about anything. The most challenging tasks may be to identify the key search terms and then interpret the quality and messages from respective articles. Authors of this collection of chapters have laid down examples of how to do this in a systematic way. Increasingly, those who wish to use physical activity interventions to promote mental health (in its broadest sense) will need these skills to present their case. It is not unrealistic to assume that there are many working and studying in the field of mental health promotion and treatment who have not even considered the implications of promoting a more physically active lifestyle. Hopefully this book will lead individuals and policy makers to re-evaluate their actions and consider a behavioral approach, at least as an adjunct. It may also challenge medical professionals, psychologists and others without an exercise specialism to evaluate their practice with greater insight by considering the physical and psychological health needs of their patients. The integration of the mind and body in prevention and treatment is fundamental.

Some medical conditions have clear contraindications, and the expertise of an exercise professional should be engaged. However, throughout the book we have seen examples of how even light to moderate intensity exercise can have beneficial effects. Practitioners need to be less concerned about "doing more harm" and more concerned with the implications of reinforcing sedentary behaviors in these populations.

In terms of research, clearly there is a long continuum (or several undefined dimensions) from research with animals on neuroanatomical and biochemical changes (associated with enhanced cognitive and emotional functioning) in response to exercise to promoting social functioning (as a component of mental health) through exercise interventions. Nevertheless, cross-fertilization of research among those leading clinical trials, experimental exercise neuroscientists, and social scientists seeking to promote physical activity in a cost-effective way, is necessary. One researcher may be somewhat isolated and make only small advances in knowledge; however, a collaboration of transdisciplinary researchers is likely to make exciting advances in our understanding of questions about efficacy, effectiveness, and efficiency.

EFFICACY VERSUS EFFECTIVENESS

It is unfortunate that most studies do not report how people get active. Such efforts may themselves include critical treatment components (Salmon, 2001) but are also informative for translating research into practice. Barlow *et al.* (1999) suggest confidence in treatment efficacy should be based on two simultaneous considerations. First, the efficacy of a given intervention should be based on results from systematic studies (ideally, RCTs) in controlled clinical research contexts. Second, we should consider the effectiveness of the intervention (does it work in real world settings) which is related to issues of feasibility (e.g., patient acceptability, probability of compliance, ease of dissemination), generalizeability (e.g., patient characteristics, contextual factors) and cost effectiveness. Arguably, we have the emerging basis for feasibility but little knowledge of generalizeability and cost-effectiveness which are critical for integrating physical activity into health service delivery. Manske *et al.* (2004) have noted, in relation to smoking cessation research:

the striking misalignment between the questions researchers have asked and the questions that service delivery organizations need to have answered . . . [researchers] have not focused on discerning who benefits from and needs [a] type of treatment, how providers should be trained, settings and contexts in which treatment has greatest impact, or how to ensure program quality during delivery.

(conclusion section, ¶9)

Given the emerging nature of the evidence presented here we have only begun to address issues of concern for practitioners. Consequently, future research should endeavour to focus on the systems of care as well as individual change (Ockene *et al.*, 1997). There is clearly a need to examine *how* physical activity is best delivered to promote mental health, and how we can help guide practitioners in their decisions to consider physical activity as a treatment option. Unfortunately, there is a long way to go. The development of formal research policies, formalized organizational and structural support, appropriate and targeted funding, formal monitoring of research activity and its dissemination, and ongoing training for both researchers and practitioners, will all be necessary for physical activity and exercise as mental health promotion strategies to gain more comprehensive acceptance (Nutbeam, 1996).

CLOSING COMMENT

Physical activity is not a panacea for all of life's ills. It is but one element of the human experience. Yet, as this collection demonstrates, there is clear and emerging evidence that "From the cradle to the grave, regular physical activity appears to be an *essential* (our emphasis) ingredient for human well-being" (Boreham and Riddoch, 2003, p. 24). The promotion of physical activity for mental health can be seen as a "win-win" situation with physical health benefits accruing for most individuals and mental health benefits for some (Mutrie and Faulkner, 2003). There is certainly very little evidence to suggest we should *not* be considering physical activity and exercise as strategies for promoting mental health. We have only begun to tap the potential that physical activity may have in improving mental health across a wide range of disease and disabilities (see the American College of Sports Medicine, 1997) and we invite all readers to play a part in exploring the potential physical activity may have for promoting mental health. The alternative is for trends in society to increasingly enable us to use less and less energy (as technology develops); thus, increasing deconditioning and related poor physical health. This text highlights how poor physical health can have important deleterious mental health consequences.

REFERENCES

American College of Sports Medicine (1997). *ACSM's Exercise Management for Persons with Chronic Disease and Disabilities*. Champaign, IL: Human Kinetics.

Barlow, D. H., Levitt, J. T., and Bufka, L. F. (1999). The dissemination of empirically supported treatments: a view to the future. *Behaviour Research and Therapy*, *37*, S147–S162.

Berry, D. (2004). *Risk, Communication and Health Psychology*. Maidenhead, UK: Open University Press.

Biddle, S. J. H., Fox, K. R., Boutcher, S. H., and Faulkner, G. (2000). The way forward for physical activity and the promotion of psychological well-being. In S. J. H. Biddle, K. R. Fox, and S. H. Boutcher (Eds). *Physical Activity and Psychological Well-being* (pp. 154–168). London: Routledge.

Blair, S. N., Kohl, H. W., Paffenbarger, R. S., Clark, D. G., Cooper, K. H., and Gibbons, L. W. (1989). Physical fitness and all-cause mortality: a prospective study of healthy men and women. *Journal of the American Medical Association*, *262*, 2395–2401.

Bock, B. C., Marcus, B. H., Rossi, J. S., and Redding, C. A. (1998). Motivational readiness for change: diet, exercise, and smoking. *American Journal of Health Behavior*, *22*, 248–258.

Boreham, C. and Riddoch, C. (2003). Physical activity and health through the lifespan. In J. McKenna and C. Riddoch (Eds). *Perspectives on Health and Exercise* (pp. 11–32). UK: Palgrave Macmillan.

Boudreaux, E. D., Francis, J. L., Carmack-Taylor, C. L., Scarinci, I. S., and Brantley, P. J. (2003). Changing multiple health behaviors: smoking and exercise. *Preventive Medicine, 36*, 471–478.

Boutcher, S. H. (2000). Cognitive performance, fitness, and aging. In S. J. H. Biddle, K. R. Fox, and S. H. Boutcher (Eds). *Physical Activity and Psychological Well-being* (pp. 118–129). London: Routledge.

Briss, P. A., Brownson, R. C., Fielding, J. E., and Zaza, S. (2004). Developing and using the guide to community preventive services: lessons learned about evidence-based public health. *Annual Review of Public Health, 25*, 281–302.

Carless, D. and Faulkner, G. (2003). Physical activity and mental health. In J. McKenna and C. Riddoch (Eds). *Perspectives on Health and Exercise* (pp. 61–82). Houndsmills: Palgrave MacMillan.

Coalter, F. (2001). *Realising the Potential of Cultural Services: The Case for Sport.* London: Local Government Association.

Cotman, C. W. and Berchtold, N. C. (2002). Exercise: a behavioural intervention to enhance brain health and plasticity. *Trends in Neurosciences, 25*, 295–301.

Cloninger, C. R., Przybeck, T. R., Svrakic, D. M., and Wetzel, R. D. (1994). *The Temperament and Character Inventory (TCI): A Guide to its Development and Use.* St Louis, MO: Washington University Press.

Department of Health (2004). *At least Five a Week. A Report from the Chief Medical Officer.* London: HMSO.

Doherty, S. C., Steptoe, A., Rink, E., Kendrick, T., and Hilton, S. (1998). Readiness to change health behaviours among patients at high risk of cardiovascular disease. *Journal of Cardiovascular Risk, 5*, 147–153.

Faulkner, G. and Biddle, S. J. H. (2001). Exercise as therapy: it's just not psychology! *Journal of Sports Sciences, 19*, 433–444.

Fox, K. R. (1999). The influence of physical activity on mental well-being. *Public Health Nutrition, 2*, 411–418.

Gray, A. M., Marshall, M., Lockwood, A., and Morris, J. (1997). Problems in conducting economic evaluations alongside clinical trials. *British Journal of Psychiatry, 170*, 47–52.

Harris, R. P., Helfand, M., Woolf, S. H., Lohr, K. N., Mulrow, C. D., Teutsch, S.M. *et al.* (2001). Current methods of the U.S. preventive services task force: a review of the process. *American Journal of Preventive Medicine, 20*(3S), 21–35.

Hatsukami, D. K., Henningfield, J. E., and Kotlyar, M. (2004). Harm reducing approaches to reducing tobacco-related mortality. *Annual Review of Public Health, 25*, 377–395.

Hays, K. F. (1999). *Working it Out: Using Exercise in Psychotherapy.* Washington, DC: American Psychological Association Books.

Hill, A. B. (1965). The environment and disease: association or causation? *Proceedings of the Royal Society of Medicine, 58*, 295–300.

Hirschhorn, N. (2002). Clearing the smoke – or spreading the fog? *Nicotine and Tobacco Research, 4*, S191–S193.

La Forge, R. (1995). Exercise-associated mood alterations: a review of interactive neurobiological mechanisms. *Medicine, Exercise, Nutrition and Health, 4*, 17–32.

Lavori, P. W., Rush, A. J., Wisniewski, S. R., Alpert, J., Fava, M., Kupfer, D. J. *et al.* (2001). Strengthening clinical effectiveness trials: equipoise-stratified randomization. *Biological Psychiatry, 50*, 792–801.

McNeill, A. (2004). ABC of smoking cessation: harm reduction. *British Medical Journal, 328*, 885–887.

Manske, S., Miller, S., Moyer, C., Phaneuf, M. R., and Cameron, R. (2004). Best practice group-based smoking cessation: results of a literature review applying effectiveness, plausibility and practicality criteria. *American Journal of Health Promotion*, *18*, 409–423.

Mutrie, N. and Faulkner, G. (2003). Physical activity and mental health. In T. Everett, M. Donaghy and S. Fever (Eds). *Physiotherapy and Occupational Therapy in Mental Health: An Evidence Based Approach* (pp. 82–97). Oxford: Butterworth Heinemann.

Myers, J., Prakash, M., Froelicher, V., Do, D., Partington, S., and Atwood, J.E. (2002). Exercise capacity and mortality among men referred for exercise testing. *New England Journal of Medicine*, *346*, 793–801.

Nutbeam, D. (1996). Improving the fit between research and practice in health promotion: overcoming structural barriers. *Canadian Journal of Public Health*, *87*(Suppl. 2), S18–S23.

Ockene, J. K., McBride, P. E., Sallis, J. F., Bonollo, D. P., and Ockene, I. S. (1997). Synthesis of lessons learned from cardiopulmonary preventive interventions in health care settings. *Annals of Epidemiology*, *7*(Suppl. 7), S32–S45.

Paffenbarger, R. S. Jr, Hyde, R. T., Wing, A. L., and Hsieh, C. C. (1986). Physical activity, all-cause mortality, and longevity of college alumni. *New England Journal of Medicine*, *314*, 605–613.

Perna, F. M. and Bryner, R. W. (2002). The psychology of exercise and immunology: Implications for HIV infection. In D. L. Mostofsky and L. D. Zaichkowsky (Eds). *Medical and Psychological Aspects of Sport and Exercise* (pp. 237–259). Morgantown, WV: Fitness Information Technology.

Ryan, R. M. and Deci, E. L. (2000). Self-determination theory and the facilitation of intrinsic motivation, social development, and well-being. *American Psychologist*, *55*, 68–78.

Salmon, P. (2001). Effects of physical exercise on anxiety, depression, and sensitivity to stress: a unifying theory. *Clinical Psychology Review*, *21*, 33–61.

Statistics Canada (2003). *Canadian Community Health Survey: Mental Health and Well-being*. Ottawa, ON: Statistics Canada.

Tai, S. S. and Iliffe, S. (2000). Considerations for the design and analysis of experimental studies in physical activity and exercise promotion: advantages of the randomised controlled trial. *British Journal of Sports Medicine*, *34*, 220–224.

Weeks, D. L. and Noteboom, J. T. (2004). Using the number needed to treat in clinical practice. *Archives of Physical Medicine and Rehabilitation*, *85*, 1729–1731.

Index

Note: Page numbers in italics refers to illustrations.

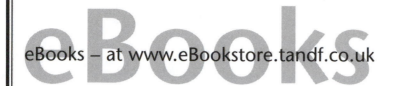